LIBRARY OF RELIGIOUS BIOGRAPHY

Edited by Mark A. Noll, Nathan O. Hatch, and Allen C. Guelzo

THE LIBRARY OF RELIGIOUS BIOGRAPHY is a series of original biographies on important religious figures throughout American and British history.

The authors are well-known historians, each a recognized authority in the period of religious history in which his or her subject lived and worked. Grounded in solid research of both published and archival sources, these volumes link the lives of their subjects — not always thought of as "religious" persons — to the broader cultural contexts and religious issues that surrounded them. Each volume includes an index to serve the needs of students, teachers, and researchers.

Marked by careful scholarship yet free of academic jargon, the books in this series are well-written narratives meant to be *read* and *enjoyed* as well as studied.

LIBRARY OF RELIGIOUS BIOGRAPHY

William Ewart Gladstone: Faith and Politics in Victorian Britain
David Bebbington

Aimee Semple McPherson: Everybody's Sister • *Edith L. Blumhofer*

Her Heart Can See: The Life and Hymns of Fanny J. Crosby
Edith L. Blumhofer

Orestes A. Brownson: American Religious Weathervane
Patrick W. Carey

Thomas Merton and the Monastic Vision • *Lawrence S. Cunningham*

Billy Sunday and the Redemption of Urban America • *Lyle W. Dorsett*

The Kingdom Is Always but Coming: A Life of Walter Rauschenbusch
Christopher H. Evans

Liberty of Conscience: Roger Williams in America • *Edwin S. Gaustad*

Sworn on the Altar of God: A Religious Biography of Thomas Jefferson
Edwin S. Gaustad

Abraham Lincoln: Redeemer President • *Allen C. Guelzo*

Charles G. Finney and the Spirit of American Evangelicalism
Charles E. Hambrick-Stowe

Emily Dickinson and the Art of Belief • *Roger Lundin*

The Puritan as Yankee: A Life of Horace Bushnell • *Robert Bruce Mullin*

Prophetess of Health: A Study of Ellen G. White • *Ronald L. Numbers*

Blaise Pascal: Reasons of the Heart • *Marvin R. O'Connell*

Occupy Until I Come: A. T. Pierson and the Evangelization of the World
Dana L. Robert

God's Strange Work: William Miller and the End of the World
David L. Rowe

The Divine Dramatist: George Whitefield and the
Rise of Modern Evangelicalism • *Harry S. Stout*

Assist Me to Proclaim: The Life and Hymns of Charles Wesley
John R. Tyson

PROPHETESS OF HEALTH

A Study of Ellen G. White

• •

THIRD EDITION

Ronald L. Numbers

WILLIAM B. EERDMANS PUBLISHING COMPANY
GRAND RAPIDS, MICHIGAN / CAMBRIDGE, U.K.

© 1976, 1992, 2008 by Ronald L. Numbers
All rights reserved

First edition published 1976 by Harper & Row, New York

Second revised and enlarged edition published 1992
by the University of Tennessee Press, Knoxville

This third edition published 2008 by
Wm. B. Eerdmans Publishing Co.
2140 Oak Industrial Drive N.E., Grand Rapids, Michigan 49505 /
P.O. Box 163, Cambridge CB3 9PU U.K.

Library of Congress Cataloging-in-Publication Data

Numbers, Ronald L.
Prophetess of health: a study of Ellen G. White /
Ronald L. Numbers. — 3rd ed.
p.   cm.   — (Library of religious biography)
Includes bibliographical references and index.
ISBN 978-0-8028-0395-5 (pbk.: alk. paper)
1. White, Ellen Gould Harmon, 1827-1915.
2. Women health reformers — United States — Biography.
3. Diet.   4. Hydrotherapy.   5. Medicine — Religious aspects.
I. Title.

BX6193.W5N85   2008
286.7092 — dc22
[B]
                                        2008006080

www.eerdmans.com

To My Friends
Vern and Barbara Carner

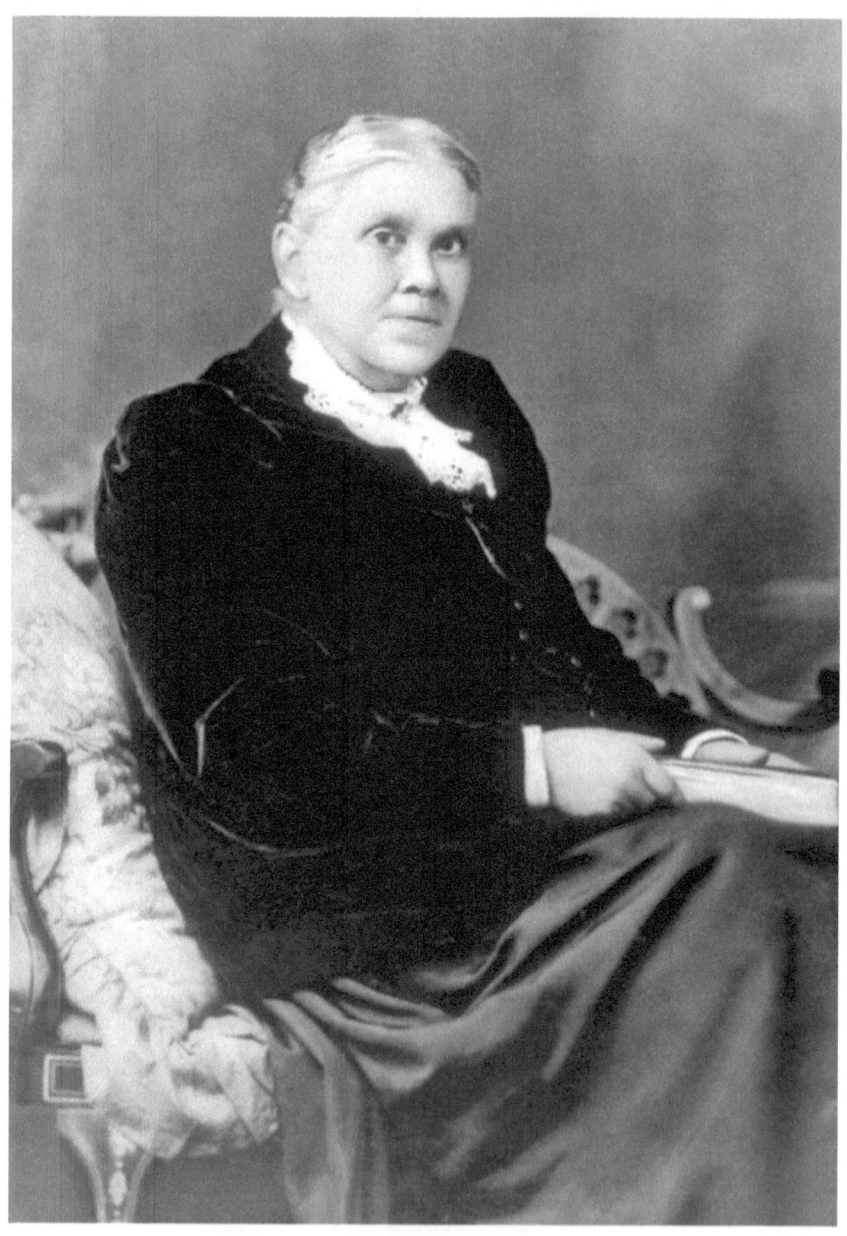

Ellen G. White
Courtesy Ellen G. White Estate, Inc.

Contents

List of Illustrations	ix
Abbreviations	x
Preface to the Third Edition	xi
Preface to the Second Edition	xxvi
Preface to the First Edition	xxx
Introduction: The Historian as Heretic, by Jonathan M. Butler	1
1. A Prophetess Is Born	43
2. In Sickness and in Health	76
3. The Health Reformers	95
4. Dansville Days	127
5. The Western Health Reform Institute	156
6. Short Skirts and Sex	184
7. Whatsoever Ye Eat or Drink	219
8. Fighting the Good Fight	239
Afterword: Ellen White on the Mind and the Mind of Ellen White, by Ronald L. Numbers and Janet S. Numbers	267

Contents

Appendix 1: Physical and Psychological Experiences of Ellen G. White: Related in Her Own Words   291

Appendix 2: The 1864 Dansville Visit   320

Appendix 3: The Trial of Elder I. Dammon   326

Appendix 4: The Secret 1919 Bible Conferences   344

Index   402

Illustrations

Ellen G. White	Frontispiece
Ellen G. White and Elizabeth Bangs	46
Sylvester Graham	98
William A. Alcott	104
Russell T. Trall	116
Phrenological Illustrations	118
James C. Jackson	122
Our Home on the Hillside	129
White Family and Adelia Patten	142
Title Page, *How to Live*	147
Original Western Health Reform Institute	158
Horatio S. Lay	161
Phoebe Lamson	163
Trall's Hygeian Home	178
John Harvey Kellogg	180
New Western Health Reform Institute	182
Elizabeth Smith Miller in Short Skirt	186
Amelia Bloomer	187
Harriet N. Austin in the American Costume	189
Ellen White in Short Skirt and Pants	194
Two Adventist Sisters in Reform Dresses	199
Model Reform Dress	201
Title Page, *An Appeal to Mothers*	209
Water Treatments, Battle Creek Sanitarium	248

Abbreviations

EGW	Ellen G. White
HR	*Health Reformer*
LLU-HR	Heritage Room, Loma Linda University Library
MHC	Michigan Historical Collections, University of Michigan
MSU	Michigan State University Archives and Historical Collections
R&H	*Advent Review and Sabbath Herald*
SDA	Seventh-day Adventist

Preface to the Third Edition

When I began toying with the possibility of writing a book about Ellen White, in 1972, I feared that the exercise might prove in vain. I knew that the Seventh-day Adventist church would never publish anything critical of the founding mother, and I suspected that no non-Adventist publisher would be interested in such a parochial topic. However, when my friend Vern Carner — a cross-wearing provocateur on the religion faculty at Loma Linda University — "guaranteed" that he would find a publisher for me, I plunged ahead, confident that at least I would benefit from the experience. True to his word, Carner talked Harper and Row into looking at my manuscript (after an editor at Eerdmans politely brushed me off). The story of the book's reception and my experience is well told in Jonathan M. Butler's essay that appears in this edition of *Prophetess of Health*. To my great satisfaction, the book not only contributed to a reevaluation of White within Adventism but elevated her from a virtually unknown historical actor to a minor star on the stage of American religious history.

The current quest for the historical Ellen White began in the late 1960s.[1] Although I joined the project early on, I can take no credit for having launched it. That recognition goes largely to a clique of criti-

---

1. This section is based in part on my talk "The Quest for the Historical Ellen White," delivered on May 26, 2001, as the Second Richard Hammill Memorial Lecture, Loma Linda University, co-sponsored by the Adventist Today Foundation and the Association of Adventist Forums.

cally trained young scholars then on the faculty of Andrews University — Roy Branson (Christian ethics, Harvard), Herold Weiss (New Testament, Duke), Bill Peterson (Victorian literature, Northwestern), and Don McAdams (European history, Duke) — who set about to deconstruct the iconic Ellen White that her family and apologists had carefully crafted over the preceding century. I began interacting with the group in the summer of 1969, when, fresh out of graduate school at Berkeley, I took a job in the Andrews history department.

A few years earlier, Branson (a cousin of mine) and I had helped to organize the Association of Adventists Forums, an independent organization of educated Seventh-day Adventists, which began publishing a new journal called *Spectrum*. The autumn 1970 issue carried the first rumblings of the historiographical revolution in the making. In "Ellen White: A Subject for Adventist Scholarship," Branson and Weiss called for uncovering "the *real* Ellen White." Their agenda comprised discovering "the nature of Mrs. White's relationship to other authors," recovering "the social and intellectual milieu in which she lived and wrote," and examining "the development of Ellen White's writings within her own lifetime." They naively (or perhaps ironically) promised that such an approach would reveal a "more vibrant Ellen White . . . a more believable person," who would become "actually more authoritative." The same issue of *Spectrum* included an article by Peterson that served up a concrete example of what the unmasking process might reveal: a self-described inspired writer who owed a greater debt to unacknowledged historical sources than to divinely sent visions.[2]

In the thirty years since *Prophetess of Health* first appeared, two

---

2. Roy Branson and Herold D. Weiss, "Ellen White: A Subject for Adventist Scholarship," *Spectrum*, II (Autumn 1970): 30-33; William S. Peterson, "A Textual and Historical Study of Ellen G. White's Account of the French Revolution," *Spectrum*, II (Autumn 1970): 57-69. At the time McAdams chose an administrative career in the church over publishing his 250-page document "Ellen G. White and the Protestant Historians"; but for a belated summary of his findings, which demonstrated extensive plagiarism, see Eric Anderson, "Ellen White and Reformation Historians," *Spectrum*, IX (July 1978): 23-26. Anderson, a former student of McAdams's, contrasted McAdams's "caution" with "the icon-busting gusto that some readers saw in Ronald L. Numbers' *Prophetess of Health,* though both works portray an Ellen White heavily influenced by her environment."

key documents — reprinted here in abridged form — have come to light that contribute greatly to our understanding of White's early ministry and the ways her contemporaries viewed her claims to divine inspiration. In 1987 the Adventist historian Frederick W. Hoyt finally mustered the courage to make public a historical bombshell that he had discovered several years earlier: the published (but long forgotten) transcript of a trial in early 1845 of a Millerite elder in Maine, Israel Dammon, accused of vagrancy and disturbing the peace. The trial record shows seventeen-year-old Ellen Harmon, accompanied by James White (her future husband), caught up in the very "fanaticism" that she would later denounce: kissing, touching, crawling, and shouting. During the trial some three-dozen witnesses testified about the activities of Dammon and his rambunctious Adventist associates. They portrayed Ellen Harmon as a young trance medium who went by the name of "Imitation of Christ" and who lay on the floor for hours with a pillow under her head, receiving and relating her visions. This image hardly comported with the decorous picture of the fledgling prophetess later painted by the Whites and their supporters.[3]

In 1979 the editor of *Spectrum,* Molleurus Couperus, published the hitherto unreleased transcript of an innocently named "Bible Conference" for church leaders, held in 1919, just four years after White's death. For two days the custodians of White's reputation wrestled with such potentially explosive questions as "How should we use the writings of the spirit of prophecy [that is, the writings of Mrs. White] as an authority to settle historical questions?" Arthur G. Daniells, longtime president of the church and confidant of the late prophetess, identified the two most pressing public-relations problems facing the church: "One is on infallibility and the other is on

---

3. Frederick G. Hoyt, "Trial of Elder I. Dammon, Reported for the *Piscataquis Farmer,*" *Spectrum,* XVII (August 1987): 29-36; reprinted in *The Disappointed: Millerism and Millenarianism in the Nineteenth Century,* ed. Ronald L. Numbers and Jonathan M. Butler, rev. ed. (Knoxville: University of Tennessee Press, 1993), pp. 227-40. See also Bruce Weaver, "Incident in Atkinson: The Arrest and Trial of Israel Dammon," *Adventist Currents,* III (April 1988): 16-35; and Rennie Schoepflin, ed., "Scandal or Rite of Passage? Historians on the Dammon Trial," *Spectrum,* XVII (August 1987): 37-50. For Hoyt's latest contribution to White scholarship, see "Wrestling with Venerable Manuscripts," *Adventist Today,* XII, no. 3 (2004): 10-13, 21.

Preface to the Third Edition

verbal inspiration." He — and other participants — identified specific instances of plagiarism as well as the process by which "a lot of things got into the Testimonies," widely believed to have come directly from White's visions. Daniells knew from personal experience that it would be fruitless "for anybody to stand up and talk about the verbal inspiration of the Testimonies, because everybody who has ever seen the work done knows better, and we might as well dismiss it." He suspected that James White had long ago anticipated the difficulties now facing the church:

> He knew that he took Sister White's testimonies and helped to write them out and make them clear and grammatical and plain. He knew that he was doing that right along. And he knew that the secretaries they employed took them and put them into grammatical condition, transposed sentences, completed sentences, and used words that Sister White did not herself write in her original copy.

"If that explanation had been accepted and passed on down," he said wistfully, "we would have been free from a great many perplexities that we have now." But instead of bravely educating church members about White's practices, he and his colleagues timidly suppressed the proceedings of their remarkably candid conference.[4]

During the decade or so after 1976 the effort to determine just how much White had copied from other sources grew in intensity. *Prophetess of Health* had received considerable attention — both positive and negative — for identifying small amounts of copying, laid out in parallel columns. Partly inspired by my revelations, Walter T. Rea, a senior Adventist pastor and longtime admirer of White, undertook a diligent search for more parallels. The publication in 1982 of his iconoclastic book, *The White Lie,* shocked the Adventist community by exposing the vast extent of White's copying. Rea's later work on White's *Conflict of the Ages* series proved, in his words, "beyond any reasonable doubt that far more than 80% of the material enclosed within the covers of these books was taken from others."[5]

---

4. Molleurus Couperus, "The Bible Conference of 1919," *Spectrum,* X (May 1979): 23-57.

5. Walter T. Rea, *The White Lie* (Turlock, Calif.: M & R Publications, 1982). Rea

Preface to the Third Edition

To determine for themselves the extent of the problem, church leaders spent hundreds of thousands of dollars to pay a New Testament scholar at Pacific Union College, Fred Veltman, to assess exactly how White had constructed the books she claimed to have written. After meticulously examining 15 of the 87 chapters of *The Desire of Ages (DA)*, White's much-revered life of Jesus, Veltman concluded that "On an average we may say that 31.4 percent of the *DA* text is dependent to some extent on literary sources." In contrast to scholars who had blamed White's assistants for the plagiarisms in her books, Veltman concluded that "Ellen White, not her literary assistants, did the literary borrowing." His research had shown "that Ellen White at times felt free to take verbatim expressions from the writings of others but that for the most part she paraphrased her sources. Generally the closer one is able to move back through the textual tradition to Ellen White's own hand, the greater is the degree of literary dependency."[6] After such revelations, including the previously unimaginable fact that White had borrowed from works of fiction, it hardly made any difference whether future investigations uncovered one or a hundred more instances of plagiarism. White's reputation for literary excellence and originality lay in shambles, and her honesty was under challenge.

A second church-financed study of the prophetess, this one by the White Estate historian Ronald Graybill, also boomeranged.

---

showed that Ellen White had borrowed extensively from other sources in writing *Testimonies to the Church*, vols. 1-9 (1868-1909), *The Spirit of Prophecy* (1877-84), *Steps to Christ* (1892), *Sketches from the Life of Paul* (1883), *The Great Controversy* (1884 and later editions), *Patriarchs and Prophets* (1890), *Thoughts from the Mount of Blessing* (1896), *The Desire of Ages* (1898), *Christ's Object Lessons* (1900), *Education* (1903), *The Ministry of Healing* (1905), *Counsels to Teachers* (1913), *The Acts of the Apostles* (1911), and the posthumously published *Prophets and Kings* (1916). See also Rea, Letter to the Editor, *Spectrum*, XIV (October 1983): 63-64, where he gives the 80 percent estimate.

6. Fred Veltman, "Full Report of the Life of Christ Research Project" (unpublished MS, November 1988), pp. 882, 890, 911, 913. For an abstract of this work, see Veltman, "The *Desire of Ages* Project," *Ministry*, LXII (October 1990): 4-7; (December 1990): 11-15. See also Walter Rea, "The Making of a Prophet," *Adventist Currents*, II (March 1987): 30-33. On White's use of literary assistants, see Alice Elizabeth Gregg, "The Unfinished Story of Fannie Bolton and Marian Davis," *Adventist Currents*, I (October 1983): 21-27, 34-35; (February 1984): 23-25, 29. I am indebted to J. B. Goodner for a copy of Veltman's full report.

Preface to the Third Edition

While working at the Estate in Takoma Park, Maryland, Graybill had simultaneously pursued a doctorate in American religious history at the nearby Johns Hopkins University. Given his free access to White's unpublished manuscripts, he decided to focus on the private life of the prophetess, as wife and mother. The resulting portrait was not pretty. Graybill revealed that by the 1870s the Whites' marriage had deteriorated so badly that they occasionally lived separately. "If they had to 'walk apart the rest of the way,'" Graybill describes her writing to James in 1874, "she hoped that at least they would not try to 'pull each other down. . . . I do believe it is best for our labors to be disconnected and we each lean upon God for ourselves.'" While visiting in California two years later, Ellen confided to her friend Lucinda Hall that James was trying to control her — at the same time that he, in Michigan, was complaining about her attempts to control him. "My husband is now happy. Blessed news!" Ellen announced sarcastically in a letter to Hall. "If he will only remain happy I would be willing to ever remain from him. If my presence is detrimental to his happiness God forbid I should ever be connected with him. . . . I do not think my husband really desired my society." To her husband she wrote sharply: "I shall use the old head God gave me until he reveals that I am wrong. Your head won't fit my shoulders. Keep it where it belongs, and I will try to honor God in using my own. I shall be glad to hear from you but don't waste your precious time and strength in lecturing me on matters of mere opinions." At times Ellen experienced dreams or visions in which her heavenly guide would point out James's defects, while assuring her that she deserved more credit for what they had achieved. She undiplomatically reminded James that he had been "highly favored in being connected with one whom God is leading, counseling, and teaching." In 1880 she forbade him from joining her on the West Coast. The next year he died.[7]

Although she loved her children and frequently fretted about

---

7. Ronald D. Graybill, "The Power of Prophecy: Ellen G. White and the Women Religious Founders of the Nineteenth Century" (Ph.D. dissertation, Johns Hopkins University, 1983), pp. 38-48. Graybill's earlier contributions to White scholarship include *Ellen G. White and Church Race Relations* (Washington, D.C.: Review and Herald Publishing Assn., 1970); and "How Did Ellen White Choose and Use Historical Sources? The French Revolution Chapter of *The Great Controversy*," *Spectrum*, IV (Summer 1972): 49-53.

Preface to the Third Edition

their spiritual and physical health, she was not above manipulating them with appeals to her heavenly authority. "I have written you letters dictated by the spirit of God, and I beg you not to disregard my efforts," she admonished son Edson on one occasion. On another she wrote: "God has taught your mother, and she has taught you your wrongs." Frequently, she played favorites, heaping praise on Willie — her "best boy," her "sunshine" — while reminding Edson "that his life was 'a mistake,' 'worse than useless,' and 'a failure.'"[8]

Regrettably for Graybill, he tried to outsmart church leaders by submitting two versions of his dissertation: a complete one to his committee at Johns Hopkins and a sanitized one to his bosses at the White Estate. The discovery of Graybill's duplicity created a minor scandal. As one distressed church leader noted, the Hopkins version of the dissertation "leaves the wrong impression of Ellen White. It seems to suggest that she was a power-hungry woman who had visions on command. It suggests, for example, when James White got into trouble with other church leaders, Mrs. White would have a vision to help him out." Not surprisingly, Graybill lost his job — and his standing as the church's most scholarly defender of White.[9]

The Adventist leadership did not look kindly on those who wrote critically about the prophetess. Immediately after complet-

---

8. Graybill, "The Power of Prophecy," pp. 63-66.

9. J. R. Spangler, "The Graybill Dissertation," unpublished MS originally written for *Ministry*, ca. January 1984. In a quaint announcement of Graybill's firing from the White Estate, the president of the General Conference informed church members that Graybill had first been placed on "administrative leave" and then "reassigned" to Home Study International, a correspondence school, in part because he approached "the study of Ellen White from the perspective of a secular historian who attempts to explain her role . . . from an exclusively humanistic point of view"; Neal C. Wilson, "White Estate Staffer Reassigned," *Adventist Review*, Feb. 2, 1984, p. 31. See also Douglas Hackleman, "The 'Greening' of Graybill," *Adventist Currents*, I (February 1984): 11-15, 28; and Bonnie L. Casey, "Graybill's Exit: Turning Point at the White Estate?" *Spectrum*, XIV (March 1984): 2-8. After a troubled stint on the history faculty at what is now La Sierra University, Graybill moved on to the Loma Linda University Medical Center, where he now works as community outreach coordinator. In recent years he has critiqued the claim, made by a prominent black Adventist minister, that White was a mulatto. See Ronald D. Graybill, "That 'Great African-American Woman,' Ellen Gould Harmon White," *Spectrum*, XXVIII (Autumn 2000): 71, a review of Charles Edward Dudley Sr., *The Genealogy of Ellen Gould Harmon White: The Prophetess of the Seventh-day Adventist Church* (Nashville: Dudley Publishing Services, 1999).

ing his controversial essay on White's historical scholarship — but before he could be dismissed — Bill Peterson escaped from Andrews University to the University of Maryland. Herold Weiss, under pressure from the president of the General Conference, who urged the university to fire him, fled from Andrews to nearby St. Mary's College in South Bend. Roy Branson lost his bid for tenure at Andrews and his chances for ordination as a minister; for years church leaders blackballed attempts to hire him in the denomination's educational system (though he now teaches at Columbia Union College, an Adventist school in Maryland). Loma Linda University terminated Jonathan Butler just as he was beginning to write a full-scale biography of White (for reasons largely unrelated to his scholarship), forced Vern Carner off the faculty, and got rid of me without a formal firing by promising a year's severance pay in return for a letter of resignation. Walter Rae lost his job and (temporarily) his pension after thirty-six years in the ministry. By suppressing publication of his research (and requesting that I not even mention it in *Prophetess of Health*), Don McAdams for a time prospered as an administrator in the Adventist educational system, though he later left church employment.

Butler's promised biography never materialized, but he did publish several insightful studies of White. For a church still enthralled by White's vivid descriptions of end-time events — and still expecting the imminent return of Jesus to earth — Butler's 1979 essay on "The World of E. G. White and the End of the World" undermined the eschatological foundations of Seventh-day Adventism. In it Butler argued that White's "predictions of the future appeared as projections on a screen which only enlarged, dramatized and intensified the scenes of her contemporary world," not scenes revealed to her in vision. Even more provocatively, he insisted that "What Seventh-day Adventists must fully acknowledge . . . is the element of *prophetic disconfirmation.* The prophetess predicted that Protestant America would end with the passage of Sunday legislation, the repudiation of constitutional government, the persecution of the Saturday-keeping minority, resulting finally in the Second Coming." But none of these predictions had come to pass. In 1991 Butler published a reassessment of White's childhood and youth, emphasizing her formative experiences with the "shouting" Methodists, the fa-

Preface to the Third Edition

natical wing of Millerism, and the visionary culture of New England.[10]

Before the appearance of *Prophetess of Health* Ellen White remained largely hidden in the shadows of American religious history. If mainstream historians deigned to mention Adventists at all, they typically paired William Miller with Joseph Smith and Mary Baker Eddy as founders of innovative American religious movements.[11] After 1976 this neglect gave way to featured roles, as *Prophetess of Health* established itself, in the judgment of Martin E. Marty, as "the standard biography" of White.[12] In short order White became a fix-

---

10. Jonathan M. Butler, "Adventism and the American Experience," in *The Rise of Adventism: Religion and Society in Mid-Nineteenth-Century America*, ed. Edwin S. Gaustad (New York: Harper & Row, 1974), pp. 173-206; "The World of E. G. White and the End of the World," *Spectrum*, X (August 1979): 2-13; Butler, "Prophecy, Gender, and Culture: Ellen Gould Harmon [White] and the Roots of Seventh-day Adventism," *Religion and American Culture*, I (1991): 3-29. On White and eschatology, see also Douglas Morgan, *Adventism and the American Republic: The Public Involvement of a Major Apocalyptic Movement* (Knoxville: University of Tennessee Press, 2001).

11. See, e.g., William Warren Sweet, *The Story of Religion in America* (New York: Harper and Brothers, 1939); Alice Felt Tyler, *Freedom's Ferment: Phases of American Social History to 1860* (Minneapolis: University of Minnesota Press, 1944); Sweet, *Religion in the Development of American Culture, 1765-1840* (New York: Charles Scribner's Sons, 1952); Jerald C. Brauer, *Protestantism in America: A Narrative History* (Philadelphia: Westminster Press, 1953); and Edwin Scott Gaustad, *A Religious History of America* (New York: Harper and Row, 1966). The following mentioned her name in passing: Whitney R. Cross, *The Burned-over District: The Social and Intellectual History of Enthusiastic Religion in Western New York, 1800-1850* (Ithaca, N.Y.: Cornell University Press, 1950), p. 316; Winthrop S. Hudson, *Religion in America* (New York: Charles Scribner's Sons, 1965), p. 196; Martin E. Marty, *Righteous Empire: The Protestant Experience in America* (New York: Dial Press, 1970), p. 124; and Robert T. Handy, *A History of the Churches in the United States and Canada* (New York: Oxford University Press, 1976), p. 294. The exceptions were Sydney E. Ahlstrom, *A Religious History of the American People* (New Haven: Yale University Press, 1972), p. 481, which devoted a couple of paragraphs to White, "the 'Adventist Prophetess,'" and her Seventh-day Adventist followers; and C. C. Goen, "Ellen Gould Harmon White," in *Notable American Women, 1607-1950: A Biographical Dictionary*, 3 vols. (Cambridge, Mass.: Harvard University Press, 1971), 3: 585-88, which noted that "No critical biography of Ellen White exists, and few writers outside the Seventh-Day Adventist Church have treated her career."

12. Martin E. Marty, *Pilgrims in Their Own Land: 500 Years of Religion in America* (Boston: Little, Brown, 1984), p. 485.

Preface to the Third Edition

ture in accounts of women and religion in America.[13] She replaced Miller as the archetypical Adventist, often appearing bracketed with Smith or Eddy or some other reformer to illustrate the fecund nature of the spiritual marketplace in America.[14] Peter W. Williams declared White — along with Anne Hutchinson, Harriet Beecher Stowe, Mary Baker Eddy, and Aimee Semple McPherson — to be one of the most prominent women in American religious history.[15]

---

13. See, e.g., Janet Wilson James, "Women in American Religious History: An Overview," in *Women in American Religion,* ed. Janet Wilson James (Philadelphia: University of Pennsylvania Press, 1980), pp. 1-25, esp. pp. 8, 22; Ann Braude, "Women's History Is American Religious History," in *Retelling U.S. Religious History,* ed. Thomas A. Tweed (Berkeley and Los Angeles: University of California Press, 1997), pp, 87-107, esp. pp. 89-90; Catherine A. Brekus, *Strangers and Pilgrims: Female Preaching in America, 1740-1845* (Chapel Hill: University of North Carolina Press, 1998), pp. 307-8, 333; and Marilyn J. Westerkamp, *Women and Religion in Early America, 1600-1850: The Puritan and Evangelical Traditions* (London: Routledge, 1999), p. 181.

14. See, e.g., Catherine L. Albanese, *America: Religions and Religion* (Belmont, Calif.: Wadsworth, 1981), pp. 145-49; Martin E. Marty, *The Irony of It All, 1893-1919,* vol. 1 of *Modern American Religion* (Chicago: University of Chicago Press, 1986), pp. 256-57, 358; R. Laurence Moore, *Religious Outsiders and the Making of Americans* (New York: Oxford University Press, 1986), pp. 133-36, 225; and Jon Butler, Grant Wacker, and Randall Balmer, *Religion in American Life: A Short History* (New York: Oxford University Press, 2003), pp. 313-14. In a discussion of "sectarian innovations" in the nineteenth century, George M. Marsden, *Religion and American Culture* (Fort Worth: Harcourt Brace Jovanovich, 1990), p. 80, discusses White and Smith but substitutes John Humphrey Noyes for Eddy. R. Laurence Moore, *Selling God: American Religion in the Marketplace* (New York: Oxford University Press, 1994), p. 142, substitutes Lydia Pinkham for Smith. For other discussions of White based at least in part on *Prophetess of Health,* see Henry Warner Bowden, *Dictionary of American Religious Biography* (Westport, Conn.: Greenwood Press, 1977), pp. 503-4; Peter W. Williams, *Popular Religion in America: Symbolic Change and the Modernization Process in Historical Perspective* (Englewood Cliffs, N.J.: Prentice-Hall, 1980), pp. 128, 183-84; and Stephen J. Stein, *Alternative American Religions* (New York: Oxford University Press, 2000), pp. 81-86. See also Ronald L. Numbers and Rennie B. Schoepflin, "Ministries of Healing: Mary Baker Eddy, Ellen G. White, and the Religion of Health," in *Women and Health in America: Historical Readings,* ed. Judith Walzer Leavitt (Madison: University of Wisconsin Press, 1984), pp. 376-89; Jonathan M. Butler and Rennie B. Schoepflin, "Charismatic Women and Health: Mary Baker Eddy, Ellen G. White, and Aimee Semple McPherson," in *Women, Health, and Medicine in America: A Historical Handbook,* ed. Rima D. Apple (New York: Garland, 1990), pp. 337-65.

15. Peter W. Williams, ed., *Perspectives on American Religion and Culture* (Oxford: Blackwell, 1999), p. 289.

Preface to the Third Edition

Paul K. Conkin canonized White — with Eddy and Ann Lee of the Shakers — as one of "the great trinity of female prophets in American Christianity."[16] In similar fashion White rose to prominence in the history of American health reform.[17] And because of later work

16. Paul K. Conkin, *American Originals: Homemade Varieties of Christianity* (Chapel Hill: University of North Carolina Press, 1997), pp. 127-42, quotation on p. 269. Although most non-Adventist historians who incorporated White into their narratives simply drew on *Prophetess of Health* and the growing body of secondary literature on White, a few, such as Conkin, mined the primary sources themselves. In *Protestants and Pictures: Religion, Visual Culture, and the Age of American Mass Production* (New York: Oxford University Press, 1999), pp. 121-98, David Morgan extensively explored "Adventism and Images of the End" and White's questionable aesthetic judgment. By far the most suggestive non-Adventist analysis of White appeared in Ann Taves's *Fits, Trances, and Visions: Experiencing Religion and Explaining Experience from Wesley to James* (Princeton, N.J.: Princeton University Press, 1999), pp. 128-30, 153-65. Taves, following Butler, convincingly placed White squarely in the "Methodist shout tradition," which prized ecstatic experiences such as dreams and visions. When charged by critics with "fanaticism" and "mesmerism," explained Taves, White deflected their taunts by alleging that they would no doubt make the same accusations about Jesus. Presenting herself as the sober messenger of God, she demonized those whom she regarded as "true" fanatics and mesmerists. For a thoughtful Adventist evaluation of Taves, see A. Gregory Schneider, "The Shouting Ellen White," *Spectrum*, XXIX (Autumn 2001): 16-22.

17. See, e.g., Ronald G. Walters, *American Reformers, 1815-1860* (New York: Hill and Wang, 1978), p. 156; Stephen Nissenbaum, *Sex, Diet, and Debility in Jacksonian America: Sylvester Graham and Health Reform* (Westport, Conn.: Greenwood Press, 1980), pp. 152-53; James C. Whorton, *Crusaders for Fitness: The History of American Health Reformers* (Princeton, N.J.: Princeton University Press, 1982), pp. 201-2; Harvey Green, *Fit for America: Health, Fitness, Sport, and American Society* (New York: Pantheon, 1986), p. 135; Martha H. Verbrugge, *Able-Bodied Womanhood: Personal Health and Social Change in Nineteenth-Century Boston* (New York: Oxford University Press, 1988), p. 125; Michael S. Goldstein, *The Health Movement: Promoting Fitness in America* (New York: Twayne, 1992), pp. 27, 44; Ruth Clifford Engs, *Clean Living Movements: American Cycles of Health Reform* (Westport, Conn.: Praeger, 2000), pp. 28-32. Before 1976 John B. Blake was the lone non-Adventist to mention Ellen White's health-reform visions — in a lecture originally given in a series at Loma Linda arranged by Carner and me; John B. Blake, "Health Reform," in *The Rise of Adventism: Religion and Society in Mid-Nineteenth-Century America*, ed. Edwin S. Gaustad (New York: Harper & Row, 1974), pp. 30-49, esp. p. 30. Although Seventh-day Adventists take pride in White's success as a temperance lecturer, historians of the temperance movement never mention her. See, e.g., Ruth Bordin, *Woman and Temperance: The Quest for Power and Liberty, 1873-1900* (Philadelphia: Temple University Press, 1981); and Barbara Leslie Epstein, *The Politics of Domesticity: Women, Evangelism, and Tem-

of mine on the history of antievolutionism, she also acquired a reputation as the godmother of "scientific creationism."[18]

Not all readers appreciated or even grasped my intended message. One befuddled college freshman, having slogged through *Prophetess of Health* for a course on American religion, indulged in some historical revisionism while writing his final exam:

> When 1843 came and went, many were hugely disappointed. Ellen White was one of those. As the years passed, she realized that she could not adjust to a non-Millerite philosophy. She was dreadfully unhappy and she yearned to be re-included in a sect. From these yearnings & the teachings of Ronald Numbers emerged the foundation of Seventh-day Adventism.[19]

Some Adventists used me as a foil in their own psycho-theological struggles. One Adventist religion teacher, for example, contrasted his progressive view of Ellen White's inspiration with my assumption of "an absolute once-true-always-true model for the phenomena of revelation and inspiration, not unlike a conservative fundamentalist holding to inerrancy" — ignoring the fact that conservative Adventists (correctly) faulted me for possessing no doctrine of divine inspiration whatsoever.[20]

After some hesitation, many Adventist scholars embraced the

---

perance in Nineteenth-Century America (Middletown, Conn.: Wesleyan University Press, 1981).

18. In *The Creationists* (New York: Alfred A. Knopf, 1992) I traced the origins of so-called young-earth creationism back to Ellen White and her Adventist protégé George McCready Price. In *The Scandal of the Evangelical Mind* (Grand Rapids, Mich.: William B. Eerdmans, 1994), p. 13, the church historian Mark A. Noll follows *The Creationists* in recounting the history of creationism "from its humble beginnings in the writings of Ellen White, the founder of Seventh-day Adventism, to its current status as a gospel truth embraced by tens of millions of Bible-believing evangelicals and fundamentalists around the world." See also, for example, Michael Ruse, *The Evolution Wars: A Guide to the Debates* (Santa Barbara, Calif.: ABC-CLIO, 2000), pp. 110-15; and Ruse, *The Evolution-Creation Struggle* (Cambridge, Mass.: Harvard University Press, 2005), pp. 158, 238-40.

19. I am indebted to my friend Grant Wacker for sharing this novel interpretation.

20. Alden Thompson, *Inspiration: Hard Questions, Honest Answers* (Hagerstown, Md.: Review and Herald Publishing Assn., 1991), p. 294.

findings, if not always the implications, of *Prophetess of Health*.[21] In the mid-1990s the editorial board of *Spectrum* voted me one of the five most influential Adventists in the past quarter century.[22] However, the corporate Seventh-day Adventist church, which now claims "more than 20 million believers" worldwide, continues to portray Ellen White much as it did in the years before 1976. In 1992, for instance, the Review and Herald Publishing Association released a book titled *The Great Visions of Ellen G. White,* by Roger W. Coon, an officer of the Ellen G. White Estate. "Adventists," he declared, "have held since earliest times that her writings were inspired by the Holy Spirit in the same manner — and to the same degree — as those of the 40-plus writers of the Bible." He devoted an entire chapter to White's 1863 vision on health, assuring readers that "Science has confirmed virtually all the counsels that emanated from Ellen White's first major health reform vision of 1863." As far as Coon and the White Estate were concerned, *Prophetess of Health* did not exist.[23]

---

21. See, e.g., Gary Land, "Faith, History and Ellen White," *Spectrum,* IX (March 1978): 51-55; Benjamin McArthur, "Where Are Historians Taking the Church?" *Spectrum,* IX (March 1978): 9-14; Arthur Patrick, "Re-Visioning the Role of Ellen White beyond the Year 2000," *Adventist Today,* VI (March-April 1998): 19-21; Land, "An Ambiguous Legacy: A Retrospective Review of *Prophetess of Health,*" *Spectrum,* XXIX (Autumn 2001): 23-26. See also Gary Land, ed., *Adventism in America: A History* (Grand Rapids, Mich.: William B. Eerdmans, 1986), pp. 219-23, "Debate over Ellen White"; and Malcolm Bull and Keith Lockhart, *Seeking a Sanctuary: Seventh-day Adventism and the American Dream* (San Francisco: Harper and Row, 1989), pp. 130, 237-38. Although Richard W. Schwarz was not allowed to cite *Prophetess of Health* in *Light Bearers to the Remnant: Denominational History Textbook for Seventh-day Adventist College Classes* (Mountain View, Calif.: Pacific Press, 1979), other books from church-owned publishing houses have mentioned it. George W. Reid, *A Sound of Trumpets: Americans, Adventists, and Health Reform* (Washington, D.C.: Review and Herald Publishing Assn., 1982), based on a doctoral dissertation written at Southwestern Baptist Theological Seminary, describes *Prophetess of Health* as "a thorough, compact, and well-documented study of Ellen G. White's role in Adventist health reform. While professing objectivity, its clear tenor leans toward discrediting much of what Mrs. White claimed" (p. 171). Gary Land, ed., *The World of Ellen G. White* (Washington, D.C.: Review and Herald Publishing Assn., 1987), recommends *Prophetess of Health* "for further reading."

22. "Five Most Influential SDAs — 1969-1994," *Spectrum,* XXIV (December 1994): 7-11.

23. Roger W. Coon, *The Great Visions of Ellen G. White* (Hagerstown, Md.: Review and Herald Publishing Assn., 1992), pp. 11, 101. The number of "believers" appears

Preface to the Third Edition

The most extensive recent study of Ellen White is Herbert E. Douglass's *Messenger of the Lord: The Prophetic Ministry of Ellen G. White*, authorized as a college textbook by the board of trustees of the Ellen G. White Estate, the General Conference Department of Education, and the church's Board of Higher Education. Like Coon, Douglass highlights White's similarity to the biblical writers — and exposes the character defects of her critics, whose lack of confidence in the prophetess he attributes to the influence of Satan. Forsaking conventional biography for apologetics, Douglass addresses everything from the "shut door" to masturbation. "Modern research indicates that Ellen White's strong statements can be supported when she is properly understood," Douglass assures his readers. "Two medical specialists have suggested that in a zinc-deficient adolescent, sexual excitement and excessive masturbation might precipitate insanity." Yet despite the gulf between his views and mine, Douglass has always been a kind and friendly critic.[24] My fond hope

---

on the Seventh-day Adventist Church Web site; actual *membership* is closer to 13.5 million. In 2005 the Seventh-day Adventist publishing house in Australia published a study by the physician Don S. McMahon, *Acquired or Inspired? Exploring the Origins of the Adventist Lifestyle* (Victoria, Australia: Signs Publishing Co., 2005), aimed at proving that White's health writings were inspired, not borrowed. As the Loma Linda University biologist Leonard Brand testified in a foreword to the book, he found it difficult after reading McMahon's findings "to see how it would be possible to explain Ellen White's health principles without a definite input of information from a non-human source." Shortly thereafter, Brand collaborated with McMahon in bringing McMahon's findings to the attention of American Adventists: *The Prophet and Her Critics: A Striking New Analysis Refutes the Charges that Ellen G. White "Borrowed" the Health Message* (Nampa, Idaho: Pacific Press, 2005). The latter book devotes a chapter to exposing the perceived weaknesses of *Prophetess of Health*, especially its failure to entertain "the hypothesis of divine inspiration" (p. 44). Despite their pretense to scientific rigor, McMahon's books are riddled with pseudoscientific claims, historical errors, and misleading comparisons. For a critical appraisal of McMahon, see T. Joe Willey, "Science Defends Supernatural? Using Apologetic Science to Vindicate the Health Gospels of Ellen G. White," *Adventist Today* 16 (May-June 2008).

24. Herbert E. Douglass, *Messenger of the Lord: The Prophetic Ministry of Ellen G. White* (Nampa, Idaho: Pacific Press, 1998), pp. ix (authorized), 408-15 (biblical writers), 493-94 (masturbation), 535 (Satan); Douglass, "Reexamining the Way God Speaks to His Messengers: Rereading *Prophetess of Health*," *Spectrum*, XXIX (Autumn 2001): 27-32. For a recent account of Ellen White's initial interest in masturbation, see Ronald L. Numbers: "Sex, Science, and Salvation: The Sexual Advice of

Preface to the Third Edition

is that his irenic spirit will infuse the continuing quest to discover the historical Ellen White.

Madison, Wisconsin
February 2006

Ellen G. White and John Harvey Kellogg," in *Right Living: An Anglo-American Tradition of Self-Help Medicine and Hygiene*, ed. Charles E. Rosenberg (Baltimore: Johns Hopkins University Press, 2003), 206-26.

Preface to the Second Edition

Fifteen years have passed since I finished writing *Prophetess of Health*. During that time two and a half million new Seventh-day Adventists, mostly from Third World countries, doubled the size of the church. Adventist hospitals, reorganized collectively as the Adventist Health System/United States, grew into "the country's largest Protestant, nonprofit, nationally integrated health care delivery system." Surgeons at the Loma Linda University Medical Center captured international headlines by transplanting a baboon's heart into a premature infant known as Baby Fae. Books showing *How You Can Live Six Extra Years* heralded the abstemious Adventist lifestyle. Occasional internecine disputes, often centering on the authority of Ellen G. White, threatened at times to fracture the church, but many doubters and dissenters, like myself, chose to flee rather than to fight. The part played by *Prophetess of Health* in these debates — plus much more — is the subject of an introductory chapter by my friend and fellow Adventist expatriate Jonathan M. Butler.

Although the focus of my own work after the appearance of *Prophetess of Health* shifted away from Adventist studies, from time to time I could not resist the temptation to continue exploring the religious tradition in which I was reared. The most substantial product resulting from these occasional indulgences was *The Disappointed: Millerism and Millenarianism in the Nineteenth Century* (Bloomington: Indiana University Press, 1987), coedited with Jonathan M. Butler. This collection of historical essays included an essay, written with Janet S. Numbers, titled "Millerism and Madness:

Preface to the Second Edition

A Study of 'Religious Insanity' in Nineteenth-Century America." Janet and I also joined forces to write "The Psychological World of Ellen White," *Spectrum,* XIV (August 1983), 21-31, parts of which are recycled in the Afterword. David R. Larson, an Adventist ethicist, and I contributed an essay on "The Adventist Tradition" to *Caring and Curing: Health and Medicine in the Western Religious Traditions,* ed. Ronald L. Numbers and Darrel W. Amundsen (New York: Macmillan Publishing Co., 1986), pp. 447-67. In it we sketched the history of Adventist beliefs and practices in the domain of health, paying particular attention to ethical issues. With the collaboration of Rennie B. Schoepflin, an expert on the history of Christian Science healing, I was able to expand the one-paragraph comparison of Ellen White and Mary Baker Eddy that appears on pp. 264-65 of this volume into a full article: "Ministries of Healing: Mary Baker Eddy, Ellen G. White, and the Religion of Health," in *Women and Health in America: Historical Readings,* ed. Judith Walzer Leavitt (Madison: University of Wisconsin Press, 1984), pp. 372-89. And I have devoted much of the past decade to writing a history of "scientific creationism," a movement indirectly inspired by the geological speculations of Ellen White. This work will be published by Alfred A. Knopf in 1992 under the title *The Creationists.*

The past decade and a half have witnessed a veritable explosion of publications on Ellen White, Seventh-day Adventism, and popular health reform. Fortunately for me, none of these new works necessitates abandoning the conclusions I reached in *Prophetess of Health.* If anything, they have made me look too timid rather than too bold. I have thus elected not to tamper with the existing text, except to correct a number of minor typographical errors, many of them spotted by William D. Conklin. I have, however, added a new Afterword, an essay on "Ellen White on the Mind and the Mind of Ellen White," and a new appendix containing a chronology of White's numerous physical and mental complaints, taken almost entirely from her own writings. In the preface to the original edition I wrote that "In trying to understand Ellen White, I have consciously shied away from extended analyses of her mental health and psychic abilities. Someday this should be done. . . . " I decided to undertake this treacherous task myself only because my wife, Janet S. Numbers, a clinical psychologist, agreed to collaborate with me on the project,

Preface to the Second Edition

and because a two-year stint as a Fellow in Interdisciplinary Studies at the Menninger Foundation in Topeka, Kansas, bolstered my confidence that we might have something of value to say on the subject.

When I acknowledged my intellectual debts in the first edition of *Prophetess of Health,* I twice failed to give adequate credit, once by accident, a second time by design. William S. Peterson, briefly a colleague of mine at Andrews University and now a professor of English at the University of Maryland, played a key role in sensitizing me to problems in Ellen White scholarship, both in conversations and through his pioneering essay "A Textual and Historical Study of Ellen G. White's Account of the French Revolution," *Spectrum,* II (Autumn 1970), 57-69. Bill, please accept my apologies and belated thanks.

During the 1973-74 school year I learned much about Ellen White and the resources of the Ellen G. White Estate from weekly conversations with Ron Graybill, then a research associate at the Estate. He was just beginning his doctoral studies in history at Johns Hopkins University, and I was spending a year there as a postdoctoral fellow in the history of medicine. At the insistence of his boss, Arthur L. White, Ron requested that I delete any mention of his name, a request to which I reluctantly acceded. I can now thank not only Ron but the entire staff of the White Estate for their help in spotting errors of fact and interpretation in the penultimate draft of *Prophetess of Health.* In an effort to prevent publication of the book by exposing my biased and sloppy research, the White Estate assembled a team of investigators to track down every source I had cited and to check every statement for accuracy. The White Estate detectives discovered not only an embarrassing number of slips but several pertinent documents I had either overlooked or had been prevented from seeing. Thanks to their indefatigable industry, I was able to correct these errors before publication and in some instances to augment the documentation for my claims. At the time, I detested what they were doing to me; I now wish I could submit every one of my manuscripts to such prepublication scrutiny.

I must confess, however, that one misstatement, one outright error, and one oversight slipped through this fine sieve. I alluded to the resentment some followers felt in 1851 toward Ellen White's "habit of publishing private testimonies revealing their secret sins

Preface to the Second Edition

— and names." I should not have used the word "habit." Although she published testimonies exposing individual errors before 1851, this practice did not become habitual until later. In the years up to 1851 she merely publicized the "errors and sins" of others, which gave ample cause for dissatisfaction. On p. 63, note 32, I inadvertently gave the date of Merritt Kellogg's letter as June 3 (my birthday!) rather than June 18, 1906.

Years after writing *Prophetess of Health,* I discovered one day that I had said nothing about the origin of the now-crucial Adventist distinction, derived from the Levitical law, between "clean" and "unclean" flesh. (Clean animals have cloven hooves and chew their cuds; clean fish have fins and scales.) After her 1863 vision Ellen White condemned the eating of all meat, especially pork, but she said little until late in the century about the clean-unclean dichotomy. By 1890, however she was arguing that the Old Testament distinction between "articles of food as clean and unclean" was not "a merely ceremonial and arbitrary regulation, but was based upon sanitary principles." Nevertheless, except for pork, she did not proscribe any particular meats on this basis, and the church did not formally ban unclean meats until much later. Readers interested in obtaining additional information on this point should consult Ron Graybill's pamphlet on "The Development of Adventist Thinking on Clean and Unclean Meats," issued by the White Estate in 1981.

Finally, I wish to thank Jane B. Donegan for her help in preparing this revised edition.

Madison, Wisconsin
February 1991

Preface to the First Edition

Ellen G. White, Seventh-day Adventist prophetess, ranks with the Mormon Joseph Smith, the Christian Scientist Mary Baker Eddy, and Charles Taze Russell of the Jehovah's Witnesses as one of four nineteenth-century founders of a major American religious sect.[1] Yet, outside her own church of two and a half million members, she is probably the least known. Her comparatively unsensational life and her church's reticence to expose her private papers to the scrutiny of critical scholars have contributed to this undeserved obscurity. By her death in 1915 she had founded one of the nation's largest indigenous denominations, created a string of sanitariums and hospitals stretching from Scandinavia to the South Pacific, and inspired an educational system without peer in the Protestant world today. She had traveled widely, lectured extensively, and written dozens of books on a variety of subjects. Few contemporaries, male or female, accomplished more.

Her charisma sprang largely from frequent "visions," which she began to experience in 1844 at the age of seventeen. In dramatic trances lasting from a few minutes to several hours she received heavenly messages regarding events past and present, celestial and terrestrial. Her disciples accepted her "testimonies" as genuine revelations from God and, with her encouragement, accorded her a status equal to the biblical prophets.

---

1. Ellen White always used the initial from her middle name Gould rather than from her maiden name Harmon. One of her second cousins, Agnes Coolbrith, married Joseph Smith.

Preface to the First Edition

On the evening of June 5, 1863, in the little Michigan town of Otsego, Ellen White had a special vision on health. There God revealed his hygienic laws, to be kept as faithfully as the Ten Commandments given to Moses. Seventh-day Adventists, Mrs. White learned, were to give up eating meat and other stimulating foods, shun alcohol and tobacco, and avoid drug-dispensing doctors. When sick, they were to rely solely on Nature's remedies: fresh air, sunshine, rest, exercise, proper diet, and — above all — water. Adventist sisters were to give up their fashionable dresses for "short" skirts and pantaloons similar to the Bloomer costume, and all believers were to curb their "animal passions." The terrible consequences of masturbation, to which Mrs. White devoted her first book on health, the Lord illustrated in graphic detail. "Everywhere I looked," she reported, "I saw imbecility, dwarfed forms, crippled limbs, misshapen heads, and deformity of every description."

The content of this vision was hardly new. Since the 1830s Sylvester Graham and his fellow health reformers had been preaching virtually the same thing, extolling vegetarianism and damning drugs, corsets, and intemperance of every kind. The following decade many water enthusiasts, called hydropaths, joined the hygienic crusade, offering baths, packs, and douches as the way to health. Within a few years water-cure establishments fairly littered the American landscape, and health-reform books and magazines could be found in countless homes from Maine to California. Mrs. White steadfastly denied being influenced by these works; but, as we shall see, her writings often betray more than a passing acquaintance with contemporary authors.

This study of Ellen White's activities as a health reformer began in the summer of 1972, while I was teaching the history of medicine at Loma Linda University. In an effort to find material that might interest my students, I turned to the health writings of Mrs. White, whose visions were responsible for the founding of the school and whose influence could still be seen. Modern drugs had long ago replaced water therapy, but such items as meat, tea, and coffee still made only surreptitious appearances.

My initial goal was modest: to look at Mrs. White's major writings within the context of nineteenth-century health reform. My scope expanded, however, when I accidentally ran across a copy of

Preface to the First Edition

Dr. L. B. Coles's *Philosophy of Health* in the Loma Linda medical library. Scattered throughout the margins of this book were shorthand notes and page numbers in the hand of Dr. John Harvey Kellogg, former owner of the volume and a onetime protégé of the prophetess. Unable to find anyone who could decipher the shorthand, but suspicious that the page numbers referred to one of Mrs. White's works, I began a volume-by-volume search for a correlation. A check of her *Christian Temperance and Bible Hygiene* finally revealed what Dr. Kellogg had discovered three-quarters of a century before: a strikingly close similarity between Dr. Coles's language and Mrs. White's. This serendipitous discovery spurred me to undertake a thorough examination of Ellen White's development as a health reformer, the result of which is this book.

Although this work at times ranges beyond her health-related activities, it falls far short of a full-fledged biography. Detailed studies of her endeavors in education and theology, for example, remain to be done. Nevertheless, this is, I believe, the first book about her that seeks neither to defend nor to damn but simply to understand. As one raised and educated within Adventism, I admittedly have more than an academic interest in Mrs. White's historical fate; but I have tried to be as objective as possible. Thus I have refrained from using divine inspiration as an historical explanation.

In so doing, I have parted company with those Adventist scholars who insist on the following presuppositions: (1) that the Holy Spirit has guided the Advent movement since the early 1840s, (2) "that Ellen Harmon White was chosen by God as his messenger and her work embodied that of a prophet," (3) "that as a sincere, dedicated Christian and a prophet, Ellen White would not and did not falsify," and (4) that the testimony of Mrs. White's fellow-believers "may be accepted as true and correct to the best of the memory of the individuals who reported."[2] It seems to me that such statements, particularly the last two, are more properly conclusions than presuppositions.

I have also departed from traditional Adventist scholarship in oc-

---

2. Arthur L. White, "Ellen G. White and the Shut Door Question" (mimeographed copy of a statement to appear in his forthcoming biography of Ellen G. White), pp. 4-5.

Preface to the First Edition

casionally using the testimony of individuals who rejected Mrs. White's claim to inspiration. I have done so — with some hesitance and much care — because to ignore them on *a priori* grounds seemed methodologically irresponsible. These individuals offer a perspective of Mrs. White not found in the writings of her followers. While some of them may have placed undue emphasis on the negative aspects of her life, their inclination to do so seems to have been no greater than the tendency of her disciples to emphasize the positive. Certainly no Adventist would hesitate to use critical accounts of Joseph Smith or Mary Baker Eddy; Mrs. White should be treated no differently.

In trying to understand Ellen White, I have consciously shied away from extended analyses of her mental health and psychic abilities. Someday this should be done, but the present does not seem like an appropriate time. First, my training has not qualified me to make anything like a retrospective diagnosis; and second, I do not want discussions of this work to focus on such controversial and emotionally laden issues.

It is no exaggeration to say that this book never could — or would — have been written without the assistance of numerous institutions and individuals, only a few of whom can be named here. To each I offer my sincere thanks, but hasten to add that none bears any responsibility for the views I have expressed. (Some of my benefactors I know disagree strongly with my interpretations.) Despite extraordinary efforts — by my critics as well as by myself — to catch all possible errors, some mistakes undoubtedly have slipped by. For these I have only myself to blame; however, I would appreciate their being brought to my attention.

During the summer of 1972 a grant from the Walter E. Macpherson Society of the Alumni Association of the Loma Linda University School of Medicine enabled me to travel East collecting documentation. One of the greatest pleasures of this trip was meeting William D. Conklin of Dansville, New York, who generously (and repeatedly) shared both his time and his unparalleled knowledge of Our Home on the Hillside. The staff of the Ellen G. White Estate in Washington, D.C., assisted me in locating and using the unpublished Ellen White papers housed in their vault. Kenneth P. Scheffel provided similar assistance with the records of John Harvey Kellogg in the Michigan Historical Collections at the University of Michigan.

Preface to the First Edition

The Loma Linda University School of Medicine granted me the entire 1972-73 school year to complete this study. I am especially grateful to former Dean David B. Hinshaw, who valued history and believed in the principle of academic freedom. In the Heritage Room of the Loma Linda University Library, James R. Nix served as an invaluable guide, while in nearby Riverside, Donald E. Mote permitted me to examine his unique files of Adventist documents.

In the final stages of preparing this book, I benefited greatly from the criticisms and suggestions of friends and colleagues, some of whom waded through multiple drafts. Lengthy discussions with Richard W. Schwarz of Andrews University saved me from a number of embarrassing errors and proved once again that honest persons can look at the same evidence and see fundamentally different things. Three of my sternest — and most helpful — critics were my cousins Roy Branson of Georgetown University, Bruce Branson of Loma Linda University, and Donald Bozarth of Columbia Union College. William Frederick Norwood, my predecessor at Loma Linda, was a constant source of wisdom and encouragement.

Among the others who contributed beneficial suggestions were: Molleurus Couperus, Loma Linda University; Gary Land, Andrews University; Regina Markell Morantz, University of Kansas; David Musto, Yale University; Neil Wayne Northey, Mariposa, California; Patricia Spain Ward, University of Wisconsin; T. Joe Willey, Loma Linda University.

John B. Blake kindly allowed me to borrow the title "Prophetess of Health" from an earlier article of his on Mary Cove Nichols. Janet Schulze provided moral support and editorial assistance. Charlotte McGirr typed and retyped the manuscript, and Kathryn Shain typed it again.

Finally, this volume is dedicated to Vern Carner, friend and former colleague at Loma Linda University, who convinced me to write this book one fateful Saturday afternoon and who shared fully the pain and excitement that resulted from that decision.

Madison, Wisconsin
November 1975

INTRODUCTION

The Historian as Heretic

JONATHAN M. BUTLER

"When the historian and the believer are the same person, the writing of a book can become an enterprise fraught with tension and, occasionally, agony. One must be an obtuse reader, indeed, not to see this tension and even feel this agony in the pages of Numbers' book."

Ernest R. Sandeen
"The State of a Church's Soul"

Nothing more poignantly illustrates the conflict between the historian and the believer than the trouble it can cause within families. When Ronald L. Numbers, recently hired as a historian at the University of Wisconsin, neared the completion of his manuscript on the Seventh-day Adventist prophet Ellen G. White, his father, Ray-

---

This study relies on both the "outer" history found in key published sources and the "inner" history uncovered in personal letters, memoranda of conversations, reports, oral tapes, and transcriptions of lectures. These latter unpublished materials were generously provided me by Ronald L. Numbers from his own extensive collection. Unless otherwise designated below, the unpublished sources may be found among his papers in Madison, Wisconsin. The personal conversations between Numbers and others are reported in memos by Numbers. In addition to drawing on these materials, I also interviewed several of the principals. My most important and extensive interviews were of Numbers himself, February 26, March 5, and April 19-21, 1990. But I benefited as well from conversations with Eric Anderson, Roy Branson, Vern Carner, and Ronald Graybill.

Introduction

mond W. Numbers, the pastor of an Adventist church in Las Vegas, was approaching the end of his ministerial career. Pastor Numbers prayed that his son would not publish the book. After *Prophetess of Health* nevertheless appeared in print in mid-1976, a broken father, unable to write his son directly, wrote to his daughter, Carolyn. Recalling the many times their mother and he had prayed over their children's cribs to dedicate them "to the giving of the Last Message of Mercy to the World," he added, "Satan has no right to steal you or Ronnie away from what you were born for." He concluded the letter by claiming a promise in Ellen White's *Child Guidance:* "The seed sown with tears and prayers may have seemed to be sown in vain, but their harvest is reaped with joy at last. Their children have been redeemed."[1]

The publication of his son's book had been a shattering experience for Ray Numbers as a father; and, curiously enough, it was just as devastating for Pastor Numbers as a son. More than forty years before, when Ray had been a ministerial major at the Adventist college near Washington, D.C., his own father, Ernest R. Numbers, himself a minister, had abandoned his family and faith in Ellen White after being publicly exposed in a brief lapse into adultery. The fact that Ray's father had held a middle-level administrative post in the church's General Conference ensured far-slung knowledge of the scandal. For the sensitive young theology student, this shameful experience had been at once damaging and formative. He devoted his life and career to redeeming the sullied family name. But after forty years of blameless toil in the Lord's vineyard, his restoration had been undone. Ironically, the son of an apostate was now also the father of an apostate. Having spent a lifetime restoring his name, there was too little time to do so again. Earlier than planned the disheartened pastor retired.[2]

When *Prophetess of Health* was first published, Adventist academics thought it chic to provide psychological explanations for Ron Numbers's slant. They spoke of unresolved conflicts with his inflexibly fundamentalist father or hostility to his father's version of

---

1. R. W. Numbers to Carolyn [Numbers] Remmers, July 20, 1976.
2. Interview of Ronald L. Numbers, March 5, 1990; R. W. Numbers to Charles Houck, May 13, 1979.

the church. This tack played well among the cultivated Adventists in educational and medical centers. No thought was given, however, to the way such pop psychology could as easily have been turned on the apologists themselves. Nor did the defense suggest that psychology or psychohistory might serve as a suitable tool for understanding the Adventist prophet as well as her detractors. Psychohistory only served to account for prophets of other traditions — Joseph Smith or Mary Baker Eddy — not Ellen White.[3]

Such apologetics understandably piqued Numbers as a historian, who wanted his work analyzed, not his life psychoanalyzed. But a rebuttal to Ron Numbers that cast reflections not only on the rebellious preacher's son but, to no small degree, on the preacher-father deeply disturbed Ray Numbers, too. He spoke plaintively to his son about it. (They had generally never had problems speaking to each other, even when speaking on opposite sides of a question.) While Pastor Numbers wondered if he had, unwittingly, prompted his son's book, his concern went deeper, to the way he might have affected his son's soul. The father wanted to know, candidly, if he had been a rigid and unreasonable authority figure at whom his son now hurled his book. Ron assured his father that he had been a wonderful, caring parent, more flexible than many of his contemporaries and, while his son had grown up to disagree with him on many points of faith, he had always respected him. Thus, whatever the strains that had been placed on father and son as believer and historian, the openness and affection between them, through it all, seemed to belie the psychological reductionism of *their* critics.[4]

The effort to explain away *Prophetess of Health* by way of the psychological problems of its author was neither more dignified nor less dubious than the mere *ad hominem* attack. In fact, the intensely personal nature of responses to Numbers's book within

---

3. Jack Provonsha, an ethicist, and Brian Bull, a pathologist, discussed *Prophetess of Health: A Study of Ellen G. White* (New York: Harper & Row, Publishers, 1976) in taped Sabbath School classes at Loma Linda University in the spring of 1976, in which they attributed flaws in the book to the personal and theological inadequacies of its author. General reference to such responses, itself critical of them, is found in Fritz Guy, "What Should We Expect from a Prophet?" *Spectrum*, VIII (January, 1977), 22.

4. Interview of Ronald Numbers, February 26, 1990.

INTRODUCTION

the Adventist church smacked of a family quarrel. As something of an extended family, Adventists usually prove more generous to non-family members than errant relatives. When Numbers, at thirty, began his research on the Adventist prophet at the Ellen G. White Estate, Arthur L. White, grandson of the prophet and head of the archives, welcomed him not only as a respected young scholar from the Loma Linda University School of Medicine but as good Adventist stock. Numbers's maternal grandfather, W. H. Branson, had been the church's General Conference president and the author of a classic apologetic answer to the charges of the church's most notorious apostate, Dudley M. Canright.[5] For this favorite son of the church to have gone sour, then, was taken as something akin to a betrayal of the family.

Two of Numbers's uncles, husbands of his father's sisters, did what they could to rein in their nephew. Roger Wilcox, who served as General Field Secretary of the General Conference, proved less avuncular than officious in relation to Ron. Named as chair of a committee at G.C. headquarters to deal with the book, Wilcox planned strategy for minimizing its damage. Another uncle, Glenn Coon, an evangelist who headed the ABC Prayer Crusade ("Ask, Believe, Claim"), implored Ronnie not even to publish his manuscript and offered to repay him whatever expenses he had incurred in the writing of it, "whether it is a thousand or ten thousand dollars." Admitting he was not able to afford such an offer, he promised to pray for a miracle and then pay in installments. As an alternative to his nephew's manuscript, he suggested that the two of them co-author a more positive book on Ellen White. Though Coon remained Numbers's favorite uncle, his effort to abort publication of the book obviously failed. But the ABC's-of-prayer crusader consoled himself with the thought that his prayer had not failed. For, as Uncle Glenn later pointed out, he could find no Bible promise which said, "Ron will not write a book against [Sister] White."[6]

---

5. Canright lambasted Adventism and its prophet in two works: *Seventh-day Adventism Renounced* (New York: Fleming H. Revell Co., 1889); and *Life of Mrs. E. G. White, Seventh-day Adventist Prophet: Her False Claims Refuted* (Cincinnati: Standard Publishing Co., 1919). Branson's refutation was *Reply to Canright: The Truth About Seventh-day Adventists* (Washington: Review and Herald Publishing Assn., 1933).

6. Glenn and Ethel Coon to Ronald and Diane Numbers, January 28, 1975; Ron-

Neither of these relatives was the least bit persuasive with Numbers. However, his cousin, Roy Branson, an ethicist at the S.D.A. Theological Seminary, had exerted an earlier influence on him when the two taught together at Andrews University in 1969-70. In that year, Branson co-wrote with Herold Weiss, a New Testament scholar, a brief, provocative essay on "Ellen White: A Subject for Adventist Scholarship." Published in *Spectrum,* a new, independent journal largely for Adventist academics and professionals, for which Branson and Numbers had been among the founding fathers, the essay called for Adventists "to discover the nature of Mrs. White's relationship to other authors," "to recover the social and intellectual milieu in which she lived and wrote," and "to give close attention to the development of Ellen White's writings within her own lifetime, and also to the development of the church." Two years later, at Loma Linda University, Numbers began his study of Ellen White as a health reformer for which the Branson-Weiss essay, in general terms, could have served as a prospectus.[7]

In this retrospective on *Prophetess of Health,* I hope to assess the impact of the book on Seventh-day Adventists, without overlooking its reception beyond the circle of Adventism. In a sense, this introduction echoes the book's two underlying themes: milieu and change. First, in regard to cultural and intellectual milieu, Numbers, like the subject of his study, did not write *in vacuo*. His work may be the single most important example — but by no means the extent — of a historiographical coming of age within Adventism since 1970. While the focus here is on Numbers, it is revealing to view the way in which his work fits into the larger landscape of contemporary Adventism. Second, just as the prophet and her church underwent changes in the nineteenth century, perceptions of the prophet and the church's self-understanding have undergone profound development over the past two decades, at least among educated Adventists. How did Numbers contribute to these changes and what was the nature of the changes?

---

ald Numbers to Glenn and Ethel Coon, February 15, 1975; Glenn and Ethel Coon to Raymond and Lois Numbers, December 13, 1976; Roger A. Wilcox to R. W. Numbers, June 15, 1976.

7. *Spectrum,* II (Autumn, 1970), 30-33.

INTRODUCTION

Until Numbers's book on Ellen White, the Adventist prophet was among the better-kept secrets in American religious history. Seventh-day Adventists themselves seemed to hide their founding mother from the public. In his mapping of American religion, Martin E. Marty writes that ethnicity is the "framework or skeleton of religion in America; around 1960 that skeleton was taken out of the closet." For Adventists, who are at once a religion and a kind of ethnic group, Ellen White has served as a "skeleton" in the two ways Marty suggests: First, she has been the framework for the movement, holding life and limb together in every area of the church's thinking and behavior. All of Adventism stands in her debt for its understanding of the Sabbath, the Second Coming of Christ, justification and sanctification, health reform and medicine, child nurture and education. But, second, she has been a "skeleton in the closet" in that Adventists have hidden her from the non-Adventist public, as if to talk too openly about their "mother" betrays an unnatural dependence on her. Likewise, over the years, the church's ministers and teachers have concealed facts about her career from an *Adventist* public, as if the children were not mature enough to see their spiritual mother as an imperfect human being.[8]

Like other religious minorities, Adventists can be quite sensitive about their public image. In their recent historical and sociological study of the church, Malcolm Bull and Keith Lockhart concluded that there have been, historically, two public perceptions of Adventists: as apocalyptic fanatics and as philanthropic physicians, symbolized respectively by William Miller at the entrance to the movement and John Harvey Kellogg at its exit. Hidden from view is

---

8. In encyclopedia entries on Seventh-day Adventists, the earlier generation of Adventist apologists ignored or played down Ellen White's role in the church. The prophet is not mentioned in the following encyclopedia articles: *Collier's Encyclopedia,* 1960 ed., s.v. "Seventh-day Adventists," by LeRoy E. Froom; *The World Book Encyclopedia,* 1967 ed., s.v. "Seventh-day Adventists," also by Froom; and *Merit Student's Encyclopedia,* 1967 ed., s.v. "Seventh-day Adventists," by Francis D. Nichol. For another entry in which Ellen White is noted but not as a prophet, see *Encyclopedia Britannica,* 1962 ed., s.v. "Seventh-day Adventists," by Nichol. For his comments on ethnic religion, see Martin E. Marty, *A Nation of Behavers* (Chicago: University of Chicago Press, 1976), pp. 158-77; quotation on p. 160; I first applied Marty's view of ethnicity to Ellen White and the Adventists in Jonathan Butler, "Reporting on Ellen White," *The View,* I (Winter, 1981), 1, 11.

the complex, internal existence of the church out of which most Adventists live. Ellen White characterizes this Adventism.[9] If she has been faceless to the public, within the movement she — not Miller or Kellogg — serves as the mirror in which Adventism sees its own face. Millerism represents something of an embarrassment, the debacle from which a now superior Seventh-day Adventism once extricated itself. And because Kellogg left Adventism after growing too big for it, he imposes on the church a sense of inferiority. With a self-image that combines both feelings of superiority and of inferiority, Adventists display both pride and insecurity regarding public images of their prophet. In general, they prefer no association of Ellen White with the apocalyptic fanaticism of her origins. They emphasize, instead, the universality of her health writings and medical institutions.

For Adventists, Numbers had chosen the right topic — health — in introducing their prophet to the public, but this made it all the more disappointing when he identified her with marginal aspects of health reform. Adventists had known all along of skeletons in the closet with respect to their millenarian beginnings, but they had not suspected that similar skeletons could be found in their origins as health reformers. Numbers had hauled them out. This unnerved church members who were not used to seeing their prophet through other people's eyes. They complained that where her writings appeared bizarre, White had been quoted "out of context." This was both untrue and true. It was not true that the documents had been generally misread or misinterpreted. It was true, however, for perhaps the first time, that White's statements were being handled by secular hands. That is, as a result of Numbers's work, White's life and writings were being viewed in their context, but from the perspective of *another context*. Adventists were most unsettled to find her in *Time* magazine. Indeed, they seemed as disturbed by *Time*'s coverage of *Prophetess of Health* as they were by the book itself. For in its review-story, the national weekly had portrayed White to its huge readership as a visionary who, as Numbers had shown, linked mas-

---

9. Malcolm Bull and Keith Lockhart, *Seeking a Sanctuary: Seventh-day Adventism and the American Dream* (San Francisco: Harper & Row, Publishers, 1989), p. 268.

turbation to "imbecility, dwarfed forms, crippled limbs, misshapen heads, and deformity of every description."[10]

Confronted by what they took to be bad press on Ellen White, some Adventists could still remain blasé. After all, the prophet had prophesied of future attempts to nullify her writings, which transformed every criticism of her into another prophetic fulfillment.[11] Her predictions of the future actually reflected her contemporary experience. For she had faced severe threats to her authority throughout her lifetime. The first serious challenge occurred in the 1840s and 1850s, when she and her husband, James White, co-founded Seventh-day Adventism; the next one came around the turn of the century, when the widowed matriarch sought to re-found the church in her own image.

In the early period, Adventists focused on the nature and authenticity of her visions as well as the relationships of her visions to the authority of the Scriptures. Her visions served as a kind of *urim* and *thummim* that endorsed various biblical interpretations of the pioneers. In Adventist orthodoxy, White assumed a modest, confirmatory role relative to the Bible, much as she subordinated herself in her marriage to her dominant husband James. The 1860s and 1870s, however, saw the visionary's influence increase as her husband's power decreased. By the time of her husband's death in 1881, White enjoyed a more expansive role in the church. Her relationship to her devoted son Willie, who came to oversee her affairs, formed the paradigm of her matriarchal leadership at the turn of the century, much as her marriage had done for early Adventism. No longer the subservient wife, she now imperiously mothered a new generation of Adventist leaders and their followers. Her dramatic public visions had ended, but her no less dramatic literary output had replaced it. And where her authority had once been secured by merely confirming the biblical interpretations of various brethren, she now claimed divine authority for her statements on the basis of

---

10. The book was reviewed in "Prophet or Plagiarist?" *Time*, CVIII (August 2, 1976), 43; a three-part response to *Time* by Kenneth H. Wood appeared in Adventism's official church organ, *R&H*, CLIII (August 19, 1976), 2-3; (August 26, 1976), 2, 11-16; and (September 2, 1976), 2, 13-14.

11. See, for example, EGW, *Selected Messages* (Washington: Review and Herald Publishing Assn., 1958), vol. I, pp. 41-42.

their originality. Thus, her writings shifted for Adventists from mere commentary on the Scriptures to something of a new Scriptures.[12]

Assaults on White's authority have been aimed at either the prophet as visionary or as writer. To charge that Seventh-day Adventists, despite their claims, have relied on White's visions or writings as more authoritative than the Scriptures implicates both the early and later prophet. To account for her visions in psychopathological terms, as hypnotism or hysteria for example, grapples with the trance phenomena of her early life. To debunk her as a plagiarist goes to the heart of her literary identity. Canright, an Adventist evangelist who had been a close friend of the prophet before his defection, produced the most comprehensive and sophisticated polemic against her, as he took on both the visionary and the writer. His book was, however, no more than the polemic of a disillusioned ex-believer, which limited its credibility and its public.[13]

Adventist leaders initially dismissed Numbers as another Canright. In establishing and protecting its borders, the church has always found in the defector a familiar, easy, and probably necessary target. In the church's mind, Ellen White could be viewed only in the extreme, as either prophet or fraud, divinely inspired or satanically controlled; little middle ground existed between hagiography and heresy. But in seeking "neither to defend nor to damn but simply to understand" Ellen White, Numbers confronted the church with something new, and ultimately more challenging than the polemic. He also ensured a larger reading public for his efforts. Numbers, after all, was the product not only of a complete Adventist parochial education but of the graduate degrees beyond Adventism that the church encouraged for its brightest youth before they returned, ideally, to teach in the Adventist system. He represented, then, not a fail-

---

12. Both White's domestic life and her public career are dealt with in Ronald Graybill, "The Power of Prophecy: Ellen G. White and the Women Religious Founders of the Nineteenth Century" (Ph.D. diss., Johns Hopkins University, 1983); see also Steven Daily, "The Irony of Adventism: The Role of Ellen White and Other Adventist Women in Nineteenth Century America" (D.Min. diss., School of Theology at Claremont, 1985).

13. Canright's *Life of Mrs. E. G. White* prompted a systematic rebuttal from the church's best-known apologist more than three decades later in F. D. Nichol, *Ellen G. White and Her Critics* (Washington: Review and Herald Publishing Assn., 1951).

Introduction

ure of Adventism's religious and educational vision but a noteworthy success. With a freshly minted Ph.D. in the history of science from the University of California, Berkeley, and teaching appointments at the two Adventist universities — first Andrews, then Loma Linda — Numbers had finished revisions of his dissertation on Laplace's nebular hypothesis before turning to an Adventist topic. This was hardly the pinched or unschooled profile of the typical polemicist, concerned less with exploring a subject than exposing it. This is not to say that Numbers came to his study of Ellen White devoid of animus. Few intellectual Adventists can reflect honestly on their religious background without some element of anger. To those within the church or outside it, however, Numbers seemed superbly suited, by both religious background and professional training, to produce as fair a study as any of the health-minded Adventist prophet.[14]

His resultant monograph had an astonishing impact on Seventh-day Adventists. One Adventist religion scholar commented that *Prophetess of Health* "constitutes the most serious criticism of the prophetic powers of E. G. White ever to appear in print." For the sheer explosiveness of its historiographical challenge, Numbers did for White what Fawn Brodie had done for Joseph Smith.[15] Indeed, nothing like it had happened among Adventists before, and proba-

---

14. Kenneth Wood believed that the church's answer to Numbers had been already rendered in its answer to Canright a quarter of a century earlier, *R&H*, CLIII (August 19, 1976), 3; Numbers's expressed intent to write non-polemical history appeared in his preface to *Prophetess of Health*, p. xi; Numbers's three books were not published in the order they had been written: *Prophetess of Health* appeared first, in 1976; the dissertation, which had been written earlier, was released as *Creation by Natural Law: Laplace's Nebular Hypothesis in American Thought* (Seattle: University of Washington Press, 1977); his third book, begun on a fellowship at Johns Hopkins while revising his Ellen White book, was entitled *Almost Persuaded: American Physicians and Compulsory Health Insurance, 1912-1920* (Baltimore: Johns Hopkins University Press, 1978). The quick succession of two scholarly books after *Prophetess of Health* made it difficult for Adventists to categorize Numbers as an in-house polemicist.

15. Jerry Gladson, then an assistant professor of religion at Southern Missionary College, Numbers's alma mater, remarked on the book in *Unlock Your Potential*, XI (October-December, 1976), 6; Numbers provoked a more systematic response to his study from within Adventism than Fawn M. Brodie did from Mormons for her *No Man Knows My History: The Life of Joseph Smith, the Mormon Prophet* (2nd ed.; New York: Alfred A. Knopf, 1971).

bly nothing like it can happen again. The explanation for this resides largely in the fact that in his book Numbers addressed an Adventist agenda. To be sure, in making his case as a first-rate historian, he avoided both apologetic and exposé. But in his study he did not transcend the prophet-fraud framework.

What preoccupied Numbers were Adventism's historical and scientific claims for the "prophetess of health" and how those claims held up under the scrutiny of a historian of science. At the same time, he laid aside the question of supernatural claims regarding her, as a matter for faith, not historical explanation. As a throwback to a nineteenth-century Baconianism in which nature and the Bible complemented rather than contradicted one another, Seventh-day Adventists had found in White's health teachings a "scientific" basis for belief in her divine inspiration. Two somewhat contrary models had served the church here. On the one hand, most Adventists saw White's health writings as singularly original and well in advance of modern scientific medicine; only lately had medical research been able to confirm what Adventists had known all along from inspiration. On the other hand, even those few educated Adventists who acknowledged that their prophet had been an eclectic indebted for her health views to her context found the "proof" of her inspiration compelling: with much fallacious health science available to her, she had always taken the correct position.[16]

Numbers demolished both these models of explanation. More than that, in undermining White's own claims of intellectual independence as a health reformer, he called into question her integrity. Though he had largely concentrated his study on the scope of White's health teachings, Numbers could not have raised more far-reaching questions in regard to the prophet's life and charismatic leadership. Shedding light on her entrée into health reform in the late 1860s, he illumined the critical transition for the prophet from young visionary to middle-aged writer, marked by a shift from confirmatory to initiatory inspiration. Her claims to originality were

16. Prior to Numbers's book the latter view remained largely the unexpressed opinion of a handful of heretical Adventist academics. The former view, of a prophet ahead of her times, was the openly orthodox position offered to the Adventist public; see *Medical Science and the Spirit of Prophecy* (Washington: Review and Herald Publishing Assn., 1971).

sabotaged, of course, where Numbers pointed up cases of her literary borrowing. He stopped short of tagging her a plagiarist, however, because he felt that plagiarism implied the conscious intent to deceive.[17]

In his book, Numbers's achievement was clear. He had probed a period of White's career in which myths had been born, and he had debunked them. This was at once a strength and a limitation of the study. In favor of the approach was that it offered a long-overdue counterbalance to Adventist hagiography. Numbers had moved Ellen White from an icon within the Adventist household of faith to an accessible historical figure of more universal significance. In order to accomplish this, he had played the iconoclast. He can be faulted for the fact that to topple a venerated image, however necessary, seems by itself unsatisfying and incomplete. One non-Adventist reviewer critiqued him, for example, for "failing to convey adequately the charisma that Ellen White must have possessed to permit her ... to overcome considerable opposition to her health ideas and fasten them as articles of faith upon her expanding body of disciples."[18]

Not surprisingly, Numbers's book occasioned a full-blown historical debate within Adventism. But before discussion of the book had reached anything close to the refinement of a debate, in fact while the "book" was still a manuscript, it provoked something akin to a hagiographical "holy war." Arthur White, as the chief guardian of his grandmother's papers, ensured that the conflict over Numbers's study would elicit this sanguinary reaction. After all, White had devoted his life to protecting the persona of the prophet, and, at sixty-five, was writing the official biography of his grandmother. Like his father before him, he had operated the White Estate as a closed archives. Then, in the mid-1960s, he allowed limited access to primary materials, but with formal trustee approval required for the quotation of any heretofore unreleased documents. Ostensibly, this policy was designed to protect the privacy of individuals to whom Ellen White had written personal and pointed "testimonies."

17. In an interview after the book's publication, Numbers conjectured that White may have copied other writers and denied it due to mental problems; *Wisconsin State Journal,* July 31, 1976.

18. From the review of *Prophetess of Health* by James Harvey Young in *American Historical Review,* LXXXII (April, 1977), 464.

In fact, however, the White Estate seemed most concerned with protecting the image of the prophet herself.[19]

Just two years before Numbers arrived at the White Estate for his research, Arthur White had been "burned" by an Adventist English professor, William Peterson, whose textual and historical study of an Ellen White chapter on the French Revolution marked the first instance of a modern critical study of the prophet's writings. In a brief scholarly article, Peterson found White to be a poor historian in that her use of historical materials betrayed bias and inaccuracy. But the acrimonious debate that followed implied that Peterson's findings had been for Adventists less a study than a desecration.[20]

When Numbers submitted his request for document releases, Arthur White became alarmed that the Peterson problem could repeat itself, or worse. Speaking for the White Estate board, he refused five requests of Numbers's on the following sensitive subjects: the phrenological exam of Edson and Willie White, Ellen White's two sons; John Harvey Kellogg's reference to James White as a "monomaniac in money matters"; James's mental health; Ellen White's insistence on an anti-meat pledge for the church as a whole; and the prophet's account of dining on wild duck. In a low point in relations between Arthur White and Numbers, the archivist also denied knowledge of a sensitive document that had been recently brought to his attention. By this time, White had become deeply agitated by

---

19. For Arthur White's discussion of the custody of Ellen White's writings, see his *Ellen G. White: Messenger to the Remnant* (Washington: Review and Herald Publishing Assn., 1969), pp. 68-98; the entire episode of Numbers coming up against the White Estate is reminiscent of Janet Malcolm, *In the Freud Archives* (New York: Alfred A. Knopf, 1984).

20. Peterson's study, which appeared in the same issue of *Spectrum* as the Branson-Weiss article, proved so controversial that it eclipsed an important theoretical discussion of Ellen White and revelation, also in that issue, by Frederick E. J. Harder, "Divine Revelation: A Review of Some of Ellen White's Concepts," II (Autumn, 1970), 35-56. For Peterson's article and the various replies and counter-replies in *Spectrum*, see Peterson, "A Textual and Historical Study of Ellen White's Account of the French Revolution," II (Autumn, 1970), 57-69; W. Paul Bradley, "Ellen G. White and Her Writings," III (Spring, 1971), 43-64; Peterson, "An Imaginary Conversation on Ellen G. White: A One-Act Play for Seventh-day Adventists," III (Summer, 1971), 85-91; John W. Wood, Jr., "The Bible and the French Revolution: An Answer," III (Autumn, 1971), 55-72.

INTRODUCTION

"the Ron Numbers matter." Before cooperating any further with the historian on his research efforts, then, White flew from Washington to Loma Linda and spent an entire afternoon grilling Numbers on his faith in Ellen White. At one point he drew from his briefcase the small booklet *Appeal to Mothers,* in which the prophet described her revelations on masturbation. White asked, "Brother Numbers, do you believe this?" Still dependent on the White Estate for materials, Numbers replied, diplomatically, that "this would be one of the most difficult documents to substantiate today."[21]

Uneasy about Numbers's work, White had assigned Ronald Graybill, a White Estate researcher in his late twenties, to aid Numbers with desired revisions. He had hoped a young historian, about to enroll as a part-time graduate student in American history at Johns Hopkins University, could represent the Estate's interests to Numbers even better than he. Graybill had earned the respect not only of churchmen, such as White, but of lay and academic audiences within the church for his popular historical writing and speaking on Ellen White. In this position, Graybill seemed to do no wrong. In response to Peterson's article, for example, he dredged up the fact that Ellen White's use of historians had involved reliance on only a single Adventist writer who had anthologized a number of historical quotations. The fact that this exposed White to be an even worse historian than Peterson had supposed was lost on Graybill's church audience; it was more important that he had undercut Peterson's research. A meticulous young scholar had used historical method to serve Ellen White rather than debunk her. As a result, within Adventism's intellectual community at least, he increasingly set the timetable for the church's new historical awakening to its prophet-founder.[22]

Graybill naturally resented any suggestion that he was the Es-

---

21. For Numbers's account of these events, see the transcript of his San Bernardino County Museum lecture, May 29, 1976; see also Arthur L. White, "A Review of the Ron Numbers Matter" (unpublished typescript, Ellen G. White Estate, n.d.); White to Numbers, July 3, 1973; and Numbers to White, July 15, 1973.

22. Graybill's response to Peterson appeared in "How Did Ellen White Choose and Use Historical Sources? The French Revolution Chapter of Great Controversy," *Spectrum,* IV (Summer, 1972), 49-53; Graybill ingratiated himself to Arthur White, and earned a position at the White Estate, with his sympathetic treatment of *E. G. White and Church Race Relations* (Washington: Review and Herald Publishing Assn., 1970).

tate's apologist-for-hire. Indeed, his major professor, Timothy L. Smith, cautioned him against becoming a "kept historian." For his part Numbers believed that when it came to the study of Ellen White, one could not indefinitely serve two masters. Not even Graybill's considerable finesse could satisfy the unyielding and, basically, contradictory demands of both historical scholarship and church diplomacy. Trying his own hand at prophecy, Numbers once wrote Graybill: "You may be the White Estate's fair-haired boy today, but I'd be willing to bet you won't be tomorrow." Numbers himself had not scorned all accommodation to an Adventist audience. With his friend Vern Carner, he had founded and edited *Adventist Heritage: A Magazine of Adventist History,* popularly written and illustrated to recast new historical scholarship on the church in terms palatable to Adventists. In hopes of providing still another publishing outlet for Adventist historians, he had also launched a projected multivolume series of "Studies in Adventist History." Moreover, he had turned to his study of the Adventist prophet's health views in order to make his lectures more appealing to Loma Linda medical students. But his deepest reason for the research was less pragmatic. For him, "the ultimate cause prompting me to write what I did was, I think, to discover the truth."[23]

In 1973-74 Numbers took a fellowship year at Johns Hopkins, during which he revised his White manuscript while beginning a new book. Before coming east, he sent Graybill a preliminary draft of *Prophetess of Health.* This first exposure to Numbers's work shocked Graybill. He fretted to the author about "the tone of the material, the selection and emphasis and the kinds of sources you accepted," and he foresaw in Adventism "a crisis of the first magnitude" over the book. Though differing in their approach to Ellen White, when Numbers arrived for his fellowship year the two developed a rapport based on their common interest in the prophet. Numbers invited Graybill to share his apartment in Baltimore the one night a week he stayed over. In proximity to Numbers, and a

23. Numbers's memo of conversations with Graybill, July 26, June 28, and September 29, 1976; Numbers to Graybill, May 11, 1976; the first volume of "Studies in Adventist History" belatedly appeared as Gary Land, ed., *Adventism in America* (Grand Rapids: William B. Eerdmans Publishing Co., 1986); Numbers gave his reasons for writing the book in his lecture of May 29, 1976.

world away from the White Estate, Graybill felt the pull of single-minded historical inquiry. At times he daydreamed aloud of how, after Arthur White's departure, he could write his own critical biography of Ellen White. For now, however, Graybill allowed himself no more than a vicarious involvement in *Prophetess of Health*. But he enhanced the book's argument by feeding Numbers provocative historical materials that the White Estate had uncovered in readying its reply to the author. This happened so often that Numbers, in the midst of the Watergate era, referred to Graybill's role at the White Estate as that of a "Deep Throat."[24]

By the time the book was published in mid-1976, however, Graybill had assumed the role of arch-apologist on whom many in the church relied for the definitive answer to Numbers. In fact, one distinguished Adventist historian, even before a rebuttal had been prepared, expected that "Ron Graybill's indefatigible scholarship will come close to plugging the 'leaks'" in White's authority caused by *Prophetess of Health*. Meanwhile, Numbers, now the "apostate," had been cast into the "outer darkness" of the University of Wisconsin, with almost no access to Adventists. Owing to the profound disparity between Graybill and Numbers in the mind of the Adventist public, one denominational editor quipped, "Two Rons don't make a White." In reality, however, their relationship had always involved a deep level of reciprocity, personifying the interdependence of orthodoxy and heresy.[25]

Throughout the polishing of his manuscript, Numbers benefited enormously from Graybill's intense scrutiny of the work. For an Adventist historian writing on Ellen White the Seventh-day Adventist millennial metaphor of an "investigative judgment" proves applicable. In an image suggested to them by the biblical notion of the sanctuary, Adventists believe that all of heaven, at the "end of time," sits in judgment on earthlings below by recording every good deed and misdeed. In an analogy to this, Numbers sensed the eyes of an invisible spiritual community on him as he wrote his book. At

---

24. Graybill to Numbers, June 10, 1973; Numbers's memos of conversations with Graybill, January 22, and February 10, 1975; and June 9, 1976.

25. Walter C. Utt, "Utt Critiques New E. G. White Book," *Campus Chronicle*, LII (May 20, 1976), 3; Judy Rittenhouse made the comment about the "two Rons" in conversation with the author in 1974.

the White Estate this metaphor took on flesh and blood; Graybill acted as a recording angel. Because factual errors in *Prophetess of Health* were therefore significantly reduced, Graybill had been an advantage to Numbers; but the controversial historian had, in turn, helped Graybill. In taking a heretical position, Numbers had moved "left" of Graybill, and therefore created more space for him — between Numbers and Arthur White — in which to establish a new, more moderate stance. But this only worked as a symbiotic relationship so long as the two organisms, so to speak, both remained alive and mutually supportive of each other. Should Numbers become dead to the Adventist community, more moderate positions would then be the furthest left, and therefore vulnerable. In a return letter to the same historian who had looked for him to plug leaks, Graybill warned that if Numbers were not credited with having made "some genuine points, people will never see any need to adjust their concept of inspiration accordingly." He added, "We can't offer people solutions to problems that they don't have."[26]

From Numbers's point of view, however, Graybill had often been duplicitous by exacerbating relations between the historian of science and the White Estate and, in turn, the church, in order to appear all the more indispensable in a redemptive, mediating role. Numbers came to believe that Graybill had sacrificed him to further his own interests. Historical points that Graybill seemed to have found persuasive in private conversations, he later faulted before an Adventist public. Numbers knew the White Estate researcher was internally conflicted over many of the historical issues raised by *Prophetess of Health*. He felt betrayed when Graybill projected the conflict onto an Adventist stage as a morality play in which Numbers wore the black hat and he donned a white one.[27]

Ironically, Graybill, the historian of religion, often saw his role in more pragmatic, less moral terms than did Numbers, the historian of science. He saw himself, if not as a hired gun, at least as the attorney representing a client. He might not have been fully convinced of the validity of all the White Estate positions, but he was willing to offer them the best defense available. He was not just a defense attor-

---

26. Graybill to Walter C. Utt, July 7, 1976.
27. Numbers's memo of conversation with Graybill, February 10, 1975.

ney, however. He also had a pastoral concern for church members, whom he was trying to lead to a better understanding of their heritage without, at the same time, threatening their faith. It was not until several years later, when work on his dissertation forced him to synthesize what he knew about Ellen White into a coherent whole, that he discovered how impossible it was to deal with her life objectively without being accused of adopting a negative tone.[28]

If the strife at the White Estate over Numbers's book took on aspects of a morality play, at Loma Linda University, where the author held an academic appointment from 1970 to 1974, it seemed more like a farce. During his year's leave of absence at Johns Hopkins, Numbers circulated the first draft of his manuscript, in confidence, among five colleagues. But somehow the document reached a duplicating machine, and soon purloined copies, at five dollars apiece, were making the rounds. In this stage Numbers's manuscript resonated more irreverence than the later finished product, and it still may be the case that Adventist perceptions of the historian's work have been shaped more by the first draft than the published version. The pre-publication fallout led, by July of 1974, to the loss of Numbers's job at Loma Linda. It is still not clear, however, whether he resigned or was fired. In fact, both occurred about the same time. In an informal, but crucial spring meeting between the university president and the board chairman, Neal Wilson, it had been determined that the young medical historian would not be allowed to return to campus after his fellowship year in Baltimore. In the same period, too, board members of the Loma Linda University Church discussed whether he ought not be disfellowshipped. On the East Coast, Numbers learned that he had become a political liability to David Hinshaw, the dean of the medical school who had hired him, and out of a sense of personal loyalty to him offered to resign if his salary could be continued through the following year. Not until later did he learn from Wilson that he had been "fired."[29]

Incredibly, however, the issue of academic freedom relative to

---

28. See note 57 below.

29. Joe Willey to Numbers, n.d.; "Three Elder's Report" (Society of Concerned Adventists Nonrestricted and International, n.d.), p. 14; Numbers's memo of conversation with Neal Wilson, July 4, 1974.

his case never surfaced at Loma Linda. No faculty member or administrator in the university, or elsewhere in Adventist education for that matter, publicly protested Numbers's termination. Instead, the university community became engrossed in clearing the names of faculty members accused of aiding and abetting the historian in his research and writing. Months after Numbers had left the campus, a conspiracy theory, which linked various university personnel to the book, took hold in the highest echelons of church leadership. Rumors circulated that a local pastor had filched financial records on Numbers and others at Loma Linda and delivered them at a local motel room to the church's General Conference president, Robert Pierson, and Wilson. The pastor and a colleague sought to establish a conspiracy between Numbers and Dean Hinshaw, Carner, who taught religion at LLU, and A. Graham Maxwell, chairman of the division of religion. They charged that *Prophetess of Health* could not have been written alone; the book was too detailed, with too many footnotes. Thus they concocted a story in which the alleged co-conspirators had met together in various cities throughout the country to lay plans to destroy Ellen White and the church. In support of Numbers's research Maxwell had supposedly contributed from twenty to forty thousand dollars of his own money; and in one instance, in Chicago, plans had been made "in the presence of prostitutes."[30]

It was ludicrous, of course, that so isolated an act as writing a book could be explained as a conspiracy. Nor did it make any sense that several colleagues in the same institution would travel to distant cities in order to meet with one another, when they were free to lunch together any day of the week in Loma Linda. Despite the far-fetched nature of these charges, however, the targets of them within the university felt themselves to be in real jeopardy. Hinshaw and Maxwell seemed to have fallen victim to vendettas, with the controversial book providing a convenient excuse to get rid of them. Though the district attorney was queried in regard to

---

30. This entire squalid if by now somewhat humorous episode is detailed in "The Three Elder's Report"; a meeting called by Neal Wilson on August 31, 1976, with most of the principals was summarized in "Notes of Harvey Elder"; a conversation among Gary Stanhiser, Arnold Trujillo, J. W. Lehman, and A. Graham Maxwell may be found in a synopsis by David R. Larson.

taking legal action against the accusers, because of the circumstantial nature of the case no charges were brought. But if nothing reached a court of law, the episode did reach the court of public opinion. Because analogies to Watergate abounded, the affair was termed a "stained-glass window Watergate." After all, there had been, allegedly, a "break-in" and a pilfering of documents. A chief executive of the church had been implicated. A "cover-up" had ensued, followed by a full-scale investigation and exposure. As a result, a fatuous conspiracy theory had been laid bare by evidence of a real conspiracy.[31]

After moving to Madison in the summer of 1974 to join the department of the history of medicine at the University of Wisconsin, Numbers found that the Adventist hysteria over his projected volume, though largely out of sight, was not out of mind. The White Estate enlisted the support of Rene Noorbergen, once a writer for *The National Enquirer* who had recently published popular and sympathetic biographies of "psychics" Jeane Dixon and Ellen White, to investigate Numbers's motives for writing his study. Noorbergen planned to question Numbers by telephone about his book while surreptitiously recording his responses with a sophisticated polygraph. But Numbers had been forewarned (by Graybill) of the chicanery and rebuffed Noorbergen when he called. The White Estate also sent a staff member, Robert Olson, to the Madison Adventist church for a weekend series on the prophet in order to counteract any negative influence the historian might have on the local membership. He urged church members to ostracize Numbers. By this time the historian was philosophically estranged from Adventism but still hoped to remain tied to the church as a cultural Adventist. Once Olson had alerted local Adventists to him, however, he saw no point in returning to the Madison church.[32]

---

31. In addition to "The Three Elder's Report," the story was covered by Mike Quinn in "Book Criticizing Adventist Founder Fires Controversy at Loma Linda," *Riverside Press Enterprise* (September 19, 1976), B-1, B-4. See also memo of conversation between Numbers and Bruce Branson, November 2, 1976; and Bruce Branson to Numbers, February 15, 1977.

32. Rene Noorbergen, *Jeane Dixon: My Life and Prophecies* (New York: William Morrow and Co., 1969), and *Prophet of Destiny* (Canaan, Conn.: Keats Publishing Co., 1972); memo of conversation between Roy Branson and Numbers, November 4,

The Historian as Heretic

Numbers's first months in Madison marked a dark period for him. Not only was he spent physically and emotionally, but he was alone. Alienated from Adventists, he had not yet adjusted to life beyond Adventism. Moreover, his marriage was ending, and his wife's betrayal at the root of the breakup seemed emblematic of the way his Adventist colleagues had betrayed him. Though expecting his work on Ellen White to be controversial among the Adventist rank and file, he counted on Adventist historians to rally to his defense. But with the circulation of his manuscript Numbers had become a pariah. Despite the fact that this had resulted from their colleague's historical research in his area of specialty, Adventist historians (with a few exceptions) had been no more supportive of him than were Adventist academics in general. Loma Linda University had not only dropped him from its staff but, in the following year, had dumped him from the masthead of *Adventist Heritage,* the journal he had founded, without a single public outcry from his historian colleagues.[33]

If Numbers saw himself as betrayed by his fellow scholars, they could interpret his iconoclastic study as a betrayal of them, though the explanation for this is somewhat oblique. In recent years an increasingly sophisticated class of academics had joined the ranks of Adventist higher education. Brandishing Ph.D.'s from big-name, secular universities, this new breed of Adventist professor had often found itself at odds with the vast majority of conservative church members, who supported the colleges and universities. The only way to survive in so precarious a position was by way of complete discretion. Almost anything could be said in private. But Adventist academics who publicly dared to break the informal code of silence on controversial issues did so on their own. Numbers certainly had his silent partners. From time to time colleagues quietly voiced their personal approval of his work. But none of them wanted to be driven from cover by their more outspoken colleague. In a sense, Numbers had betrayed *them* by forcing them into a diffi-

---

1974; memo of conversation between Numbers and Noorbergen, November 7, 1974; memo on discussion between Numbers and Robert Olson, October 26, 1974.

33. Note 14 above recounts when Numbers wrote his three books; Numbers to Jonathan Butler, June 10, 1975; James R. Nix to Numbers, July 9, 1975.

cult position. Either they endorsed him and lost their jobs, or they exaggerated the distance between themselves and him and lost a piece of their souls.[34]

Concern for job security at Adventist colleges no doubt had been a factor in the lack of support for Numbers on the part of disingenuous colleagues. But Adventist historians also had genuine reservations about Numbers's study. The church's historians had not resolved their own distinctive version of the believer-historian conflict. They complained about the tone of Numbers's writing. One senior historian commented, for example, that he could accept everything about the book but the disrespectful conclusion to the reform dress story where Numbers wrote, "Journeying to California, Mrs. White discreetly left her pants behind."[35] But their concerns ran deeper than literary packaging to the very basis of the argument.

Adventist historians adhered to the secular canons of historiography, except with regard to Ellen White. She occupied a supernaturalist preserve off-limits to naturalist history. In teaching or writing history on any other topic, Adventist historians generally would find it naive to evoke "the hand of God" as a cause. Notwithstanding the occasional old-guard historian who saw evidence of angels at the Battle of Bull Run (and only there because Ellen White had said so), virtually all of them explained the American Revolution or the Civil War, Women's Suffrage or the New Deal as other historians did. But the historical study of Ellen White was a different matter. Because Adventist historians ruled out exploring the visionary's life with the same methods that governed their study of an Abigail Adams or an Elizabeth Cady Stanton, they chose *qua* historians to ignore her altogether. They often brushed close to the prophet with studies of other figures or events in Adventist history that served, indirectly, to humanize her. But Numbers, unforgivably, had gone in where angels had feared to tread. To draw again upon an Adventist metaphor, he had torn apart the last veil, historiographically speaking, between the holy and most

---

34. Bull and Lockhart describe the vocational conflicts of an Adventist educator in *Seeking a Sanctuary*, pp. 230-43; on the criticisms of Numbers by his fellow academics, see p. 237.

35. Godfrey T. Anderson registered this criticism to me and to Numbers on separate occasions; the infamous line appears below on p. 202.

holy places. He had entered the inner sanctum of the prophet's life, not as a believer but as a historian.[36]

Numbers saw the equivocal posture of Adventist historians as far less tolerable than the straightforward opposition of the White Estate's churchmen. By temperament, he favored total candor. He saw the issues in the same stark terms that Arthur White did: he simply found himself at odds with him. But relations between Numbers and the Estate's administrative personnel remained civil, if not cordial. This made sense to both parties. Numbers, after all, needed approval from the archives to quote its sources in his manuscript, and the White Estate staff hoped that a good rapport between them and the historian would ensure a book more favorable to the prophet. It became all the clearer that a book was actually in the offing when, in May of 1974, Numbers signed a contract to publish his manuscript through Harper and Row. Numbers had arranged with the White Estate to critique his work in manuscript, and now Clayton Carlson, head of Harper and Row's religious books department, looked forward to the Estate's comments as well, if only to minimize factual errors in the book.[37]

Once Numbers had produced his revised manuscript in the fall, however, it was not always clear that Arthur White saw the Estate's critique as a means of improving the future publication. Rather, he seemed bent on so discrediting Numbers with Harper and Row that the publisher would abort the project altogether. To this end, White flew to New York in January of 1975 and spent a day with Carlson poring over a notebook full of documents. In several months of preparing its formal response to Numbers, the White Estate staff had divided the labor as follows: White on dress, Olson on sex, and Graybill on phrenology. These three then went to New York in February with a 223-page reply for Carlson's eyes only. By this time, rela-

---

36. To counter this mindset among his colleagues as well as church members at large, a junior Adventist historian argued, in the year Numbers published *Prophetess of Health,* that historical and theological explanations of a phenomenon, even with reference to a prophet, need not exclude one another; Gary Land, "Providence and Earthly Affairs: The Christian and the Study of History," *Spectrum,* VII (April, 1976), 2-6.

37. Numbers describes this aspect of his relationship with the White Estate in his lecture of May 29, 1976.

tions between Numbers and the White Estate had deteriorated to the point that some at the Estate now believed Satan had "gained control" of the historian. Arthur White did not want Numbers to have access to the response because it would only provide "grist for his mill." But there was another reason to keep him from seeing it; the document was riddled with *ad hominem* barbs that were bound to offend him. Carlson, however, flatly refused to accept the White Estate response if the person most able to make use of it were not allowed to see it. So, White gathered up the manuscript and returned with it to Washington, D.C.[38]

By the end of the month, however, he had changed his stance and forwarded a copy of the Estate's reply to Numbers. Graybill then called the historian and asked to meet with him. On a weekend in early March, Graybill and Richard Schwarz, chair of the history department at Andrews University, traveled to Madison for extensive discussions with Numbers about his manuscript. Numbers was still on good terms with Graybill, and he counted Schwarz a close friend. The senior Adventist historian had hired him out of graduate school and still called him "Ronnie." If Graybill was fast becoming the church's leading authority on Ellen White, Schwarz was its premier denominational historian. The threesome planned a three-day working weekend at a motel in Madison. They moved a six-foot banquet table into Graybill's room. Schwarz had brought a microfiche reader and a box of Ellen White's books and the works of denominational historians. They also had an IBM typewriter.

At the outset of the weekend, Numbers complained that in places the critique was too weak to be useful; he also found it insulting. Graybill admitted its shortcomings, apologizing especially for the personal attacks. On their weekend together, however, the three men found a good deal of common ground. They combed through every scintilla of Numbers's manuscript, and the author agreed to change both factual and interpretive points. Single words that carried emotional or negative connotations were exchanged for more agreeable terms. Numbers also solicited help in finding more heart-

---

38. Numbers's memo of conversation with Graybill, December 29, 1974; two letters crisscrossed in the mail from Arthur White to Clayton Carlson, February 6, 1975; and Carlson to White, February 6, 1975.

warming episodes in the prophet's life in order to build empathy for her as a historical figure. No one ended the weekend under the illusion that his book was anything less than a major revision of the traditional Adventist view of Ellen White. Numbers had accounted for the visionary's life in strictly naturalistic terms; the average Adventist would find this shocking. But given the firestorm of criticism that Numbers would face for his book, one remarkable aspect of these Madison discussions deserves notice. In a report to his White Estate colleagues, Graybill stated, "On virtually every occasion where Dr. Schwarz and I felt the evidence was strong and clear, Dr. Numbers agreed to change his manuscript." Or, where one of them sided with him, Numbers stuck with his original interpretation. The subsequent published criticisms of *Prophetess of Health*, then, even those of Graybill or Schwarz, more than likely faulted not just Numbers but one or the other of his companions on that Madison weekend.[39]

The 258-page book appeared in print in May of 1976. The even longer White Estate critique of it came out in the fall. Just prior to the publication of his book, Numbers and the White Estate had blamed each other for many of the same sins. The Estate believed that the historian had mishandled the prophet by way of sweeping generalizations, a sneering attitude, quotations taken out of context, and, most important, dishonesty. Numbers thought the Estate had treated him in much the same way. If the two had sometimes mirrored each other, in an ironic twist, Numbers found himself, in the late spring, in a similar position to the White Estate in regard to releasing materials. To people who were "misrepresenting" her, the Estate had always refused permission to quote the prophet. But when it came to publishing their reply to Numbers, which copiously quoted his book, the Estate needed the historian's permission. It would be necessary for him, of course, to judge whether *he* had been misrepresented in its document. Numbers may never have had any intention of finally declining the White Estate request, but he did let the matter hang for a while. Arthur White wrote several solicitous

---

39. The Madison weekend is described in a memo from Graybill to Arthur White and the White Estate Board of Trustees, May 11, 1975. See also Numbers's lecture of May 29, 1976; Schwarz to Pastor and Mrs. Raymond W. Numbers, March 11, 1975.

letters to the author beginning in late April. After seeing the critique, however, Numbers caustically responded that he found it to be "grossly unfair." As late as mid June he still withheld permission, for he had expected the Estate staff to be as fair in evaluating his work as they wanted him to be in evaluating Ellen White. "But apparently," he concluded, "we have a double standard."[40]

Spectrum provided the most important public forum within the church for evaluating the published book. Roy Branson, as editor, had invited a review by noted church historian Ernest Sandeen. Himself from a fundamentalist background, Sandeen understood the torturous conflict between believer and historian, especially when they inhabited the same person. But he also knew that, as if by some historiographical law, the skeptical believer produces the best historical scholarship. Though it had obviously been a deeply painful experience for the young historian, Numbers had made an invaluable contribution to his church and to the scholarly world beyond it. If Seventh-day Adventists were not too defensive to come to terms with Numbers's view of Ellen White (and, in this regard, Sandeen had every confidence in Adventists), they would avoid the pitfall of Christian Scientists, who had rejected historical scrutiny of Mary Baker Eddy. Thus, Sandeen saw Numbers's essay as more than simply "a valuable work of social history"; it was also "a moving personal document and a report on the state of one American denomination's soul." Upon reading the review in manuscript, Branson thought it would be good for his cousin's soul to hear it, so he called him and read it to him over the phone. For more than two years, Numbers had faced almost nothing but criticism for his work on Ellen White. This essay, from a historian he greatly respected, expressed profound gratitude for his efforts. He broke down and sobbed.[41]

The Adventist commentators in *Spectrum*, for the most part, took a dimmer view of Numbers's book than Sandeen expected of them.

---

40. Longer in words, not pages, the reply of the Ellen G. White Estate appeared as *A Critique of the Book Prophetess of Health* (Washington: Ellen G. White Estate, 1976); for the exchanges on permission to cite Numbers's book, see Arthur White to Numbers, April 21, 1976; White to Numbers, April 29, 1976; Numbers to White, May 6, 1976; White to Numbers, May 24, 1976; and Numbers to White, June 18, 1976.

41. Ernest R. Sandeen, "The State of a Church's Soul," *Spectrum*, VIII (January, 1977), 15-16.

Only one Adventist historian, Numbers's predecessor in the history of medicine at Loma Linda, W. Frederick Norwood, embraced the book. He insisted that it would disturb only those who had exalted Ellen White "to a pedestal of inerrancy and infallibility, a position she did not claim for herself or even for the Bible writers." But two other Adventist scholars rebutted the book with finely spun apologetics. Warning readers that Numbers wrote history from an entirely naturalistic slant, Schwarz argued that the raw historical facts called for a supernaturalistic explanation. He admitted that White may have borrowed from other health reformers, but he suggested that both the prophet and her secular informants may have been inspired by the same Spirit. He contended, too, that Numbers had obtained his facts from unreliable, hostile witnesses such as Canright and Kellogg. Fritz Guy, an Adventist theologian, faulted the book for its unbalanced view of White, its naturalistic approach to her, and its skepticism with regard to her integrity. But he regarded all this as a negative virtue. For a limited or faulty perspective on the prophet might spur further investigation of her and also provide an opportunity to correct theological misperceptions among Adventists regarding inspiration.[42] Numbers believed that Schwarz's comments on the writing of history tended to "caricature rather than clarify the art." With reference to Schwarz's defense of multiple revelations, Numbers professed to admire such "valiant efforts to rescue Mrs. White from some embarrassing situations." But he pointed out that if the church accepted these explanations, "its doctrine of inspiration [would] never be the same." The criticism that he had lent too much credence to Adventist defectors Numbers found potentially the most damaging. He counted roughly 1,185 citations in his book, however, and found that nearly two-thirds came from pro-Ellen White materials, while a mere 3.9 percent were from those hostile to the visionary. The differences between Schwarz and Numbers, as it turned out, were more apparent in the pages of *Spectrum* than they were in reality. For Schwarz, incredibly, had based at least some of his critique on an earlier draft of Numbers's manuscript, not the

42. W. Frederick Norwood, "The Prophet and Her Contemporaries," *Spectrum*, VIII (January, 1977), 2-4; R. W. Schwarz, "On Writing and Reading History," ibid., 20-27.

published book. When he later read the book, Schwarz apologized to him for rebutting "errors" that had been changed in the final version, in part at Schwarz's own urging. Guy, presumably, had read the book, but to make his key historical points, in Numbers's view, he had drawn uncritically on the White Estate's reply.[43]

Under the title "A Biased, Disappointing Book," the White Estate presented in this same issue of *Spectrum* a synopsis of its longer response to Numbers. The fundamental difference between the White Estate and the historian (and perhaps, finally, their only difference) was that the Estate believed Ellen White's divine inspiration could be historically proven; Numbers insisted it could not. The Estate asked: "Did Ellen White receive her health message from the Lord or from earthly sources?" Arguing that the prophet, prior to her health vision of 1863, had no more than a limited, fragmentary knowledge of health reform, the Estate said that White's intellectual independence implied her supernatural inspiration. But in establishing White's independence, the Estate hurt its case at one point by proving too much. When the White's son Henry was stricken in December of 1863 with a fatal illness, it recounted, the frantic parents called a local physician instead of employing Dr. Jackson's system of water cure. This argument proved an embarrassment, however, because the prophet had received a divine endorsement of the water-cure system six months prior to this in her health vision of June 5. In its zeal to prove White's obliviousness to earthly sources, then, the Estate had inadvertently suggested that the prophet ignored her heavenly source as well. Numbers, of course, had made his case for the derivative nature of White's health writings by showing how knowledgeable early Adventist leaders were of the health-reform movement and by citing close literary parallels between White's work and that of other health reformers. But Numbers added, "Even if Mrs. White were unique, it would add no *historical* evidence to her claim of inspiration."[44]

---

43. Ronald L. Numbers, "An Author Replies to His Critics," ibid., esp. 34-36; and memo of conversation among Numbers, Schwarz, and Gary Land, September 17, 1977.

44. The Estate's summary comment appears in *Spectrum*, VIII (January, 1977), 4-13; it condenses a 24-page document entitled "A Discussion and Review of *Prophetess of Health*," as well as its longer study, *A Critique of the Book Prophetess of Health*. For Numbers's comment, see *Spectrum*, VIII (January, 1977), 29.

In every aspect of the debate between the Estate and Numbers, it seemed clear that they resided in separate universes. Given the gaping void between them, it is surprising that the two parties remained in close enough proximity to carry on such an extended quarrel. It is an important commentary on the nature of Seventh-day Adventism, however, that its intellectuals and its clerical leadership remain keenly aware of each other. Numbers could not be dismissed out of hand; he had to be dealt with. But church officials were miffed that the *Spectrum* issue devoted to Numbers had, by and large, taken his work seriously. And an article written by another of its guest reviewers had, in their view, gone too far. Fawn Brodie, best known to Adventists for her highly regarded biography of Mormon prophet Joseph Smith, contributed perhaps the most provocative reflections on White's life that Adventists had ever read. Noting that Numbers had left a psychobiographical analysis of the visionary to future writers, Brodie proceeded to highlight material in the narrative that could inform such a clinical study. Church leaders were enraged. They threatened to censure or shut down *Spectrum*. General Conference executives, including President Pierson and Vice-President Wilson, along with White Estate officials, met in an emotionally charged meeting in Philadelphia with members of *Spectrum*'s editorial board. The session's most riveting moment captured the depth of feeling with regard to the Brodie essay. A White Estate official silenced the room with the following vivid remark: "It's as if Mrs. White had been stripped naked, stripped naked!"[45]

Throughout the year of its publication, church officials orchestrated a concerted campaign against *Prophetess of Health*. Along with its twenty-four-page reply and full-length *Critique,* the church highly promoted an inexpensive, paperback edition of *The Story of Our Health Message,* a sympathetic study by Dores E. Robinson, a secretary and grandson-in-law to the prophet. Study aids designed to answer questions raised by Numbers now accompanied this book. Other apologetic books on Adventism and health followed. In

---

45. Fawn M. Brodie, "Ellen White's Emotional Life," ibid., 13-15. *Spectrum* continued as an independent journal within Adventism, but its editor, Roy Branson, on leave from the SDA Theological Seminary at the Kennedy Center for Bioethics, subsequently lost his seminary appointment and his ministerial credentials.

reactionary fashion, these did not so much respond to *Prophetess of Health* as retell the Adventist health story as if Numbers's book had never been written. But in a series of Prophetic Guidance Workshops, each conducted for two weeks on four Adventist college campuses, Robert Olson and other White Estate officials sharply denounced specific points in the book. *Time*'s review of it in August, entitled "Prophet or Plagiarist?," called for a rejoinder in the workshops. At Andrews University in southern Michigan, the weekend after the article hit the newsstands, Olson reported that not a *Time* could be had within fifty miles of the campus. Numbers's book itself could not be conveniently obtained at Andrews. The university bookstore would not display it, but did sell it on request. The book was treated as contraband, carefully wrapped in plain paper, so customers could leave the store with it undetected.[46]

This atmosphere throughout the church made it difficult for Adventist historians to come to terms with Numbers's book in their own way. But gradually they did. An important early step in this process was a review in *Spectrum* by Gary Land, a historian at Andrews University, of the White Estate's full-length *Critique*. With some trepidation, as "a denominational employee, whose job may depend on adhering to orthodoxy," Land underscored numerous examples of "how the White Estate's adoption in practice, although not in theory, of the inerrancy approach to inspiration has led it to make arguments that do not fit the facts." But, for generations, the church had lived with the "practice" of Mrs. White's inerrancy. And Adventist historians felt a duty to integrate the new historical thinking with the old faith in such a way that Adventism might be transformed without being destroyed. In 1979, one young Adventist historian, Benjamin

---

46. D. E. Robinson, *The Story of Our Health Message* (3rd ed.; Nashville: Southern Publishing Assn., 1965); Ellen G. White Estate, "Twelve Outline Studies for The Story of Our Health Message" (Nashville: Southern Publishing Assn., 1976). For traditional Adventist studies of health after Numbers's book, see Richard A. Schafer, *Legacy: The Heritage of a Unique International Medical Outreach* (Mountain View, Calif.: Pacific Press, 1977), and George W. Reid, *A Sound of Trumpets: Americans, Adventists and Health Reform* (Washington: Review and Herald Publishing Assn., 1982). Coverage of the Prophetic Guidance Workshop at Andrews University appears in *Andrews University Focus*, XII (August-September, 1976), 9, 11; the *Time* citation is in note 10 above.

McArthur, questioned whether the church's revolution of historical consciousness, especially with regard to its prophet, might not irreparably damage the tradition, much as historical criticism had done to Judaism a century before. In a presidential address to the Association of Western Adventist Historians in the same year, Eric Anderson commented that McArthur may have been too pessimistic. But Anderson agreed that Adventist historians had to deal with the theological implications of their work. Failing to do so invited comparisons to the World War II scientist lampooned in Tom Lehrer's ditty:

> Once da rockets are up
> Who kares where dey come down?
> Dat's not my department
> Says Verner Von Braun.[47]

Non-Adventist scholars faced none of these concerns, of course. But their largely enthusiastic reception of Numbers's study, evident in a raft of favorable reviews, exerted an influence on Adventist academics. For the first time, Adventists saw Ellen White as an object of historical interest to a wider community of scholars in the fields of American social, medical, church, and women's history.[48] And the "gentiles" brought their different perspectives to the monograph. Adventists, for example, had thought of Numbers as utterly secular and naturalistic. But outsiders to the community, such as Martin E. Marty, saw him as "half-in, half-out of the Adventist church." If he was "in transit from Adventism," he had still presented an "empathic and fair story of her life." Another reviewer felt that the book reflected Numbers's "conflict between historical objectivity and commitment to religion."[49]

---

47. Gary Land, "Faith, History and Ellen White," *Spectrum*, IX (March, 1978), 51-55; Benjamin McArthur, "Where Are Historians Taking the Church?" *Spectrum*, (November, 1979), 11-14; Eric Anderson, "1979 Presidential Address, AWAH" (unpublished paper).

48. A general sampling of favorable reviews of the book may be found in *The Zetetic*, I (Spring-Summer, 1977), 100; *Christian Century*, XCIV (February 16, 1977), 157; *Isis*, LXIX (1978), 147; *Church History*, XLVII (June, 1978), 243.

49. Martin E. Marty, in *Context* (December 15, 1977), 2, and *Journal of Religion*, LVIII (1978), 340; Martin Kaufman, *Journal of American History*, LXIV (June, 1977), 179-80.

INTRODUCTION

Close to the publication of *Prophetess of Health,* Adventists certainly found no humor in, and therefore did not appreciate, the tongue-in-cheek tone of James C. Whorton, who wrote, "Numbers' 'attack' on White is subtle even by satanic standards, for he takes great care to be objective, and if his judgment errs it is on the side of charity." Whorton continued in a humorous vein in his later book on the history of American health reformers: "Although Numbers' case is convincing," he wrote, after summarizing his argument, "White perhaps did receive genuine revelations, and conceivably outraged Adventists are correct in seeing his book as a Satanic 'deception.'" If Adventists could not realistically expect outsiders to share their religious sensibilities about the book, they would have preferred a wider scope to the Adventist health story Numbers told in order to dilute revelations about their prophet. But Whorton favored the way Numbers had displayed only enough of the larger Adventist health story to tantalize readers. In doing this, it was as if he had followed the standard advice of health reformers: "to avoid gluttony, end each meal while a bit of appetite remains. One finishes *Prophetess of Health* with a feeling of satisfaction, not satiety, and a relish for future samples of related items."[50]

Adventists had complained that Numbers had been too interpretive, too biased. But some of the non-Adventists found it the sparest of narratives, understated, and lacking in an interpretive framework, for which they either lauded or faulted him. In the developing area of women's history, for example, Numbers proved potentially as controversial as he was anywhere beyond Adventist circles. Gerald Grob appreciated his narrative history as a valuable building block but complained that he had not done more to analyze White against a backdrop of the changing roles of women in the nineteenth century. Another reviewer seemed piqued by the interpretation she had found in the book of "an ignorant, hysterical, hypochondriacal female, almost without redeeming qualities, and manipulated by a few clever men." For the most part, however, as a

---

50. James C. Whorton's review appeared in *Journal of the History of Medicine,* XXXIV (1979), 239-40; he further elaborates on the book in *Crusaders for Fitness: The History of American Health Reformers* (Princeton, N.J.: Princeton University Press, 1982), pp. 201-2.

result of Numbers's effort, the Adventist visionary took her rightful place in the emergent historiography on both women and health reform. Moreover, more general and interpretive studies of American religion, society, and culture added the Ellen White of Numbers's narrative (without alterations of their own) to the historical pantheon of women religious leaders and health reformers.[51]

All of this impressed Adventist historians. Numbers, after all, was a success story. He had pulled himself up from the Adventist "ghetto" and had "made good." And if he still projected something of a diabolical persona for the average Adventist in the pew, Adventist academics found more and more to admire in him as a historian. Indeed, because secular historians had seen Ellen White as interesting and significant, a generation of Adventist historians began to view her, for the first time, as a legitimate object for their own scholarly inquiry. In this way, Numbers had inspired an escalating revolution in Adventist scholarship on the prophet. He himself had gone on to a full and productive academic life beyond Adventism. But from his lofty perch at the University of Wisconsin, he served, quite unintentionally, as a kind of conscience for Adventist historians; they were more likely to take on tough issues with candor because they felt him looking over their shoulder. They kept him apprised of develop-

---

51. For the reviews, see Gerald N. Grob, *New England Quarterly*, L (June, 1977), 361-63; John B. Blake, *Wisconsin Magazine of History*, LX (Spring, 1977), 250-51; Henry D. Shapiro, *Reviews in American History*, V (June, 1977), 242-48; Josephine F. Pacheco, *History: Review of New Books*, V (November, 1977), 39. Examples of books that draw upon Numbers are Jane B. Donegan, *"Hydropathic Highway to Health": Women and Water-Cure in Antebellum America* (New York: Greenwood Press, 1986), esp. ch. 7; Susan E. Cayleff, *Wash and Be Healed: The Water-Cure Movement and Women's Health* (Philadelphia: Temple University Press, 1987), pp. 115-17; Martha H. Verbrugge, *Able-Bodied Womanhood: Personal Health and Social Change in Nineteenth-Century Boston* (New York: Oxford University Press, 1988), p. 125; Martin E. Marty, *Pilgrims in Their Own Land* (Boston: Little, Brown and Co., 1984), pp. 321-24; Norman Gevitz, ed., *Other Healers: Unorthodox Medicine in America* (Baltimore: Johns Hopkins University Press, 1988), pp. 26, 69-70, 80; Robert C. Fuller, *Alternative Medicine and American Religious Life* (New York: Oxford University Press, 1989), pp. 33-34; Harvey Green, *Fit for America: Health, Fitness, Sport, and American Society* (New York: Pantheon Books, 1986); Catherine L. Albanese, *American Religions and Religion* (Belmont, Calif.: Wadsworth Publishing Co., 1981), pp. 146-47; Martin E. Marty, *The Irony of It All, 1893-1919*, vol. 1 of *Modern American Religion* (Chicago: University of Chicago Press, 1986), pp. 256-57.

ments within the church, sending him manuscripts for comment, kibitzing with him at scholarly meetings, even inviting him occasionally to Adventist campuses for clandestine discussions of his earlier work. A key indicator of his rehabilitation came in 1980, when West Coast Adventist historians invited Numbers to speak to them at Walla Walla College. Many of them now envied his experience with the Ellen White book — to have wrestled with the angel, to have passed through dark nights, to have felt so alive. But none of them would quite reproduce it. Much of their later historical writing confirmed Numbers's findings in other aspects of the prophet's life. Some of it went far beyond his work in radically reassessing her. None of it, however, would reach the public beyond Adventism with the impact and notoriety that Numbers had achieved. Nor would any of it create the scandal within Adventism that Numbers did. Evidently, Adventism could lose its innocence only once.

In the decade following the publication of *Prophetess of Health*, historiographical developments on Ellen White focused on her, as they had in the past, as both a visionary and a writer. Her literary identity had been first to occupy contemporary Adventist scholars, and revelations in regard to the prophet dramatically increased over time. Numbers's own modest discoveries of literary parallels between Ellen White and Larkin B. Coles, which filled no more than a page in his endnotes, soon utterly paled beside other literary finds. Donald McAdams, then a historian at Andrews University, examined a chapter on John Hus in White's revered classic, *The Great Controversy*, and found her writing to be the "selective abridgments and adaptation of historians." To his amazement, he learned that she was not just borrowing the occasional paragraph which she had run across in her reading, but was "in fact following the historians page after page, leaving out much material, but using their sequence, some of their ideas, and often their words." Indeed, the only truly original part of White's chapter in manuscript, astonishingly, had been excised by editors from the published text.[52]

---

52. Numbers's parallel columns appear in *Prophetess of Health*, pp. 134-35, n. 15; McAdams wrote a 250-page document on his discoveries, which remains unpublished and housed at the Estate. Eric Anderson provides a synopsis of his manuscript in "Ellen White and Reformation Historians," *Spectrum*, IX (July, 1978), 23-26.

For Adventists, however, McAdams's literary findings (along with those of Peterson and Numbers) were only a harbinger of worse things to come. Walter Rea, an Adventist pastor in California, had once believed that the Bible and Ellen White's writings should be the extent of a good Adventist's reading material. Indeed, he had committed vast portions of White's writings to memory. In time, though, he ranged beyond this limited reading list, deciding that it must be permissible to read books that White herself had read. But when he gained access to her library, he came upon a startling number of literary parallels between an author he had thought to be inspired and original and the writers she had read. He then spent twenty years corroborating this discovery. Drawing especially from her books *Prophets and Kings* and *The Desire of Ages* and a contemporaneous writer, Alfred Edersheim, Rea amassed a huge number of literary exhibits which he later published in a book provocatively entitled *The White Lie*. When he first presented his findings to a General Conference–appointed committee of scholars and churchmen, the committee objected to his sloppy methodology and acerbic tone, but conceded that "Ellen White, in her writing, used various sources more extensively than we had previously believed." Churchmen hoped to educate lay Adventists in regard to these troubling facts, but Rea's story reached the *Los Angeles Times* before much could be done, and the church revoked his ministerial credentials.[53]

Literary analysis of Ellen White's writings quickly gave way to even more controversial and far-reaching biblical, historical, and theological studies of her. Joseph J. Battistone, a New Testament scholar, undercut the usual Adventist use of the prophet as an author-

---

53. Rea couched his literary analysis in a provocative book entitled *The White Lie* (Turlock, Calif.: M & R Publications, 1982); his story appeared in the *Los Angeles Times* (October 23, 1980), sec. 1, pp. 1ff. For scholarly responses to Rea, see Jonathan Butler, "Prophet or Plagiarist: A False Dichotomy," *Spectrum*, XII (June, 1982), 44-48; and Alden Thompson, "The Imperfect Speech of Inspiration," ibid., pp. 48-55. The church appointed Fred Veltman, a New Testament expert in textual criticism, to do further literary analysis of Ellen White; a summary of his work may be found in Veltman, "The Desire of Ages Project: The Data," *Ministry*, LXII (October, 1990), 4-7; and "The Desire of Ages Project: The Conclusions," *Ministry*, LXII (December, 1990), 11-15; see also Robert W. Olson, "Ellen White's Denials," *Ministry*, LXIII (February, 1991), 15-18.

Introduction

itative biblical commentator. Suggesting that her writings were unreliable exegetically, he saw them as primarily homiletical in nature. No part of White's commentary on the Bible mattered more to Adventists than her interpretation of "last day events." My own article entitled "The World of E. G. White and the End of the World," which I wrote while teaching at Loma Linda University, placed White's understanding of eschatology within the context of nineteenth-century society and culture. I argued that White's scenario on the end of time, deeply formative for the Adventist identity, had been culturally conditioned. The political, social, and cultural events to which Adventists still looked in the future to signal the end of the world more properly fit conditions of her nineteenth-century world than that of the late twentieth century. In short, Adventism was an anachronism.[54]

Another key to the Adventist identity was the church's doctrine of the sanctuary and investigative judgment. For Adventists, the sanctuary served as a symbol of their special role as God's remnant at the close of human history. But an evangelical Adventist theologian, Desmond Ford, came to the conclusion that Adventism's understanding of the sanctuary was both poor exegesis and unchristian. And because Ellen White's role had been so significant in establishing the doctrine — as it had been with all basic Adventist beliefs — Ford's call for a radical overhaul of the sanctuary teaching challenged White's authority among Adventists. Indeed, in any Adventist theological debate, Ellen White's views provided the hidden agenda. Adventists preferred to place themselves, at least in theory, in the Protestant lineage of "Scripture alone," not as a nonevangelical sect based on the visions of a prophet. But, practically speaking, they were more likely defined as a group that spoke only when White spoke and were silent where she was silent. Ford's declarations on the sanctuary identified a central tenet of Adventism as rooted in White's writings rather than the Scriptures, as sectarian rather than evangelically Protestant, and, most important, as wrong rather than right. For this reason, Ford concluded that White's legacy should be seen as "pastoral" rather than "canonical." Though, at a conference in Glacier View, Colorado, church

---

54. Joseph Battistone, "Ellen White's Authority as Bible Commentator," *Spectrum*, VIII (January, 1977), 37-40; Butler, *Spectrum*, X (August, 1979), 2-13.

leaders moved considerably in Ford's direction on the sanctuary doctrine, they — almost simultaneously — stripped him of his ministerial credentials.[55]

All of these developments in Ellen White studies dealt with the prophet's writings and how they related either to the Bible or her own literary and cultural context. Another line of investigation has cut through her writings to the person behind them. Still in an initial yet promising stage, this scholarship examines the personal and social circumstances that account for White's emergence as a visionary. In writing his book on the prophet, Numbers had "consciously shied away from extended analyses of her mental health and psychic abilities." Sixteen years later, however, he and his present wife, Janet S. Numbers, a clinical psychologist, have addressed the matter of the prophet's mental health.[56]

Further inquiry on White as a visionary has widened to include the enthusiastic social environment that produced her. Graybill completed his doctoral dissertation at Johns Hopkins on Ellen White as a charismatic religious founder, and he devoted a chapter of it to her trance-visionary period in the context of an enthusiastic community. Probing her visions from both psychological and anthropological perspectives, he described the way the prophet had served as an expression of the ecstatic impulses of early Adventism. But as her community changed, she changed. Order replaced enthusiasm, and White as a more conventional religious leader took over for the trance figure. In making his case, Graybill assumed the naturalistic posture for which Numbers had been excoriated less than a decade before, and he lost his job of thirteen years at the White Estate. Shortly thereafter, an even clearer picture of the ecstatic character of early Adventism emerged with a spectacular documentary discovery by a historian at Loma Linda University. Frederick Hoyt came upon court transcripts that included testimony placing James White and Ellen Harmon, along with other Adventists, in the midst of tumultuous expressions of enthusiasm. Though Ellen White had

---

55. On the Ford controversy, see Walter Utt, "Desmond Ford Raises the Sanctuary Question," *Spectrum*, X (March, 1980), 4-5; Edward E. Plowman, "The Shaking Up of Adventism?" *Christianity Today*, XXIV (February 8, 1980), 64-67.

56. For their discussion, see "Ellen White on the Mind and the Mind of Ellen White," in this volume.

INTRODUCTION

later disavowed the more bizarre aspects of this phenomena as fanaticism, and had suppressed evidence of her own part in it, the court records told a different story.[57]

Looking back on Adventism in the 1970s and 80s, we see that the church had matured in regard to its understanding of Ellen White as both visionary and writer. And in the middle of this ferment, another astonishing primary source surfaced that went right to the heart of Adventism's spiritual agony over its prophet's authority. Shortly after White's death in 1915, Adventist Bible and history teachers met with churchmen to discuss the role of her writings in Adventist theology, education, and practice. These meetings in 1919 proved so candid and open that church leaders saw to it that a more conservative laity was kept in the dark as to what had been discussed. Sixty years later, however, transcripts of the meetings were dredged up and found compellingly relevant to the church's contemporary problems on Ellen White. What made these transcripts so remarkable was that key leaders in the church, including the General Conference president, Arthur G. Daniells, not marginal figures, were seen struggling over questions regarding the prophet. Alongside the churchmen of this earlier time the Adventist academics of the 1970s seemed far less heretical. Bemoaning the fact that Ellen White's writings had assumed canonical status among Adventists and that their new Scriptures were also held to be "verbally inerrant," one delegate insisted, to the contrary, that the value of her writing resided in "the Spiritual light it throws into our own hearts and lives [more] than in the intellectual accuracy in historical and theological matters." Another delegate offered this prescient re-

---

57. See Ronald Graybill, "The Power of Prophecy: Ellen G. White and the Women Religious Founders of the Nineteenth Century" (Ph.D. diss., Johns Hopkins University, 1983), esp. pp. 84-112. See also Bonnie L. Casey, "Graybill's Exit: Turning Point at the White Estate?" *Spectrum*, XIV (March, 1984), 2-8; the Hoyt material appears in Frederick Hoyt, ed., "Trial of Elder I. Dammon: Reported for the *Piscataquis Farmer*," *Spectrum*, XVII (August, 1987), 29-36. See also Rennie Schoepflin, ed., "Scandal or Rite of Passage? Historians on the Dammon Trial," ibid., 37-50; White's early years as a visionary within an enthusiastic context are dealt with in Butler, "Prophecy, Gender, and Culture: Ellen Gould Harmon [White] and the Roots of Seventh-day Adventism," *Religion and American Culture: A Journal of Interpretation*, I (Winter, 1991), 3-29.

mark: "Is it well to let our people in general go on holding to the verbal inspiration of [White's] Testimonies? When we do that, aren't we preparing for a crisis that will be very serious some day?"[58]

Owing in part to the failure of nerve among the leaders in 1919, Adventist academics faced a spiritual and vocational crisis in the 1970s without the benefit of knowing that at one time the movement's mainstream had experienced a similar turmoil. As a result, they had been forced into an unnecessarily peripheral and isolated position. But contemporary Adventism had undergone a real change, and profoundly altered perceptions of Ellen White lay at the heart of it. The new scholarship had established that the prophet was neither original nor inerrant, neither changeless nor timeless. To what degree this historical revolution has spread from the academic elite to the rank and file is not altogether clear. Nor is it known to what extent the vast majority of Adventists in the Third World would recognize this "new" Ellen White from North America. What has become obvious, however, is the fact that this historical consciousness-raising, unlike that of the early twentieth century, has reached a wide public, both inside and outside the church. This increases the likelihood that it will last and spread. Indeed, a survey of Adventist opinion after the revelations on White shows that fewer and fewer members equate their faith with belief in her as a prophet. Ellen White's writings can no longer be imposed as a litmus test of orthodoxy with quite the self-assurance they once were. Not even the White Estate projects the defensive posture that it did under the prophet's grandson. Since Arthur White's retirement, the Estate has steadily adopted more open policies on its holdings. In regard to critical transitions in the prophet's role among Adventists, Arthur White's passing from the scene may prove as significant as two previous events: Ellen White's death and her husband's death before hers.[59]

---

58. The published version of the minutes may be found on pp. 344-401 below.

59. Donald R. McAdams, "Shifting Views of Inspiration: Ellen White Studies in the 1970s," *Spectrum*, X (March, 1980), 27-41; and McAdams, "The Scope of Ellen White's Authority," *Spectrum*, XVI (August, 1985), 2-7; Herold Weiss, "Formative Authority, Yes; Canonization, No," ibid., 8-13. Adventists have been polled through the Valuegenesis Research Project, described in general terms in V. Bailey Gillespie, "Nurturing Our Next Generation," *Adventist Review*, CLXVII (January 3,

INTRODUCTION

But if, with the changing perceptions of Ellen White among Adventists, heresy has been the mother of orthodoxy, the heretics themselves have been largely lost to the community. A review of many of the names identified with advances in Ellen White studies — William Peterson, Roy Branson, Herold Weiss, Ronald Numbers, Donald McAdams, Ron Graybill, Jonathan Butler, Desmond Ford, Walter Rea — reveals that none of them is now employed by the church (with the exception of Graybill who was forced to change jobs within it), and most of them are no longer active church members. Within Adventism, the prophet has been lethally radioactive to many of those who have handled her. Numbers is neither a believing nor a practicing Adventist, but, because friends have urged him to, he allows his name to remain on the books of his former church at Loma Linda University. And from time to time, its pastor (under pressure from the church board) has written to him with inquiries about the disposition of his membership. Numbers also maintains a place among the consulting editors of *Spectrum*. Given his limited editorial contributions to the journal of late, he recently asked his cousin, Roy, to drop his name from the list of editors. Branson pleaded with him, however, "*Spectrum* is your one link to the church; don't make me take your name off the masthead."[60]

His father could not let him go either. As Ray Numbers read the 1919 Bible Conference transcripts, they changed his view of Ellen White in a way that his son's book could not do on its own. The testimony of past General Conference officials, as they searched their souls over prophetic authority, gave the father permission to reach out to his son. Because he never questioned his boy's honesty, yet knew he could not be telling the truth about Ellen White, he had concluded that Satan had taken possession of Ron's mind. Embarrassed by his son's apostasy, he refused for years to be seen in his

---

1991), 5-11. See also Gary Land, "Coping with Change 1961–1980," in Gary Land, ed., *Adventism in America* (Grand Rapids: William B. Eerdmans Publishing Co., 1986), pp. 219-23. For changes in White Estate policy, see Ronald Graybill, "From Z File to Compact Disk: The Democratization of Ellen White Sources," unpublished paper, 1988. Arthur White stepped down as head of the White Estate in 1978; he died on January 12, 1991.

60. Numerous letters to Numbers from successive pastors at the University Church were written between February 20, 1975, and June 23, 1983.

company if Adventists were around. Shortly after the publication of *Prophetess of Health,* Ron had chided him for sequestering his complimentary copy of the book out of sight. But after poring over the 1919 record, he finally understood his son — and proudly displayed his book in the living room. On his deathbed, he crowed to visitors about his boy "the author," who had just been awarded a prestigious "Guggenheimer" Fellowship. He was still far from seeing eye to eye with his son on the prophet. But, for the first time in his life, he acknowledged her problems. Just days before his death in 1983, he said, "Ronnie, I want you to know that I believed everything I taught you about Mrs. White. As for the mistakes in her writings and the influences on her, I recognize now that there are some problems. But *then,* I told you what I believed." With these words, a historian and a believer had never been closer.

CHAPTER ONE

A Prophetess Is Born

"a true prophet"

J. N. Loughborough[1]

"a wonderful fanatic and trance medium"

Isaac C. Wellcome[2]

She was a mere child of not more than ten when a scrap of paper and a stone altered the course of her entire life. Walking to school one morning, Ellen Harmon spied a piece of paper lying by the wayside. Picking it up, the horrified little girl read that an English preacher was predicting the end of the world, perhaps in only thirty years. "I was seized with terror," she later wrote; "the time seemed so short for the conversion and salvation of the world." For several nights she tossed and turned, hoping and praying that she might be among the saints ready to meet Christ at his Second Coming.[3] Little did she

---

1. J. N. Loughborough, *The Great Second Advent Movement: Its Rise and Progress* (Washington: Review and Herald Publishing Assn., 1909), p. 306.

2. Isaac C. Wellcome, *History of the Second Advent Message and Mission, Doctrine and People* (Yarmouth, Maine: I. C. Wellcome, 1874), p. 402.

3. This story and the account of Ellen's youth which follows are based on two editions of her autobiography: *Spiritual Gifts: My Christian Experience, Views and Labors* (Battle Creek: James White, 1860); and *Life Sketches of Ellen G. White* (Mountain View, Calif.: Pacific Press, 1915). Occasional names and dates are taken from C. C. Goen, "El-

dream that for the next seventy-five years she would work and wait expectantly for her Savior's return.

Within a short time of this frightening episode, another incident nearly ended Ellen's life. With her twin sister, Elizabeth, and a friend, Ellen was passing through a public park when an older schoolmate, angry "at some trifle," hurled a rock at the girls. Ellen was struck squarely on the nose and knocked to the ground unconscious. For three weeks she lay in a stupor, oblivious to her surroundings, while friends and relatives sadly waited for her to die. When she finally regained her senses, she suffered not only acute physical pain but also anxiety over her prospects for salvation should she die.

Somehow she passed safely through the valley of death, but time never fully erased the traces of these two childhood experiences. For the remainder of Ellen's long life, good health and Christ's Second Coming were uppermost on her mind.

Ellen Gould Harmon and her sister, Elizabeth, were born on November 26, 1827, in the village of Gorham, Maine, a few miles west of Portland. Their father, Robert, a hatter of modest means, followed the common practice of having his children, six daughters and two sons, assist him in the home industry. Mother Eunice was a pious homemaker with strong theological convictions. When the twins were still preschoolers, the Harmon family moved into the city, where the girls eventually enrolled in the Brackett Street School.

Portland in the 1830s was a picturesque New England seaport with a population approaching fifteen thousand. Horse-drawn carts and carriages filled its famous tree-lined streets, and hoop-skirted ladies could still be seen on its crowded sidewalks. The city's location on a neck of land jutting into Casco Bay made it ideal for the West Indian maritime trade that supported the economy. Ships from Maine sailed to the south loaded with lumber or marine products and returned filled with sugar, molasses, rum, and other Carib-

---

len Gould Harmon White," *Notable American Women, 1607-1950: A Biographical Dictionary,* ed. Edward T. James (Cambridge: Harvard University Press, 1971), III, 585-88; and "Ellen Gould (Harmon) White," *Seventh-day Adventist Encyclopedia,* ed. Don F. Neufeld (Washington: Review and Herald Publishing Assn., 1966), pp. 1406-14. Additional details were kindly furnished by the Ellen G. White Estate.

A Prophetess Is Born

bean goods. With so ready a supply of alcohol, it is not surprising that temperance became a burning local issue and that "intemperance" was a commonly cited cause of death. The greatest killers, however, were consumption, which accounted for over one-fourth of all mortality, and scarlet fever, which took another 20 percent. In religious matters, Portland had long been a Congregational stronghold, but Baptist and Methodist churches were beginning to attract sizable numbers.[4]

The Harmon family lived in the far southwestern outskirts of the city, not far from Ellen's school. Their neighbors on Spruce Street were working class or petty bourgeoisie. Among them were a merchant, a distiller, a truckman, a cordwainer, a shipcarpenter, a ropemaker, two stevedores, and a couple of laborers — the same type of hard-working people who later filled the Adventist ranks and became followers of Ellen White.[5]

It was in Portland, when Ellen was nine or ten, that the rock-throwing incident occurred. Despite the efforts of well-meaning physicians, Ellen's injuries continued to plague her for years. Her facial disfigurement — so bad that her own father could scarcely recognize her — caused frequent embarrassment and made breathing through her nostrils impossible for two years. Frayed nerves rebelled at simple assignments such as reading and writing. Her hands shook so badly she was unable to control her slate marks, and words became mere blurs on a page. Try as she might, she could not concentrate on her studies. Perspiration would break out on her forehead, and dizziness would overcome her.

The girl responsible for her suffering, now contrite and anxious to make amends, tried tutoring Ellen, but to no avail. Finally it became apparent to her teachers that she simply could not cope with schoolwork, and they recommended that she withdraw from classes. Later, in about 1839, she again attempted to resume her studies, at the Westbrook Seminary and Female College in Portland, but this, too, ended in disappointment and despair. "It was the

---

4. William Willis, *The History of Portland, from 1632 to 1864* (2nd ed.; Portland: Bailey & Noyes, 1865), pp. 68, 728, 769-75; *The Portland Directory* (Portland: Arthur Shirley, 1834), p. 34.

5. *The Portland Directory,* passim.

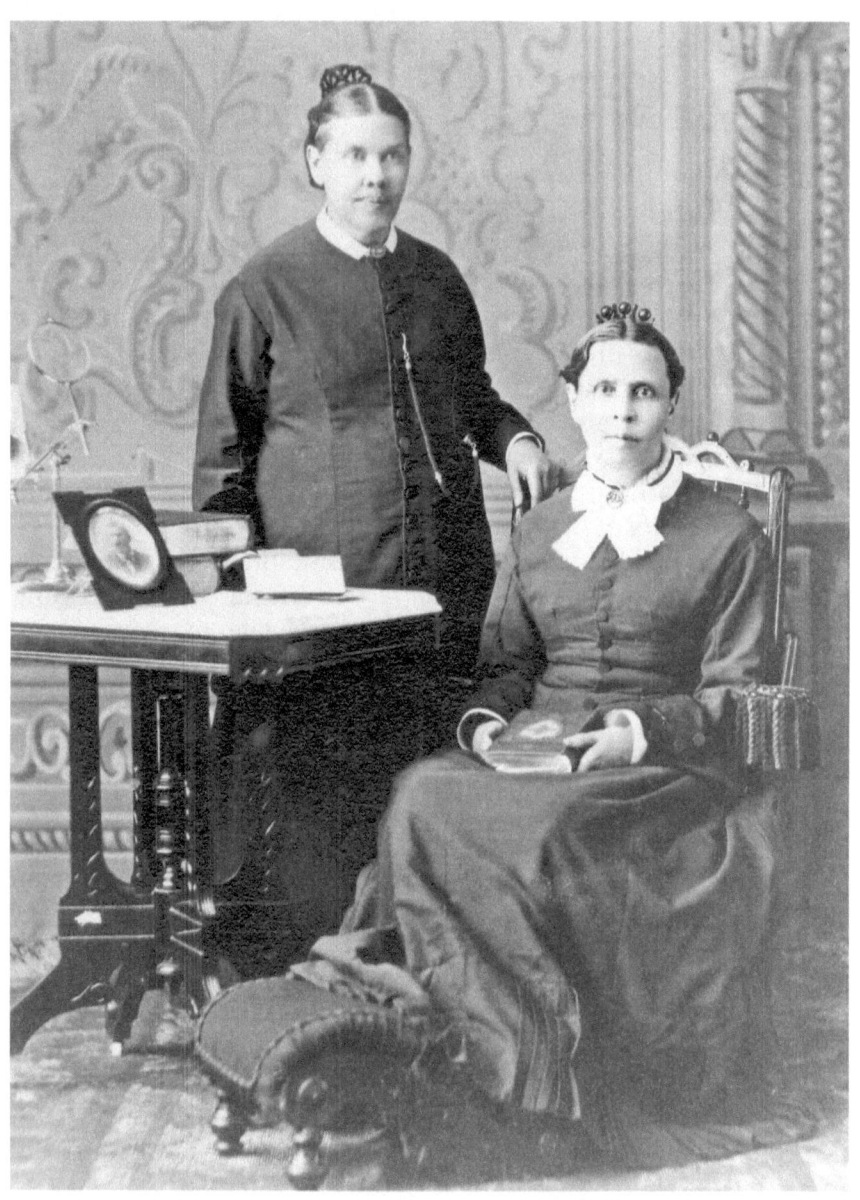

Ellen White and her twin sister, Elizabeth Bangs
Courtesy Ellen G. White Estate, Inc.

A Prophetess Is Born

hardest struggle of my young life," Ellen later lamented, "to yield to my feebleness, and decide that I must leave my studies, and give up the hope of gaining an education."

Her formal education ended, she resigned herself to the life of a semi-invalid, passing the time of day propped up in bed making hat crowns for her father or occasionally knitting a pair of stockings. In this way she could console herself with the knowledge that she was at least contributing to the family economy.

It is uncertain what effect, if any, her hat-making had upon her health. Some evidence suggests that about this time American hatters began using a mercury solution to treat the fur used in felt hats, a practice that frequently led to chronic mercurialism. This disease manifested itself in various psychic and physical disturbances: "abnormal degrees of irritability, excitability, irascible temper, timidity, depression or despondency, anxiety, discouragement without cause, inability to take orders, self-consciousness, desire for solitude, and excessive embarrassment in the presence of strangers." Tremor, making it difficult to control handwriting, was especially common. Hallucinations sometimes occurred in advanced cases. While it is impossible to know for sure if Ellen were exposed to mercury poisoning, and both unnecessary and unwise to assume that this malady would account for all of her unusual behavior, it might explain her trembling hands.[6]

In March, 1840, life took on new meaning for Ellen. In that month William Miller paid his first visit to the citizens of Portland to warn them of Christ's soon return. Miller, a captain in the War of 1812, retired from the army in 1815 to take up farming in Low

---

6. U.S. Public Health Service, *A Study of Chronic Mercurialism in the Hatters' Fur-Cutting Industry,* Public Health Bulletin No. 234 (Washington: Government Printing Office, 1937), p. 39; U.S. Public Health Service, *Mercurialism and Its Control in the Felt-Hat Industry,* Public Health Bulletin No. 263 (Washington: Government Printing Office, 1941), pp. 48-54; Ethel Browning, *Toxicity of Industrial Metals* (London: Butterworth and Co., 1961), pp. 203-4; May R. Mayers, *Occupational Health* (Baltimore: Williams and Wilkins Co., 1969), pp. 79-83; Leonard J. Goldwater, *Mercury: A History of Quicksilver* (Baltimore: York Press, 1972), pp. 270-75; J. Addison Freeman, "Mercurial Disease among Hatters," *Transactions,* Medical Society of N.J. (1860), pp. 61-64. Since so many of her contemporaries experienced religious trances similar to Ellen White's, it seems unlikely to me that mercury-induced hallucinations had anything to do with her later visions.

Hampton, New York. A decade or so earlier he had abandoned Christianity for deism, but growing concern about his fate after death drove him to intense Bible study and a return to the faith of his youth. His interest focused on the biblical prophecies, particularly Daniel 8:14: "Unto two thousand and three hundred days; then shall the sanctuary be cleansed." On the assumption that each prophetic day represented a year, that the cleansing of the sanctuary coincided with the Second Coming of Christ, and that the 2300 years began in 457 B.C., when Artaxerxes of Persia issued a decree to rebuild Jerusalem, Miller concluded that events on this earth would terminate "about the year 1843."[7]

For thirteen years Miller kept his views largely to himself, but as the end inexorably approached, he could no longer remain silent. In the summer of 1831, at the age of forty-nine, he took to the pulpit; two years later the Baptists granted him a license to preach. By mid-1839 he had delivered over eight hundred lectures in towns throughout New York and New England. His disturbing message often held audiences for prolonged periods, but aside from his earnestness and gravity he was an undistinguished speaker. "There is nothing very peculiar in the manner or appearance of Mr. Miller," wrote the editor of a Massachusetts newspaper. "Both are at least to the style and appearance of ministers in general. His gestures are easy and expressive, and his personal appearance every way decorous. His Scripture explanations and illustrations are strikingly simple, natural, and forcible...."[8]

During the early years of his ministry Miller made no attempt at organization and limited his preaching to the small churches that invited him. This changed in 1840 when Joshua V. Himes, the energetic young pastor of the Chardon Street Chapel in Boston, teamed up with Miller to coordinate a national crusade, with Himes assuming responsibility for organization and publicity. At the peak of the movement about two hundred ministers and five hundred public lecturers were spreading the Millerite message, and an estimated

---

7. Sylvester Bliss, *Memoirs of William Miller* (Boston: Joshua V. Himes, 1853); Francis D. Nichol, *The Midnight Cry* (Washington: Review and Herald Publishing Assn., 1944), pp. 17-42.

8. Bliss, *Memoirs*, pp. 137-38; Nichol, *Midnight Cry*, pp. 43-74.

fifty thousand believers were waiting expectantly for their Savior's return.⁹

Little is known about the social characteristics of these Millerites, but one historian has recently concluded that, unlike other apocalyptic millenarians, "They do not seem to have been people deprived of power, nor potential revolutionaries, nor, most significantly, threatened with destruction." Many, including Miller and Himes, were respected and influential members of their communities. Nevertheless, the Millerites were acutely aware of social unrest and religious apostasy, which they interpreted to be signs of the end. In contrast to the optimistic postmillennialists, like the popular evangelist Charles G. Finney, who expected soon to usher in a thousand years of peace and prosperity, the pessimistic Millerites saw only evidence of a world in decay.¹⁰

What they did share with the postmillennialists was a fondness for enthusiastic revivals and camp meetings, with emotional sermons, spirited songs, and fervent prayers. The Millerites held their first camp meeting in the summer of 1842 in East Kingston, New Hampshire, near the home of Ezekiel Hale, Jr., a friend of Sylvester Graham's who took care of local arrangements. A chance visitor, John Greenleaf Whittier, described the event, which attracted between ten and fifteen thousand individuals:

> Three or four years ago [he wrote in 1845], on my way eastward, I spent an hour or two at a camp-ground of the Second Advent in East Kingston. The spot was well chosen. A tall growth of pine and hemlock threw its melancholy shadow over the multitude, who were arranged upon rough seats of boards and logs. Several hundred — perhaps a thousand people — were present, and more were rapidly coming. Drawn about in a circle, forming a

---

9. Nichol, *Midnight Cry,* pp. 75-90, 217. According to David T. Arthur, the Millerites came "from nearly all Protestant groups, most especially Baptist, Congregational, Christian, Methodist, and Presbyterian churches"; "Millerism," in *The Rise of Adventism: Religion and Society in Mid-Nineteenth-Century America,* ed. Edwin S. Gaustad (New York: Harper & Row, 1974), p. 154.

10. Ernest Sandeen, "Millennialism," in *The Rise of Adventism,* pp. 111, 116; William C. McLoughlin, Jr., *Modern Revivalism: Charles Grandison Finney to Billy Graham* (New York: Ronald Press, 1959), pp. 105-6.

background of snowy whiteness to the dark masses of men and foliage, were the white tents, and back of them the provision-stalls and cook-shops. When I reached the ground, a hymn, the words of which I could not distinguish, was pealing through the dim aisles of the forest. I could readily perceive that it had its effect upon the multitude before me, kindling to higher intensity their already excited enthusiasm. The preachers were placed in a rude pulpit of rough boards, carpeted only by the dead forest-leaves and flowers, and tasselled, not with silk and velvet, but with the green boughs of the sombre hemlocks around it. One of them followed the music in an earnest exhortation on the duty of preparing for the great event. Occasionally he was really eloquent, and his description of the last day had the ghastly distinctness of Anelli's painting of the End of the World.

Suspended from the front of the rude pulpit were two broad sheets of canvas, upon one of which was the figure of a man, the head of gold, the breast and arms of silver, the belly of brass, the legs of iron, and feet of clay, — the dream of Nebuchadnezzar. On the other were depicted the wonders of the Apocalyptic vision, — the beasts, the dragons, the scarlet woman seen by the seer of Patmos, Oriental types, figures, and mystic symbols, translated into staring Yankee realities and exhibited like the beasts of a travelling menagerie. One horrible image, with its hideous heads and scaly caudal extremity, reminded me of the tremendous line of Milton, who, in speaking of the same evil dragon describes him as 'swinging the scaly horrors of his folded tail.'

"The white circle of tents; the dim wood arches; the upturned, earnest faces; the loud voices of the speakers burdened with the awful symbolic language of the Bible; the smoke from the fires, rising like incense" — all left an indelible impression on the poet and presumably struck fear in the hearts of many who attended this and similar meetings.[11]

According to Ellen White, "Terror and conviction spread through the entire city" of Portland during Miller's 1840 visit. Believers and skeptics alike packed into the Casco Street Christian

---

11. John Greenleaf Whittier, "Father Miller," in *The Stranger in Lowell* (Boston: Waite, Pierce and Co., 1845), pp. 75-83; Nichol, *Midnight Cry,* pp. 111-21.

A Prophetess Is Born

Church to hear his strange but plausible interpretations of Bible prophecy. News of Father Miller's lectures again caused fear to well up in Ellen's heart as it had that day about four years earlier when she picked up the scrap of paper announcing the impending end of the world. Yet she wanted to hear what the farmer-preacher had to say. Accompanied by several friends, Ellen made her way to the Casco Street Church and took her place among the crowds of listeners who filled the sanctuary. When Miller invited sinners to step forward to the "anxious seat," Ellen, under conviction, pressed through the congested aisles to join the "seekers" at the front. Still, she was not comforted, and doubts of her unworthiness haunted her day and night.

In the summer of 1841 she traveled with her parents to a Methodist camp meeting in Buxton. Here the constant exhortations to godliness only heightened her sense of sinfulness. Throughout the meetings she became increasingly distressed by her failure to experience an ecstatic conversion. In desperation one day she fell before the altar and pleaded for God's mercy. There, kneeling and praying, her burden of guilt suddenly vanished. The dramatic change in her countenance moved a lady nearby to exclaim, "His peace is with you, I see it in your face!" To Ellen, the whole earth now "seemed to smile under the peace of God."

Upon returning home, she decided to join her parents' Chestnut Street Methodist Church and requested baptism. After a probationary period, during which William Miller returned to Portland for a second series of lectures and reawakened Ellen's interest in the Second Advent, she and eleven other candidates were immersed in the waters of Casco Bay. On June 26, 1842, with the wind blowing and the waves running high, she symbolically buried her sins in the watery grave. She emerged from the bay emotionally spent: "When I arose out of the water, my strength was nearly gone, for the power of God rested upon me. Such a rich blessing I never experienced before. I felt dead to the world, and that my sins were all washed away."

But her beautiful day was nearly ruined in only a few hours when she went to the church to receive the official welcome into membership. There, standing next to the plainly dressed Ellen, was another candidate decked out in gold rings and a fancy bonnet. To Ellen's dismay, her minister, the Reverend John Hobart, went right on with the service without so much as mentioning the offending adornments. This experience proved to be a great trial to young Ellen, whose faith in the popular churches was already being shaken.

Even her conversion and baptism failed to bring lasting peace to Ellen's troubled mind. At times she became discouraged and sank into deep despair. With sins so grave as hers, she felt certain no forgiveness could be granted. Sermons vividly depicting the red-hot flames of hell only intensified her torment and pushed her closer to the breaking point. "While listening to these terrible descriptions, my imagination would be so wrought upon that the perspiration would start, and it was difficult to suppress a cry of anguish, for I seemed already to feel the pains of perdition."

In addition, she began experiencing terrible feelings of guilt over her timidity to witness publicly for Christ. She especially wanted to participate in the small Millerite prayer services but feared her words would not come out right. Her burden of guilt grew to such proportions that even her secret prayers seemed a mockery to God. For weeks depression engulfed her. At night she would wait until Elizabeth had fallen asleep, then crawl out of bed and silently pour out her heart to God. "I frequently remained bowed in prayer nearly all night," she wrote, "groaning and trembling with inexpressible anguish, and a hopelessness that passes all description."[12]

While in this state of mind she began having religious dreams similar to those that followed her through life. In the first one recorded she saw herself failing to gain salvation, prevented by pride from humbling herself before "a lamb all mangled and bleeding." She awoke certain that her fate had been sealed, that God had rejected her. But then she had a second dream. In this Jesus touched her head and said, "Fear not." Filled with renewed hope, Ellen at last confided in her mother, who advised talking things over with Elder Levi Stockman, a local Methodist minister who had become a Millerite. With tears in his eyes he listened to her unusual story and then said, "Ellen, you are only a child. Yours is a most singular expe-

---

12. Religious anxiety, including lying awake most of the night worrying about salvation, was not unusual among New England children Ellen's age; see Joseph F. Kett, "Growing Up in Rural New England, 1800-1840," in *Anonymous Americans: Explorations in Nineteenth-Century Social History*, ed. Tamara K. Hareven (Englewood Cliffs, N.J.: Prentice-Hall, 1971), pp. 1-16.

rience for one of your tender age. Jesus must be preparing you for some special work."

Although encouraged by Elder Stockman's words, Ellen continued to brood over her inability to pray publicly. One evening during a prayer meeting in the home of her uncle Abner Gould, she determined to break her silence. While the others prayed, she knelt, trembling, waiting her chance. Then before she really knew what was happening, she, too, was speaking. As the pent-up words spilled out, she lost touch with the world and collapsed on the floor. Those around her suggested calling a physician, but Ellen's mother assured the group that it was "the wondrous power of God" that had prostrated her daughter. Ellen herself said, "The Spirit of God rested upon me with such power that I was unable to go home that night." The next day she left her uncle's home a changed person, full of peace and happiness, and for six months she was in "perfect bliss."

Ellen launched her public ministry the night following her prayer-meeting victory. Before a congregation of Millerite believers she tearfully related her recent experience. All fear disappeared as she spoke, and before long she "seemed to be alone with God." Soon she received an invitation to speak at the Temple Street Christian Church, where her story again moved many in the audience to weep and praise God. Ellen also began holding private meetings with her friends, who she feared were not ready to meet the Lord. At first some questioned her childish enthusiasm and ridiculed her experience, but eventually she converted every one of them. Often she would pray till nearly dawn for the salvation of a lost friend, before drifting off to sleep and dreaming of another in spiritual need.

As the Millerite movement gathered momentum, more and more of its followers found themselves in doctrinal conflict with their local churches. The Harmon family was no exception. By 1843 hostility had grown to the point where members would groan audibly when Ellen got up to speak in class meetings; so she and her teen-age brother, Robert, quit attending. Finally the Reverend William F. Farrington, pastor of the Chestnut Street Methodist Church, called on the family to inform them that their divergent teachings would no longer be tolerated. He suggested that they quietly withdraw from the church and thus avoid the publicity of a trial. Mr. Harmon, seeing no reason to be ashamed of his beliefs, demanded a public hearing. Here charges of absenteeism from class meetings were brought against the Harmons, and the following Sunday seven members of the family — including Ellen — were formally dismissed from the Methodist church.

Excitement and anticipation mounted as the months and days of 1843 slipped by. Throughout March a brilliant comet hovered in the southwestern sky, like a heavenly messenger announcing the impending end of the world. Although Father Miller would say only that he expected the Lord to come sometime during the Jewish year extending from March 21, 1843, to March 21, 1844, less cautious men were all too willing to provide the faithful with specific dates for the great event. A favorite of many was April 14, the beginning of Passover and the anniversary of Christ's crucifixion. With the passing of each appointed time, a new wave of disappointment spread through the Millerite camp, allegedly driving some distraught souls to suicide or insanity.[13]

In Ellen's hometown of Portland the Millerites gathered nightly in Beethoven Hall to renew their courage and to make a final appeal to the still unconverted. Often these sessions continued late into the night as one after another Spirit-filled Millerite rose to give a spontaneous "exhortation." One evening Ellen watched in awe as the Reverend Samuel E. Brown, moved by a colleague's testimony, suddenly

---

13. Dr. Amariah Brigham, superintendent of the New York Lunatic Asylum in Utica, attributed the insanity of thirty-two patients in three northern asylums to Millerism, which he regarded as a greater threat to the country than yellow fever or cholera; "Millerism," *American Journal of Insanity*, I (January, 1845), 249-53. The accuracy of Brigham's diagnosis may be questioned, but nineteenth-century American psychiatrists generally believed that excessive religious zeal often precipitated insanity in those already predisposed to mental illness; see Norman Dain, *Concepts of Insanity in the United States, 1789-1865* (New Brunswick, N.J.: Rutgers University Press, 1964), p. 187. See also Everett N. Dick, "William Miller and the Advent Crisis, 1831-1844" (Ph.D. diss., University of Wisconsin, 1932), pp. 147-51, 194-95; Nichol, *Midnight Cry*, p. 145; and David L. Rowe, "Thunder and Trumpets: The Millerite Movement and Apocalyptic Thought in Upstate New York, 1800-1845" (Ph.D. diss., University of Virginia, 1974), pp. 201-5. In his "defense" of the Millerites, Nichol discounts the charges of insanity and suicide (pp. 355-88), while the Seventh-day Adventist historian Dick concludes that "Notwithstanding the numerous false reports it is evident that there was an increase in the number of cases of insanity from religious causes and there were numerous instances of suicides" (p. 194). Rowe's position is similar to Dick's.

turned porcelain white and fell from his chair on the platform. In a few minutes, after regaining his composure, he stood up and with his face "shining with light from the Sun of Righteousness" gave what Ellen thought was "a very impressive testimony." As they made their way home through the darkened streets of the city, the Millerites filled the night air with joyful shouts of praise to God, undoubtedly much to the annoyance of nearby sleeping residents.[14]

March 21, 1844, came and went with no sign of Christ's appearance. Obviously a mistake had been made, and on May 2, William Miller confessed that his prophetic calculations had been in error. At the same time he reassured his followers that he still believed the Second Coming was not far off. While some of the faint-hearted now deserted the movement, a surprising number, including most of the Millerite leaders, adopted an exegetical solution offered by Samuel S. Snow, a Congregational-Millerite preacher. According to Snow, a correct reading of the prophecy in Daniel upon which Miller had based his dates indicated that Christ would not come until the "tenth day of the seventh month" of the Jewish calendar, that is, October 22, 1844. Renewed energy surged through the Millerite ranks. By mid-August all hopes were pinned on October 22. No sacrifice — family, job, or fortune — seemed too great, for time on this earth would soon end. For Ellen, this was the happiest period of her life. Free from discouragement, she went from home to home earnestly praying for the salvation of those whose faith was wavering, or retired with friends to a secluded grove for quiet seasons of prayer.[15]

Few today can imagine the bitter disappointment of those devout Millerites who watched in vain through the night of October 22 for their Savior's appearance. Hiram Edson, a farmer in upstate New York, recorded those agonizing hours. He and his friends had waited hopefully until midnight, then burst into uncontrollable sobs. "It seemed that the loss of all earthly friends could have been no comparison. We wept, and wept, till the day dawn." Millerite reactions varied from resentment to puzzlement. Some bitterly renounced their former hopes in the Second Coming as a cruel delu-

---

14. EGW, *Life Sketches*, pp. 54-56.
15. Dick, "William Miller," pp. 211, 233-34, 269; Nichol, *Midnight Cry*, pp. 226-27; EGW, *Life Sketches*, pp. 59-61.

sion. Others, including a large group led by Miller and Himes, admitted their mistake but nevertheless clung to the certainty of Christ's soon return. But a resolute few insisted that their sacrifices had not been in vain, that an event of cosmic significance had taken place on October 22.[16]

This was the position of Hiram Edson. Early in the morning after the disappointment, he and some Millerite brothers had gone out to a barn to plead with God for an explanation. Their prayers were not long in being answered. After breakfast, while passing through a nearby field, Edson had a vision of heaven. He saw that the cleansing of the sanctuary foretold in Daniel 8:14 did not coincide with the Second Coming but rather with Christ's entry into the most holy place of the heavenly sanctuary just prior to his return. This view was taken a step farther by two Millerite preachers, Apollos Hale and Joseph Turner, in a paper called the *Advent Mirror*, published in January, 1845. According to Hale and Turner, Christ had ended his ministry for the world on October 22 and, upon entering the most holy place of the sanctuary, had shut the "door of mercy" on those who had rejected the Millerite warning.[17]

On a wintry day in December, 1844, seventeen-year-old Ellen Harmon met with four friends in the Portland home of a Mrs. Haines to pray for divine guidance. As the women knelt in a circle, the "Holy Spirit" rested upon Ellen in a new and dramatic way. Bathed in light, she seemed to be "rising higher and higher, far above the dark world." From her vantage point she saw the Advent people traveling a straight and narrow path toward the New Jerusalem, their way lighted by the October 22 message. When some "rashly denied the light behind them, and said that it was not God that had led them out so far," they stumbled in the darkness and fell to "the wicked world below which God had rejected." The meaning

---

16. Nichol, *Midnight Cry*, pp. 263-64; James Nix, "The Life and Work of Hiram Edson" (M.A. paper submitted to the Seventh-day Adventist Theological Seminary, Andrews University, 1971), pp. 18-19; David T. Arthur, "Come Out of Babylon: A Study of Millerite Separatism and Denominationalism, 1840-1865" (Ph.D. diss., University of Rochester, 1970), pp. 89, 97-101.

17. Nichol, *Midnight Cry*, pp. 478-81; A. Hale and J. Turner, "Has Not the Savior Come as the Bridegroom?" *Advent Mirror*, I (January, 1845), 1-4, from a copy in the Adventual Collection, Aurora College.

of her vision was clear: October 22 had been no mistake; only the event had been confused.[18]

The following February, while visiting in Exeter, Maine, Ellen received a second vision on the importance of October 22. Subsequent to the publication of the *Advent Mirror,* dissension had arisen among the Exeter Millerites over the shut-door question. Had God really closed the door of salvation to sinners on October 22? As Ellen sat listening to an Adventist sister express her doubts on the shut door, a feeling of intense agony came over her and she fell from her chair to the floor. While others in the room sang and shouted, the Lord showed Ellen that the door had indeed been closed. Most of those who witnessed this apparently heaven-sent answer "received the vision, and were settled upon the shut door." Within a day or so Ellen discussed what she had seen with Joseph Turner and was overjoyed to discover that he, too, had been proclaiming the same view. Although his *Advent Mirror* had been in the house where she was staying, she said that she had never seen a word of it prior to her vision.[19]

In the spring of 1846 Ellen met a retired sea captain named Joseph Bates, who had broken with his former Millerite brethren and was now observing the seventh-day Sabbath. At first the wary Bates doubted Ellen's reputed visionary experiences, but in November a

---

18. EGW, *Life Sketches,* pp. 64-68; James White (ed.), *A Word to the "Little Flock"* (Brunswick, Maine: Privately printed, 1847), pp. 14-18. This early tract containing Ellen's first visions is photographically reproduced in Francis D. Nichol, *Ellen G. White and Her Critics* (Washington: Review and Herald Publishing Assn., 1951), pp. 561-84.

19. EGW to Joseph Bates, July 13, 1847 (B-3-1847, White Estate). This important letter was recently discovered in the White Estate vault by Professor Ingemar Lindén. For his views on the shut door, see his *Biblicism, Apokalyptik, Utopi: Adventisemens historiska utformning i USA samt dess svenska utveckling till o. 1939* (Uppsala, 1971), pp. 71-84, 449-50; and his unpublished paper in English, "The Significance of the Shut Door Theory in Sabbatarian Adventism, 1845-ca. 1851." Arthur White in "Ellen G. White and the Shut Door Question," recently prepared as an appendix to his forthcoming biography of his grandmother, argues that Ellen White did not mean by the term "shut door" what her contemporaries meant; he ignores the fact that she herself claimed to be in agreement with Joseph Turner. The doctrine of the shut door was particularly popular among Portland Millerites. See Sylvester Bliss to William Miller, February 11, 1845; and J. V. Himes to William Miller, March 12, March 29, and April 22, 1845 (Joshua V. Himes Letters, Massachusetts Historical Society). See also Otis Nichols to William Miller, April 12, 1846 (Miller Papers, Aurora College).

special vision on astronomy, a favorite subject of his, won him over completely. In his presence Ellen described various details of the solar system and the so-called gap in the constellation Orion, then a topic of great interest because of the telescopic observations of William Parsons, the third earl of Rosse. Just months earlier, Bates himself had written a tract, "The Opening Heavens," relating Lord Rosse's discoveries, but Ellen assured him she had had no prior knowledge of astronomy.[20]

The captain's faith in the young prophetess was doubly strengthened when she had another vision, giving divine sanction to his views on the Sabbath. In heaven, she said, Jesus had allowed her to see the tables of stone on which the Ten Commandments were inscribed. To her amazement, the fourth commandment, requiring observance of the seventh day, was "in the very center of the ten precepts, with a soft halo of light encircling it." An angel kindly explained to the puzzled young woman that the Millerites must begin keeping the "true Sabbath" before Christ would come. By embracing the seventh-day Sabbath and making it a new "test," Ellen placed herself in direct opposition to the moderate wing of Millerites, who at the Albany (New York) Conference of April, 1845, had officially condemned the doctrines Ellen had come to represent: visions, the shut door, and the seventh-day Sabbath. For the next few years she and the small band of fellow believers, generally drawn from Millerites with little formal education, were designated the "sabbatarian and shut-door" Adventists.[21]

To most Millerites, Ellen's visions were simply another manifestation of the unfortunate religious drift of the times toward "fanaticism." Early nineteenth-century America abounded with "prophets" of every description, from little-known frontier seers in Ellen Harmon's own Methodist church to prominent sectarian leaders. Mother Ann Lee of the Shakers had long since passed away, but her devoted followers perpetuated her reputation as the female Mes-

---

20. Godfrey T. Anderson, *Outrider of the Apocalypse: Life and Times of Joseph Bates* (Mountain View, Calif.: Pacific Press, 1972), p. 63; Loughborough, *The Great Second Advent Movement,* pp. 257-61; Joseph Bates, *The Opening Heavens* (New Bedford, Mass.: Benjamin Lindsey, 1846), pp. 6-12.

21. EGW, *Life Sketches,* pp. 95-96; Arthur, "Come Out of Babylon," pp. 138, 144-45.

A Prophetess Is Born

siah. In the 1830s an epidemic of visions spread through the Shaker communes as young girls "began to sing, talk about angels, and describe a journey they were making, under spiritual guidance, to heavenly places." Frequently those afflicted "would be struck to the floor, where they lay as dead, or struggling in distress, until someone near lifted them up, when they would begin to speak with great clearness and composure." Jemima Wilkinson, the Publick Universal Friend who founded the religious community of Jerusalem in western New York, was known for her visions and religious dreams. Joseph Smith, the Mormon prophet from Palmyra, New York, began having visions at age fourteen and continued to receive divine revelations until his death in 1844. During the second quarter of the century the Mormons were highly visible in Missouri and Illinois, and when Ellen White went west in the 1850s, she was often mistaken for a Mormon.[22]

Even the Millerite movement in its final days was so infected with religious enthusiasm that Joshua V. Himes complained of being in "mesmerism seven feet deep."[23] The most notorious case was that of John Starkweather, assistant pastor of Himes's Chardon Street Chapel, whose "cataleptic and epileptic" fits greatly embarrassed his more subdued colleagues. Eventually he was expelled from the chapel when his spiritual gifts proved to be contagious. Despite the best efforts of Father Miller — who himself had religious dreams — to maintain decorum, his followers often got so emotionally worked up that their meetings seemed to him "more like Babel, than a solemn assembly of penitents bowing in humble reverence before a holy God."[24]

---

22. Edward Deming Andrews, *The People Called Shakers* (New ed.; New York: Dover Publications, 1963), pp. 152-53; Herbert A. Wisbey, Jr., *Pioneer Prophetess: Jemima Wilkinson, the Publick Universal Friend* (Ithaca, N.Y.: Cornell University Press, 1964), pp. 160-61; Fawn M. Brodie, *No Man Knows My History: The Life of Joseph Smith, the Mormon Prophet* (2nd ed.; New York: Alfred A. Knopf, 1971), pp. 21-22, 55; EGW, *Spiritual Gifts* (1860), p. iv.

23. Quoted in [James White], "The Gifts of the Gospel Church," *R&H*, I (April 21, 1851), 69. James White, Ellen's future husband, regarded Himes's statement as the "most heaven-daring and fatal example" of questioning the work of the Holy Spirit that he had ever heard. On Millerite attitudes toward Ellen White, see EGW, *Life Sketches*, pp. 88-89.

24. Bliss, *Memories of William Miller*, pp. 231-34, 282; David Arnold, "Dream of

Fanaticism continued to plague the Millerites even after the October 22 disappointment, and it seemed to be particularly prevalent among shut-door believers. In Springwater Valley, New York, a black shut-door advocate named Houston set up a commune called the Household of Faith and the Household of Judgment and declared that "Jesus Christ in him was judging the world." At times God spoke directly to him in visions — "no vain imagination of a crazy mind," he assured William Miller — but his authoritarian manner, irrational acts, and practice of "spiritual wifery" soon alienated even his most ardent supporters.[25] The shut-door group in Portland, Maine, was even more notorious in Millerite circles for its "*continual* introduction of *visionary nonsense*," as Himes called it. In March of 1845 Himes informed Miller that a Sister Clemons of that city "has become very visionary, and disgusted nearly all the good friends here." But only a couple of weeks later he reported that another Portland sister had received a vision showing that Miss Clemons was of the Devil. "Things are in a bad way at Portland," he concluded.[26]

Ellen Harmon may not have been involved in these episodes, but she could hardly have been unaware of them. And there were at least two persons she met in Maine whom she regarded as authentic prophets. As a girl in the early 1840s she had gone with her father to Beethoven Hall to hear a tall, light-skinned mulatto named William Foy relate his "extraordinary visions of another world." Reputable Millerites testified to his genuineness, and a physician who examined him during one of his trances found no "appearance of life, except around the heart." After the Great Disappointment, Foy turned out one evening to hear Ellen give her testimony. While she was speaking, he began jumping up and down, praising the Lord, and

---

William Miller," *Review and Herald — Extra* (n.d.), from a copy in the C. Burton Clark Collection; James White (ed.), *Brother Miller's Dream* (Oswego, N.Y.: James White, 1850), from a copy in LLU-HR. James White's account of Miller's dream also appeared in *Present Truth*, I (May, 1850), 73-75.

25. Rowe, "Thunder and Trumpets," pp. 266-68.

26. J. V. Himes to William Miller, March 12 and March 29, 1845 (Joshua V. Himes Letters, Massachusetts Historical Society). The second woman may have been Sister Durben, who witnessed Ellen's shut-door vision at Exeter in February, 1845.

insisting that he had seen exactly the same things. Ellen took this as an indication that God had chosen her as Foy's replacement.[27]

Closer to home was Ellen's relationship with Hazen Foss, her sister Mary's brother-in-law and the brother of her dear friend Louisa Foss. Shortly before October 22, 1844, Hazen had received a vision similar to Foy's, which the Lord had instructed him to relate to others. However, after the disappointment he became bitter and refused to carry out his duty. If he said anything to his family about his experience, it seems likely that Ellen learned of it by the time she had her first vision; but apparently she did not talk with him until after her third one, when she visited Mary and Samuel Foss in Poland, Maine. In the course of their long conversation Hazen told Ellen the Lord had warned him that the light would be given to someone else if he refused to share it. Upon hearing Ellen's story, he reportedly said to her, "I believe the visions are taken from me, and given to you." He died an atheist.[28]

Physically and conceptually Ellen's early visions closely resembled those of her contemporaries Foy and Foss. The episodes were unpredictable; she might be praying, addressing a large audience, or lying sick in bed, when suddenly and without warning she would be off on "a deep plunge in the glory."[29] Often there were three shouts of "Glory! G-l-o-r-y! G-l-o-r-y!" — the second and third "fainter, but more thrilling than the first, the voice resembling that of one quite a distance from you, and just going out of hearing." Then, unless caught by some alert brother nearby, she slowly sank to the floor in a swoon. After a short time in this deathlike state, new power flowed through her body, and she rose to her feet. On occasion she possessed extraordinary strength, once reportedly holding

---

27. "William Foy: A Statement by E. G. White," from an interview with D. E. Robinson, *circa* 1912 (DF 231, White Estate); William E. Foy, *The Christian Experience of William E. Foy, together with the Two Visions He Received in the Months of January and February, 1842* (Portland: J. and C. H. Pearson, 1845), from a reproduction in the White Estate.

28. EGW to Mary Harmon Foss, December 22, 1890 (F-37-1890, White Estate); EGW, *Life Sketches*, p. 77.

29. James White, *Life Incidents, in Connection with the Great Advent Movement* (Battle Creek: SDA Publishing Assn., 1868), pp. 272-73; EGW, Letter 8, 1851 (White Estate).

an eighteen-pound Teale Bible in her outstretched hand for one-half hour.[30]

During these trances, which came five or ten times a year and lasted from a few minutes to several hours, Ellen frequently described the colorful scenes she was seeing. One eyewitness recalled that

> She often uttered words singly, and sometimes sentences which expressed to those about her the nature of the view she was having, either of heaven or of earth. . . . When beholding Jesus our Saviour, she would exclaim in musical tones, low and sweet, "Lovely, lovely, lovely," many times, always with the greatest affection. . . . Sometimes she would cross her lips with her finger, meaning that she was not at that time to reveal what she saw, but later a message would perhaps go across the continent to save some individual or church from disaster. . . . When the vision was ended, and she lost sight of the heavenly light, as it were, coming back to the earth once more, she would exclaim with a long drawn sigh, as she took her first natural breath, "D-a-r-k." She was then limp and strengthless, and had to be assisted to her chair. . . .[31]

According to the testimony of numerous physicians and curiosity seekers, her vital functions slowed alarmingly, with her heart beating sluggishly and respiration becoming imperceptible. Although she was able to move about with complete freedom, not even the strongest men could forcibly budge her limbs. On occasion she was subjected to indignities. For example, her husband, James White, let one young man — later a leading Adventist minister — see if she could survive for ten minutes while he simultaneously pinched her nose and covered her mouth.[32] Many visions left Ellen

---

30. For descriptions of Ellen in vision, see Loughborough, *Great Second Advent Movement*, pp. 204-11; Martha D. Amadon, "Mrs. E. G. White in Vision," November 24, 1925 (DF 105, White Estate); Wellcome, *History of the Second Advent Message*, pp. 397-402. Although Wellcome remembered catching Ellen twice "to save her from falling upon the floor," she could not recall in later years ever being around Wellcome at the time of a vision; EGW to J. N. Loughborough, August 24, 1874 (Letter 2, 1874, White Estate).

31. Amadon, "Mrs. E. G. White in Vision," pp. 1-2.

32. Statement of D. T. Bourdeau, February 4, 1891, quoted in Loughborough, *Great Second Advent Movement*, p. 210. Loughborough (p. 205) noted that Ellen's

in total darkness for short periods, but usually her eyesight returned to normal after a few days.

The cause of her visions was a matter of dispute. Both she and her followers considered them genuine revelations from God, identical in nature to those of the biblical prophets. But skeptics offered various other explanations. Many attributed them to mesmerism, or hypnotism, which her friends attempted to refute by pointing out that "she has a number of times been taken off in vision, when in prayer alone in the grove or in the closet." Some physicians diagnosed her condition as hysteria, an ill-defined disease known sometimes to produce deathlike trances and hallucinations, especially in women. The two Kellogg doctors, Merritt and John, believed she suffered from catalepsy, which, as the latter described it, "is a nervous state allied to hysteria in which sublime visions are usually experienced. The muscles are set in such a way that ordinary tests fail to show any evidence of respiration, but the application of more delicate tests show that there are slight breathing movements sufficient to maintain life. Patients sometimes remain in this condition for several hours."[33]

A special angel always guided Ellen on her heavenly tours, directing her attention to events past and future, celestial and terrestrial. Today her descriptions of the other world might seem somewhat fanciful, but to her literalistic nineteenth-century followers they had the

---

pulse beat regularly during visions, whereas Merritt Kellogg said her pulse beat very infrequently and almost stopped; M. Kellogg to J. H. Kellogg, June 18, 1906 (Kellogg Collection, MSU). Both men witnessed many visions.

33. [Uriah Smith], *The Visions of Mrs. E. G. White: A Manifestation of Spiritual Gifts According to the Scriptures* (Battle Creek: SDA Publishing Assn., 1868); White, *Life Incidents,* p. 273; H. E. Carver, *Mrs. E. G. White's Claims to Divine Inspiration Examined* (2nd ed.; Marion, Iowa: Advent and Sabbath Advocate Press, 1877), pp. 75-76; Dr. W. J. Fairfield to D. M. Canright, December 28, 1887, in Canright, *Life of Mrs. E. G. White, Seventh-day Adventist Prophet: Her False Claims Refuted* (Cincinnati: Standard Publishing Co., 1919), p. 180; Merritt Kellogg to J. H. Kellogg, June 18, 1906; J. H. Kellogg to R. B. Tower, March 3, 1933 (Ballenger-Mote Papers). Canright (p. 181) also quotes Dr. William Russell of the Western Health Reform Institute as writing on July 12, 1869, "that Mrs. White's visions were the result of a diseased organization or condition of the brain or nervous system." According to Carver, Ellen White in 1865 said that Dr. James Caleb Jackson of Dansville, New York, had "pronounced her a subject of Hysteria." On hysteria, see Carroll Smith-Rosenberg, "The Hysterical Woman: Sex Roles and Role Conflict in 19th-Century America," *Social Research,* XXXIX (Winter, 1972), 652-78.

familiar ring of truth. Her verbal portrait of Satan, for example, was not unlike those that had terrified her as a church-going child:

> I was then shown Satan as he was, a happy, exalted angel. Then I was shown him as he now is. He still bears a kingly form. His features are still noble, for he is an angel fallen. But the expression of his countenance is full of anxiety, care, unhappiness, malice, hate, mischief, deceit, and every evil. That brow which was once so noble, I particularly noticed. His forehead commenced from his eyes to recede backward. I saw that he had demeaned himself so long, that every good quality was debased, and every evil trait was developed. His eyes were cunning, sly, and showed great penetration. His frame was large, but the flesh hung loosely about his hands and face. As I beheld him, his chin was resting upon his left hand. He appeared to be in deep thought. A smile was upon his countenance, which made me tremble, it was so full of evil, and Satanic slyness. This smile is the one he wears just before he makes sure of his victim, and as he fastens the victim in his snare, this smile grows horrible.[34]

Not all of Ellen's revelations were accompanied by physical manifestations. She often had dreams at night, especially as she grew older, which she thought were as much inspired as her daytime visions. Naturally some skeptics suspected that her dreams might not be very different from their own, but she assured them that she could tell when her dreams were of divine origin: "the same angel messenger stands by my side instructing me in the visions of the night, as stands beside me instructing me in the visions of the day."[35] Unlike the angel Moroni who appeared to the Mormon prophet Joseph Smith, Ellen's heavenly visitor never seems to have identified himself by name.

The reception of her heavenly messages was only the first step in the line of communication from God to the Advent believers. Either

---

34. EGW, *Spiritual Gifts: The Great Controversy, between Christ and His Angels, and Satan and His Angels* (Battle Creek: James White, 1858), pp. 27-28; cf. EGW, *Life Sketches*, p. 30.

35. Quoted in Arthur L. White, *Ellen G. White: Messenger to the Remnant* (Washington: Review and Herald Publishing Assn., 1969), p. 71.

orally or in writing, these had to be relayed to those for whom they were intended. Ellen steadfastly claimed that in this work she did not rely on her own faulty memory. Whenever a previous revelation was needed, the scenes she might have seen years before would come to her "sharp and clear, like a flash of lightning, bringing to mind distinctly that particular instruction." She professed to be "just as dependent upon the Spirit of the Lord in relating or writing a vision, as in having the vision. It is impossible for me to call up things which have been shown me unless the Lord brings them before me at the time that he is pleased to have me relate or write them." In this way she was able to guarantee that her words of counsel came free from any contaminating earthly influences.[36]

In her second vision, late in 1844, Ellen had been told that part of her work as God's messenger would be to travel among the scattered flock of Millerites, relating what she had seen and heard. The task might be painful at times, but God would see her through the ordeal. Although somewhat shy, Ellen was not embarrassed by her assignment. Religious work was socially acceptable for a young woman, and she was not without personal ambition. Indeed, she feared that her new responsibility might make her proud. But when an angel assured her that the Lord would preserve her humility, she determined to carry out his will. Only one obstacle stood in her way: the need for a traveling companion. Since her childhood accident, her health had never been good. At five feet, two inches, and barely eighty pounds, she was literally skin and bones. Lately an attack of "dropsical consumption" had damaged her lungs and made breathing difficult. Fatigue from long trips on steamboats and railway cars frequently brought on dangerous fainting spells, during which she might remain breathless for minutes. Obviously she could not travel alone, but who would go with her? Robert, her closest brother, was himself too feeble to be of much assistance and seemed to be self-conscious of his sister's gift. Mr. Harmon had too many mouths to feed at home even to consider chaperoning his daughter on her travels.[37]

---

36. EGW, *Spiritual Gifts* (1860), pp. 292-93; EGW, *The Writing and Sending Out of the Testimonies to the Church* (Mountain View, Calif.: Pacific Press, n.d.), p. 24.

37. EGW, *Life Sketches,* pp. 69-72; EGW, *Spiritual Gifts* (1860), p. 30; James and Ellen G. White, *Life Sketches: Ancestry, Early Life, Christian Experience, and Extensive*

Her hopes thus thwarted, Ellen once again sank into depression and wished to die. Then a miracle happened. One evening, while prayer was being offered in her behalf, "a ball of fire" struck her over the heart, knocking her to the floor helpless. As the dark cloud of oppression rolled away, an angel repeated her commission: "Make known to others what I have revealed to you." Ellen now knew that God would somehow find a way.[38]

Her first opportunity to travel came almost providentially a short time later when Samuel Foss, her brother-in-law, offered to take her to visit her sister in Poland, Maine. Thankfully she accepted this chance to give her testimony, despite her inability for the past months to speak above a whisper. Her faith was rewarded. As she related her experience to the small band of Poland Adventists, her voice cleared up perfectly. Soon she was traveling throughout New England — accompanied by her sister Sarah or by Louisa Foss, the sister of Samuel and Hazen — exhorting the disappointed Millerites to hold fast for the Lord was coming soon.[39]

One of Ellen's greatest trials as she went from place to place was the oft-repeated suggestion that her trances were mesmeric in origin. Mesmerism, or animal magnetism, originated in Germany in the 1770s with Dr. Franz Anton Mesmer's "discovery" of an invisible fluid, like electricity, that coursed through the human body. According to Mesmer, obstructions to the flow of this animal magnetism caused disease, which could be cured by the magnetic emanations from another person's hands or eyes. This treatment often put the subject in a deep trance, with unpredictable and sometimes entertaining results. Mesmer's novel therapy attracted little American interest until 1836, when a French medical school dropout named Charles Poyen landed in Portland and began lecturing, with notable success, on the topic. Among his converts was Phineas Parkhurst

---

Labors, of Elder James White, and His Wife, Mrs. Ellen G. White (Battle Creek: SDA Publishing Assn., 1880), p. 238. The career of a prophetess was in some ways similar to that of a spiritualist medium; and, as R. Laurence Moore has recently pointed out, mediumship was "one of the few career opportunities open to women in the nineteenth century." Moore, "The Spiritualist Medium: A Study of Female Professionalism in Victorian America," *American Quarterly,* XXVII (May, 1975), 202.

38. EGW, *Life Sketches,* pp. 70-71.
39. Ibid., pp. 72-73, 77.

Quimby, mentor of Mary Baker Eddy, founder of Christian Science. By the early 1840s traveling mesmerists were a popular attraction throughout New England, and Boston alone claimed "two or three hundred skilful [*sic*] magnetizers."[40]

At times even Ellen was plagued with doubts about the nature of her revelations. Were they possibly the effect of mesmerism or, worse yet, a Satanic delusion? She was somewhat comforted by her discovery that the visions continued even when she retreated to a secluded spot away from any human influence. But the doubts continued to haunt her. One morning as she knelt for family prayers, she felt a vision coming on. For an instant she wondered if this could be a mesmeric force — and was immediately struck dumb. As divine punishment for questioning, she was unable to utter a word for twenty-four hours and had to communicate by means of a pencil and slate. There was a hidden blessing in this experience; to her great delight, she was now able for the first time since her childhood accident to hold a writing instrument without shaking. The next day her speech returned, and never again did Ellen doubt the source of her visions.[41]

Her critics were not so easily silenced. Joseph Turner, with whom she had previously shared her views on the shut door, was among those convinced that mesmerism accounted for her strange behavior. He felt sure that, given the opportunity, he could put her in a mesmeric trance and control her actions. He soon had his chance when Ellen again visited her sister in Poland. While Ellen described what her angel had recently shown her, Turner sat nearby intently staring at her eyes through his spread fingers, hoping in this way to bring her under his hypnotic power. In the midst of her testimony Ellen sensed "a human influence" being exerted against her and remembered God's promise to send a second angel if ever

---

40. Robert Darnton, *Mesmerism and the End of the Enlightenment in France* (Cambridge: Harvard University Press, 1869); Eric T. Carlson, "Charles Poyen Brings Mesmerism to America," *Journal of the History of Medicine and Allied Sciences,* XV (April, 1960), 121-32; Robert Peel, *Mary Baker Eddy: The Years of Discovery* (New York: Holt, Rinehart and Winston, 1966), p. 152. Ellen White regarded mesmerists as "channels for Satan's electric currents"; EGW, "Shall We Consult Spiritualist Physicians?" *Testimonies,* V, 193.

41. EGW, *Life Sketches,* pp. 88-90.

she were in danger of falling under an earthly influence. Raising her arms heavenward, she cried, "Another angel, Father! Another angel!" At once she was freed from Turner's sinister power and went on speaking in peace. Her contemporary Mrs. Eddy was less successful in dealing with malicious animal magnetism — M.A.M. she called it — and repeatedly went to great lengths to protect herself from its influence.[42]

During a trip to eastern Maine in 1845 Ellen struck up a friendship with a twenty-three-year-old Millerite minister named James White, whom she had casually met sometime earlier in Portland. He was six years her senior, but the two young Adventists soon discovered they had much in common. Like Ellen, James came from a large New England family, being the fifth of nine children. He, too, had been a sickly child, with such poor vision that he had been unable to attend school until nineteen years of age. Then in twelve weeks of intensive study at St. Albans Academy he had obtained a teaching certificate.[43]

In September, 1842, after teaching school off and on for a couple of years and spending another seventeen weeks in attendance himself, James White listened to Miller and Himes speak at a camp meeting and soon afterward abandoned the classroom to become a full-time Millerite preacher (with credentials from the Christian Connection, the church of his parents). Borrowing a horse from his father and worn-out saddle and bridle from a minister friend, he set out that first winter "thinly clad, and without money." His assets consisted of a cloth chart illustrating the biblical prophecies, three prepared lectures, a strong voice, and plenty of determination. By April he had traveled hundreds of miles; his horse was ill, his clothes were worn, and he was still penniless. Yet he continued to proclaim the Millerite message, displaying the perseverance and fortitude that would serve him so well during the formative years of the Seventh-day Adventist church. Though apparently successful as a

---

42. EGW, *Spiritual Gifts* (1860), pp. 52, 62-63; Edwin Franden Dakin, *Mrs. Eddy: The Biography of a Virginal Mind* (New York: Charles Scribner's Sons, 1929), pp. 131-32, 159-60.

43. "James Springer White," *Seventh-day Adventist Encyclopedia*, pp. 1419-20.

A Prophetess Is Born

Millerite evangelist, young White never occupied a prominent or influential position in the movement.[44]

It did not take James long to become a firm believer in Ellen's supernatural powers — or to see the dangers of her traveling unescorted. Several times during her early ministry, warrants had been issued for her arrest, and hostile groups occasionally threatened her. As James saw it, it was "his duty" to accompany Ellen on her visits to the widely scattered Adventists of New England. Mrs. Harmon, however, saw it differently. When she got wind of the arrangement, she immediately ordered her daughter home in hopes of sparing her reputation. But James and Ellen were not to be separated, and before long they were back on the road with their friends, contacting the faithful in Maine, Vermont, and New Hampshire. With Christ coming in such a short time — possible dates were still being suggested — marriage seemed out of the question. James looked upon the idea as "a wile of the Devil" and warned another couple contemplating such a move that they would be denying their faith in the Second Coming. Unfortunately, some people misunderstood the innocent relationship between James and Ellen, and ugly rumors began to circulate. It was clear, said James to Ellen one day, that "something had got to be done." So on August 30, 1846, they set their reservations aside and presented themselves before a Portland justice of the peace to become man and wife.[45]

Married life for the newlyweds was far from glamorous. Since James's ministry did not provide him with a steady income, the nearly destitute couple was forced to move in with the Harmons, who had returned to Gorham. Here the Whites set up headquarters for about a year, until after the birth of their first child, Henry, in August, 1847. About this time an Adventist family from Topsham, Maine, the Stockbridge Howlands, took pity on the struggling young prophetess and her husband and invited them to occupy a rent-free

---

44. Ibid.; White, *Life Incidents*, pp. 25, 72-75, 96.
45. James and Ellen G. White, *Life Sketches* (1880), p. 238; Ron Graybill, "The Courtship of Ellen Harmon," *Insight*, January 23, 1973, pp. 4-7. On the warrants for Ellen's arrest, see Otis Nichols to William Miller, April 12, 1846 (Miller Papers). A few years later James White condoned disfellowshipping an Adventist couple for "traveling together to teach the third angel's message"; "Withdrawal of Fellowship," *R&H*, IV (July 7, 1853), 32.

room upstairs in their home. The Whites gratefully accepted the offer and with borrowed furniture set up housekeeping in Topsham. James put in long hours hauling rock or chopping cordwood at fifty cents a day, and with assistance from the Howlands he managed to keep food on the table. These trials and tribulations were heaven sent, the Lord explained to Ellen, to keep them from settling down to a life of ease.[46]

Before little Henry reached his first birthday, his parents reluctantly decided to leave him with friends and become itinerant preachers. The separation nearly broke Ellen's heart, but she vowed not to let her motherly affection keep her "from the path of duty." For four years, from 1848 to 1852, the Whites crisscrossed New England and New York, preaching their "sabbath and shut-door" message and living from hand to mouth on the meager contributions of their Adventist supporters. For lack of money, they "traveled on foot, in second-class cars, or on steamboat decks." The arrival of their second son, James Edson, in the summer of 1849 brought only a brief interruption to their nomadic life. He, too, was left while still a baby with a kind Millerite sister in Oswego, New York.[47]

No doubt encouraged by the more literate James, Ellen began in 1846 to publish her visions. Already one of her revelations had appeared unexpectedly in a Cincinnati paper, the *Day-Star,* edited by Enoch Jacobs, who later led a small group of Millerite defectors into a Shaker commune. Ellen had written him a private letter describing her first vision, which to her surprise he had published. It was apparent that the only way to control what got printed was for the Whites to do it themselves. So as they traveled about the country, Ellen would write out as best she could what she had seen, and then James would carefully go through the manuscript, correcting grammar and polishing style, until it came up to his standards for publication. Some critics suspected James contributed more than his editorial talents to the production of Ellen's testimonies, but she always insisted that only God influenced the content. By 1851 the

---

46. EGW, *Life Sketches,* pp. 105-6.
47. Ibid., pp. 110-41; White, *Life Incidents,* p. 292; James White to Brother and Sister Hastings, August 26, 1848, and October 2, 1848 (White Estate). The Whites possibly abandoned the shut-door doctrine shortly before 1852.

Whites had turned out three broadsides and a small pamphlet and had launched a succession of periodicals culminating in the *Advent Review and Sabbath Herald*.[48]

The year 1851 — seven years after the Great Disappointment — had special meaning for the sabbatarians. For some time Joseph Bates had been suggesting that this might be the year of their Savior's return. Early in 1849 Ellen had warned against thinking that time might "continue for a few years more," and in June of the following year her angel informed her that "Time is almost finished." The doctrines she and James had thoughtfully studied out over the past several years would now have to be learned by others "in a few months." But again Christ did not appear. Surely the Whites, who had sacrificed so much, could not be blamed for his delay. In Ellen's mind the responsibility rested squarely on the shoulders of those Millerites who, at the Albany Conference of 1845, failed to endorse the seventh-day Sabbath and visions like her own.[49]

By 1851 the Whites had abandoned much of their shut-door doctrine. They would still grant no opportunity for salvation to those who had heard and rejected the 1844 message, but they allowed the door might be cracked sufficiently to permit the entrance of children, Millerites who were willing to accept the seventh-day Sabbath, and a few other honest-hearted souls who had not rejected the October 22 message. The problem was what to do with all of Ellen's inspired testimonies indicating the door of mercy had been shut. In an attempt to take care of this embarrassment, she and James col-

---

48. Arthur, "Come Out of Babylon," p. 142; EGW, *Writing and Sending Out of the Testimonies*, p. 4; EGW, "The Testimonies Slighted," *Testimonies*, V, 63-64. For a virtually complete EGW bibliography, see Nichol, *Ellen G. White and Her Critics*, pp. 691-703.

49. EGW, "To Those Who Are Receiving the Seal of the Living God" (broadside dated January 31, 1849, Topsham, Maine), from a copy in LLU-HR; EGW, *Early Writings* (Washington: Review and Herald Publishing Assn., 1945), pp. 64-67; EGW, MS 4, 1883, quoted in A. L. White, *Ellen G. White*, p. 32. Bates's prediction of the Second Coming in 1851 is found in his *Explanation of the Typical and Anti-Typical Sanctuary* (New Bedford, Mass.: Benjamin Lindsey, 1850), p. 10. The meager evidence available suggests that Ellen privately accepted Bates's view but gave it up no later than June, 1851, when she spoke out against setting dates for the return of Christ. See the testimony of her nephew R. E. Belden to W. A. Colcord, October 17, 1929 (Ballenger-Mote Papers); and A. L. White, *Ellen G. White*, pp. 41-43.

lected her early writings, systematically deleted passages that might be construed as supporting the shut door, and published the edited version as Ellen's first book, *A Sketch of the Christian Experience and Views of Ellen G. White* (1851). From then on the Whites publicly denied that Ellen had ever been shown that the door was shut, although James apparently admitted on occasion that perhaps young Ellen had been unduly influenced by shut-door advocates at the time of her first vision.[50]

A crisis over Ellen's visions also developed in 1851. In July she wrote her friends, the Dodges: "The visions trouble many. They [know] not what to make of them." The causes for this dissatisfaction are complex. Among the sabbatarian Adventists, some were doubtless puzzled by her changing stand on the shut door, while others resented her habit of publishing private testimonies revealing their secret sins — and names. Nonbelievers frequently charged that the visions were being elevated above the Bible. This criticism particularly galled James. In an effort to keep the visions as inconspicuous as possible, he decided in the summer of 1851 not to print his wife's testimonies in the widely distributed *Review and Herald*. In the future her prophetic writings were to be confined to an "Extra," for limited circulation among "those who believe that God can fulfill his word and give visions *'in the last days.'"* The "Extras" were scheduled for every two weeks, but only one issue ever appeared. For the next four years Ellen White lived in virtual exile among her own people, being allowed to publish only seven *Review and Herald* articles, none relating a vision. Most of these brief communications admonished readers to shun worldliness in dress, speech, and action.[51]

---

50. [James White], "Reply to Bro. Trueldell," *R&H*, I (April 7, 1851), 64. A complete list of the deleted passages from the early visions is found in Nichol, *Ellen G. White and Her Critics*, pp. 619-43. James White's admission is reported in H. E. Carver, *Mrs. E. G. White's Claims to Divine Inspiration Examined* (2nd ed.; Marion, Iowa: Advent and Sabbath Advocate Press, 1877), pp. 10-11. A different view of the White-Carver conversation is given in J. N. Loughborough, "Response," *R&H*, XXVIII (September 25, 1866), 133-34.

51. EGW to Brother and Sister Dodge, July 21, 1851 (D-4-1851, White Estate); EGW, *Spiritual Gifts* (1860), p. 294; *Second Advent Review and Sabbath Herald . . . Extra*, II (July 21, 1851), 4. For a typical statement by James White on the independence of his theology from the visions, see "Palsshaw, Mich.," *R&H*, XXIV (August 23, 1864), 100. Mrs. White's seven articles appeared in the following issues of the *R&H:* III

A Prophetess Is Born

Her visions unappreciated, Ellen White again grew discouraged. The divine revelations came less and less frequently, until she feared her gift was gone. Since her public ministry had depended almost entirely on the visions, she now resigned herself simply to being a Christian wife and mother, a role to which she always attached great significance. James provided little or no encouragement. Over the years he had become increasingly resentful of accusations that he had made his wife's visions a "test" among the Advent Sabbathkeepers and that his *Review and Herald* promoted her views. Finally, in October, 1855, he exploded. "What has the REVIEW to do with Mrs. W.'s views?" he asked angrily. "The sentiments published in its columns are all drawn from the Holy Scriptures. No writer of the REVIEW has ever referred to them as authority on any point. The REVIEW for five years has not published one of them. Its motto has been, 'The Bible, and the Bible alone, the only rule of faith and duty.'" It was nobody's business, he went on, whether or not he accepted his wife's testimonies.[52]

The same issue of the *Review and Herald* containing this outburst also announced that a group of Battle Creek Adventists were taking over publication of the paper, ostensibly because James White's heavy responsibilities had broken his constitution. In recent months he had come to fear that his editorial burdens were threatening his health, and he had publicly expressed a desire to relinquish his position. He especially wanted to free himself from the "whinning complaints" of critics who were writing "poisonous letters" against him. The content of these letters is unknown, but they probably criticized him for his attitude toward the visions. We do know that a short time later he was asked in the *Review and Herald* to apologize for his low estimate of his wife's gift.[53]

(June 10, 1852), 21; III (February 17, 1853), 155-56; III (April 14, 1853), 192; IV (August 11, 1853), 53; V (July 25, 1854), 197; VI (September 19, 1854), 45-46; VI (June 12, 1855), 246. Her April 14, 1853, note, in which she compares herself with the writers of the Bible, corrects an error regarding one of her visions.

52. EGW, "Communication from Sister White," *R&H,* VII (January 10, 1856), 118; J[ames] W[hite], "A Test," *R&H,* VII (October 16, 1855), 61-62.

53. "To the Church of God," *R&H,* VII (October 16, 1855), 60; J[ames] W[hite], "The Cause," *R&H,* VII (August 7, 1855), 20; Hiram Bingham to James White, *R&H,* VII (February 14, 1856), 158.

With Ellen White in the shadows during the early 1850s, the sabbatarian Adventists had not prospered; and her husband's outspokenness made him a likely scapegoat. At a general meeting of sabbatarian leaders in November, 1855, his colleagues replaced him with a twenty-three-year-old convert, Uriah Smith. Then a committee of elders went before the assembly and sorrowfully confessed the church's unfaithfulness in ignoring God's chosen messenger. They made a special point of repudiating James's position on the vision: "To say they are of God, and yet we will not be tested by them, is to say that God's will is not a test or rule for Christians, which is inconsistent and absurd." One of Smith's first acts as the new editor was to reopen the journal's pages to Mrs. White, who happily predicted that God would now smile on the church and "graciously and mercifully revive the gifts." Her humiliation was over; her prophetic role, now secure.[54]

The lessons of this experience were not lost on Ellen White, who was now emerging as the dominant force among the sabbatarians. In the future the mere threat of divine displeasure helped to sustain her influence. "I saw that God would soon remove all light given through visions unless they were appreciated," she warned the Roosevelt, New York, church in 1861.[55] Through the remainder of Ellen's life Adventist leaders coveted her approval and submitted, in public at least, to the authority of her testimonies. Despite her occasional inconsistency and insensitivity, most members clung to the belief that she represented a divine channel of communication. To them, dramatic visions, supernatural healings, and revelations of secret sins were persuasive evidences of a true prophet.

Domestic life for the Whites was scarcely more tranquil than their public life. In April, 1852, the impoverished couple, worn out by years on the road, settled down to a semipermanent home in Rochester, New York, a popular "way station for westward migrants." With the opening of the Erie Canal in the 1820s, thousands of families like the Whites moved into Rochester, stayed for a short

54. "Business Proceedings of the Conference at Battle Creek, Mich.," *R&H,* VII (December 4, 1855), 76; Joseph Bates, J. H. Waggoner, and M. E. Cornell, "Address," ibid., 78-79; EGW, "Communication from Sister White," p. 118.

55. EGW to the Church in Roosevelt and Vicinity, August 3, 1861 (R-16a-1861, White Estate).

time, and then pushed on toward the West. Here, in an old rented house, James and Ellen collected their children about them and set up headquarters for their fledgling church. There were no luxuries. One room housed the press; the others were furnished with pieces of junk Ellen repaired. Food was cheap and simple — turnips instead of potatoes, sauce in place of butter.[56]

In August, 1854, Ellen's responsibilities increased with the birth of her third child, Willie. After the years of separation she was thankful to be with her children, but their occasional misdeeds caused her so much anxiety her health suffered. For over three years the Whites "toiled on in Rochester through much perplexity and discouragement," receiving little help or sympathy from their erstwhile friends in upstate New York. Their cause was not prospering, but the bills continued to mount. At times James seemed near death, and Ellen feared he might leave her with three children to raise and a debt of two or three thousand dollars. Two visits to Michigan convinced them there were greener pastures to the West; so in the fall of 1855 they shipped press and belongings around Lake Erie to the little town of Battle Creek, thus ending what Ellen called their "captivity." The years of struggle now lay largely in the past; days of fulfillment were just ahead.[57]

---

56. EGW, *Spiritual Gifts* (1860), pp. 160-61; Blake McKelvey, *Rochester: The Water-Power City, 1821-1854* (Cambridge: Harvard University Press, 1945), pp. 163, 334.

57. EGW, *Spiritual Gifts* (1860), pp. 165, 192-203; James and Ellen White, *Life Sketches* (1880), pp. 323-24; EGW, *Life Sketches*, p. 157; *Defense of Eld. James White and Wife: Vindication of Their Moral and Christian Character* (Battle Creek: SDA Publishing Assn., 1870), p. 4.

CHAPTER TWO

In Sickness and in Health

"If any among us are sick, let us not dishonor God by applying to earthly physicians, but apply to the God of Israel. If we follow his directions (James 5:14, 15) the sick will be healed. God's promise cannot fail. Have faith in God, and trust wholly in him."

Ellen G. White[1]

Through the years of uncertainty and hardship one constant in Ellen White's life was poor health. From childhood to middle age she enjoyed few periods without some physical or mental suffering. The story of her life fairly abounds with one sickness after another. She began her public ministry in 1844 with shattered nerves and broken body, "and to all appearance had but a short time to live." Her lungs were racked with consumption, her throat so sore she could barely speak above a whisper. On her extended travels through New England she frequently fainted and remained breathless "several minutes." Her mind on one occasion wandered aimlessly for two weeks. Accidents added to her misery; on one excursion to New Hampshire she fell from the wagon and injured her side so badly she had to be carried into the house that night.[2]

---

1. EGW, "To Those Who Are Receiving the Seal of the Living God" (broadside dated January 31, 1849, Topsham, Maine). From a copy in LLU-HR.
2. EGW, *Life Sketches of Ellen G. White* (Mountain View, Calif.: Pacific Press,

In Sickness and in Health

On several occasions seemingly miraculous healings saved her from imminent death. Not long after her marriage to James in 1846 she became so violently ill for three weeks that "every breath came with a groan." While she hovered between this world and the next, her friends gathered around her bed to pray for divine healing. As one young man, Henry Nichols, pleaded with God on her behalf, a supernatural power seemed to possess him. Ellen described what happened next: He "rose from his knees, came across the room, and laid his hands upon my head, saying, 'Sister Ellen, Jesus Christ maketh thee whole,' and fell back prostrated by the power of God." The following day, while solicitous neighbors inquired about her funeral, she rode thirty-eight miles through a storm to Topsham.[3]

During a visit to New York City in the summer of 1848 Ellen's cough grew so serious she knew she "must have relief, or sink beneath disease." For weeks she had not slept peacefully through a single night. In desperation she remembered the biblical instructions found in the fifth chapter of James: "Is one of you ill? He should send for the elders of the congregation to pray over him and anoint him with oil in the name of the Lord. The prayer offered in faith will save the sick man, the Lord will raise him from his bed, and any sins he may have committed will be forgiven." In accordance with these directions, she called in some Adventist brethren and asked for anointing and prayer. The next morning her cough was gone — and did not return until the end of her journey.[4]

With divine help so readily available, Ellen saw no reason to resort to physicians. In the concluding paragraph to an 1849 broadside "To Those Who Are Receiving the Seal of the Living God," she counseled her readers not to seek medical assistance:

> If any among us are sick, let us not dishonor God by applying to earthly physicians, but apply to the God of Israel. If we follow his directions (James 5:14, 15) the sick will be healed. God's

---

1915), pp. 69-73; James and Ellen G. White, *Life Sketches: Ancestry, Early Life, Christian Experience, and Extensive Labors, of Elder James White, and His Wife, Mrs. Ellen G. White* (Battle Creek: SDA Publishing Assn., 1880), p. 238; EGW, *Spiritual Gifts: My Christian Experience, Views and Labors* (Battle Creek: James White, 1860), pp. 48, 51.

3. EGW, *Spiritual Gifts* (1860), pp. 84-85.
4. Ibid., p. 97; James 5:14, 15 (NEB).

promise cannot fail. Have faith in God, and trust wholly in him, that when Christ who is our life shall appear we may appear with him in glory.[5]

Given the low state of the medical arts at the time, her advice probably did little harm. But it was not the poor quality of medical care that prompted her to write what she did; she simply believed it was a denial of faith and a dishonor to God to go to physicians when God's promise was so explicit.

For at least a few years Ellen White had nothing to do with physicians of any persuasion, regular or irregular. In times of sickness, which were frequent, she trustingly placed her life and the lives of her children in the hands of God. Once, during a temporary stay in Centerport, New York, little Edson became so gravely ill that he fell unconscious and the "death dampness" appeared on his brow. Prayers were offered, but with little apparent effect. His mother grew increasingly concerned. Her greatest fear was not that her baby might die — if that were the Lord's will — but that her enemies would taunt her with cries of "Where is their God?" At last she said to James, "There is but one thing more that we can do, that is to follow the Bible rule, call for the elders." Unfortunately, the only available elder (besides James) had just departed for Port Gibson on the Erie Canal. Undaunted, Ellen sent her husband racing down the towpath five miles to catch him. The good brother willingly got off the boat, returned to the house, and anointed Edson, who responded by regaining consciousness. His thankful mother reported that "A light shone upon his features, and the blessing of God rested upon us all."[6]

Relying on prayer instead of physicians became common practice among sabbatarian Adventists of the early 1850s. In 1853 Anna White, who assisted her brother James in editing the *Youth's Instructor,* wrote: "I am now living with a people who believe that God is able and willing to heal the sick now, and who when sick, apply nowhere else for aid." The experience of L. V. Masten, a non-Adventist hired by James White to take charge of printing the *Re-*

---

5. EGW, "To Those Who Are Receiving the Seal of the Living God."
6. EGW, *Spiritual Gifts* (1860), pp. 136-37.

view and Herald, illustrates this characteristic. In the summer of 1852 he was dying from cholera under the care of a regular physician when the Whites rescued him and took him into their own home. There he vowed to become an Adventist if God would heal him. He discharged his doctor and "held fast the arm of God and the faith of Jesus." Recovery soon followed. In relating his experience in the *Review and Herald,* Masten noted the large number of Sabbath-keepers who had "already been snatched from the jaws of death, and in a very short time restored to perfect health, by no other means than by the prayer of faith!" With great passion he urged his new brethren and sisters to have complete faith in God's healing power and to shun even roots and herbs when ill.[7]

In condemning the use of simple botanic remedies, Masten was going to a greater extreme than Ellen White, though there were times when she refused to administer any medication at all. When her first child, Henry, became very sick as a baby, friends recommended Townsend's sarsaparilla, a popular patent medicine. Ellen retired to her room alone and asked for divine guidance. In a vision the Lord showed her that no earthly medicine could save her little boy; so she "decided to venture the life of the child upon the promise of God." When James entered the room and asked if he should send a man for the sarsaparilla, she replied: "No. Tell him we will try the strength of God's promises." That evening Henry was anointed, and the next day he was up on his feet.[8]

Many times during her early public career Ellen White was blessed with the power to heal. Often members of her family were the beneficiaries of her gift. Both her husband, James, and her son Edson, for example, recovered from some form of "cholera" after Ellen had laid her hands on their heads and rebuked the disease in the name of Jesus. But perhaps her most satisfying miracle was the spectacular healing of her ailing mother. In late September, 1849, Mrs. Harmon accidentally ran a rusty nail through her foot and de-

---

7. Anna White to Brother and Sister Tenny, March 6, 1853 (White Estate); L. V. Masten, "Experience of Bro. Masten," *R&H,* III (September 30, 1852), 86; "Communication from Bro. Masten," *R&H,* III (November 25, 1852), 108; Masten, "Faith," *R&H,* IV (October 4, 1853), 101. On March 1, 1854, Masten died of consumption at about twenty-five years of age; "Obituary," *R&H,* V (March 14, 1854), 63.

8. EGW, *Spiritual Gifts* (1860), pp. 104-6.

veloped a nasty wound. The limb swelled frighteningly and lockjaw seemed certain. Upon hearing of the mishap, Ellen hastened to her mother's side. There, she wrote, "With the Spirit of the Lord resting upon me, I bid her in the name of the Lord rise and walk. His power was in the room, and shouts of praise went up to God. Mother arose and walked the room declaring the work was done, all the soreness gone, and that she was entirely relieved from pain."[9]

Sometime in the early 1850s Ellen's attitude toward physicians underwent a marked change. The first indication of a move toward a more moderate position came in 1851 with the publication of her first book, *Experience and Views,* which brought together her earlier writings. Deleted, along with the embarrassing shut-door passages, was the admonition from her 1849 broadside never to apply to earthly physicians. No explanation was given.[10]

A few years later a tragic incident in Camden, New York, led Ellen White publicly to repudiate her former stand. It seems that a devout Adventist from that town, Sister Prior, had been allowed to die without receiving medical aid of any kind. Immediately rumors began circulating that responsibility for the death lay with Mrs. White, who was known to have counseled against going to doctors of medicine. When word of the incident reached the prophetess, she vehemently protested that she could not possibly be accountable for the sister's death since at the time in question she had been in Rochester, over a hundred miles away. On her next visit to Camden she received a vision, indicating that poor judgment had been used in not obtaining medical help for Sister Prior. "I saw," she said, "that they [the Adventists attending the sister] had carried matters to extremes, and that the cause of God was wounded and our faith reproached, on account of such things, which were fanatical in the extreme."[11]

In 1860, in the second volume of her *Spiritual Gifts,* Ellen White carefully articulated her new posture on medical care:

---

9. Ibid., pp. 138, 117-18, 165-66. Other instances of healing are scattered throughout this volume.

10. To my knowledge, the 1849 statement has never been reprinted in any of EGW's works.

11. Ibid., p. 134. The date of Sister Prior's death is uncertain, but circumstantial evidence suggests sometime in 1853 or 1854.

In Sickness and in Health

> We believe in the prayer of faith; but some have carried this matter too far, especially those who have been affected with fanaticism. Some have taken the strong ground that it was wrong to use simple remedies. We have never taken this position, but have opposed it. We believe it to be perfectly right to use the remedies God has placed in our reach, and if these fail, apply to the great Physician, and in some cases the counsel of an earthly physician is very necessary. This position we have always held.[12]

In view of her counsel just eleven years earlier, the last sentence of this statement is puzzling.

Indicative of Ellen White's changing attitude was her visit to an itinerant doctor in early 1854, apparently her first consultation with a physician since childhood. Throughout the previous winter she had suffered miserably from a variety of complaints: heart problems, inability to breathe while lying down, recurrent fainting spells, and a cancerlike inflammation on her left eyelid. The pain was so intense she had not experienced "one joyful feeling" for months. When a "celebrated physician" came to Rochester offering free examinations, she set aside her reservations and went to see him. The doctor was most discouraging; in three weeks, he predicted, she would suffer paralysis and then apoplexy. His prognosis was not far off the mark. In about three weeks she fainted and was unconscious for a day and a half. A week later an apparent stroke left the left side of her body paralyzed, her head cold and numb, and her speech impaired. She thought this time she would surely die, but after a fervent season of prayer one night, she awoke the next morning free from pain and paralysis. Her physician, upon seeing her, could only exclaim: "Her case is a mystery. I do not understand it."[13]

---

12. Ibid., p. 135.
13. Ibid., pp. 184-88. In a letter to Mrs. C. W. Sperry, September 26, 1861, Ellen White reports having placed Edson, afflicted with dysentery, under a doctor's care (S-8-1861, White Estate). The "celebrated physician" was probably a quack "cancer doctor" or some other "specialist"; see Edward C. Atwater, "The Medical Profession in a New Society: Rochester, New York (1811-60)," *Bulletin of the History of Medicine*, XLVII (May-June, 1973), 228. It seems unlikely that Mrs. White suffered a real stroke, as we understand the term today. Nineteenth-century physicians probably would have attributed her symptoms to hysteria.

Despite Ellen White's softening attitude toward physicians, the leading sabbatarian Adventists continued for many years to shun the medical profession.[14] Their preference for prayer over medicine is more understandable if we bear in mind that many of them — including the Whites — regarded illness as sometimes satanic in origin. For instance, when Mrs. White in the spring of 1858 suffered her third "stroke" shortly after receiving a vision on the "great controversy between Christ and his angels and Satan and his angels," she was shown that Satan had tried to take her life to prevent her from writing out what she had seen about him. Against such diabolical attacks, prayer was obviously more efficacious than any medicine.[15]

Like so many women reformers in America, Ellen White was an enthusiastic advocate of temperance and healthful living — and with good reason. Both at home and abroad Americans were notorious for their hard drinking. Cider flowed as freely as water, and every farmer was at liberty to distill his own spirits. "While the means of intoxication were so abundant," observed one critic, "the gregarious and social habits of the people tended to foster drunkenness." In response to this problem, a growing number of Americans joined local and national societies to promote temperance either by persuasion or by legislation. Among the most successful and colorful of such organizations was the Washingtonian Temperance Society, created in 1840 by six reformed drinkers in Baltimore. In cities and towns across the country Washingtonian orators "mounted upturned rum-kegs from which vantage point they related their numerous experiences with the demon, rum." Their ap-

14. Evidence of this practice can be readily found in both Ellen's writings and the pages of the *Review and Herald*. See, for example, EGW, *Spiritual Gifts* (1860), pp. 206-7; EGW, "Communication from Sister White," *R&H*, VII (January 10, 1856), 118; and Joseph Bates, "Obituary," *R&H*, XII (September 2, 1858), 127. By the early 1860s many Battle Creek Adventists were patronizing a woman physician, Miss M. N. Purple; "Remarkable Answer to Prayer," *R&H*, XIX (April 22, 1862), 164.

15. EGW, *Spiritual Gifts* (1860), pp. 271-72. Ellen's vision was first published as *Spiritual Gifts: The Great Controversy, between Christ and His Angels, and Satan and His Angels* (Battle Creek: James White, 1858). Just a few months earlier a "first-day" Adventist from Rochester, H. L. Hastings, had published a similar volume entitled *The Great Controversy between God and Man, Its Origin, Progress, and End* (Rochester: H. L. Hastings, 1858).

proach proved effective; within a few years hundreds of thousands of well-intentioned drinkers had signed the Washingtonian total abstinence pledge.[16]

Given her background, Ellen White could scarcely have avoided joining the temperance crusade. Her home town of Portland, an import center for West Indian rum, was a hotbed of reform activity; Elizabeth Oakes Smith once called it a "pet City to the divine eye." During Ellen's childhood, the indefatigable Neal Dow kept the city astir with his campaign against "Demon Rum," which culminated in 1851 in the passage of the Maine Liquor Law, the first of many statewide prohibition laws in America. Her church, the Methodist, was likewise swept up in the temperance movement. By the 1840s no "good" Methodist would touch a drop of alcohol, and the very pious had left off tobacco as well. Young Ellen would no more have taken a drink or a smoke than she would have uttered a word of profanity.[17]

The Millerite movement exemplified the natural affinity between revivalism and temperance in nineteenth-century America. Father Miller, who saw the hand of the Lord in the temperance societies springing up around the country, warned the expectant saints that those who drank would be "wholly unprepared" for the Second Coming. Among his followers were reformers of every stripe, including many temperance enthusiasts. As a young Millerite preacher, James White never touched alcohol, tobacco, tea, or coffee, and a Cincinnati believer went even further by adding flesh foods to the list of forbidden articles.[18]

---

16. John Allen Krout, *The Origins of Prohibition* (New York: Alfred A. Knopf, 1925), pp. 98, 182-85; Thomas L. Nichols, *Forty Years of American Life* (London: John Maxwell and Co., 1864), I, 86-87; Gilbert Seldes, *The Stammering Century* (New York: Harper & Row, 1965), p. 279.

17. Elizabeth Oakes Smith, MS Autobiography (New York Public Library), quoted in Andrew Sinclair, *The Emancipation of the American Woman* (New York: Harper and Row, 1966), p. xiii; Frank L. Byrne, *Prophet of Prohibition: Neal Dow and His Crusade* (Madison: State Historical Society of Wisconsin, 1961); Richard M. Cameron, *Methodism and Society in Historical Perspective* (Nashville: Abingdon Press, 1961), pp. 131-39.

18. Krout, *Origins of Prohibition*, pp. 103-4; William Miller, *Evidence from Scripture and History of the Second Coming of Christ, about the Year 1843* (Boston: Joshua V. Himes, 1842), p. 247; *Cincinnati Gazette*, November 15, 1844, quoted in Everett N. Dick, "William Miller and the Advent Crisis, 1831-1844" (Ph.D. diss., Uni-

One of the most committed Millerite advocates of temperance and dietetic reform was Captain Joseph Bates, who later united with the Whites in founding the Seventh-day Adventist Church. In 1821, while returning from a voyage to South America, he resolved never again to drink a glass of ardent spirits. Over the next few years he swore off wine, then tobacco, and finally even beer and cider. In 1827 during a visit to his home in Fairhaven, Massachusetts, he was caught up in a local revival and joined the Christian church. The day of his baptism he proposed the formation of a temperance society and before long had twelve or thirteen names on his list of subscribers. On his next, and final, voyage the teetotaling captain announced to his shocked crew that there would be no intoxicating drinks on board and invited them instead to morning and evening prayers. Following his retirement from the sea Bates continued his personal reformation by espousing the cause of Sylvester Graham, a popular health reformer, and laying aside tea and coffee, meat, butter, cheese, greasy foods, and rich pastries. Although he never pushed his peculiar views on his Adventist friends, his healthy life was a constant reminder to those around him of the possible benefits of abstemious living. It seems probable that he was a major factor in leading Ellen White in 1848 to begin speaking out against the use of tobacco, tea, and coffee.[19]

In the fall of 1848 Mrs. White received the first of her many visions on healthful living. According to her husband's testimony twenty-two years later, she was then shown that tobacco, tea, and coffee should be put away by those looking for the Second Coming of Christ. (Apparently alcohol was such an obvious evil, or so little abused, it was not mentioned.)[20] Ellen did not identify this vision

---

versity of Wisconsin, 1932), pp. 257-58; James and Ellen White, *Life Sketches* (1880), p. 15.

19. Joseph Bates, *The Autobiography of Elder Joseph Bates* (Battle Creek: SDA Publishing Assn., 1868), pp. 143, 150, 172, 204-11, 234-35; Bates, "Experience in Health Reform," *HR*, VI (July, 1871), 20-21. See also Godfrey T. Anderson's two recent studies of Bates: *Outrider of the Apocalypse: Life and Times of Joseph Bates* (Mountain View, Calif.: Pacific Press, 1972); and "The Captain Lays Down the Law," *New England Quarterly*, XLIV (June, 1971), 305-9.

20. The drinking habits of Adventists in this period are difficult to determine. John H. Kellogg once recalled that in the early 1860s "some good ministers, saintly

specifically, but presumably she was referring to it when she wrote: "I saw all those who are indulging self by using the filthy weed [tobacco], should lay it aside, and put their means to a better use.... And if all would study to be more economical in their articles of dress, and deprive themselves of some things which are not actually necessary, and lay aside such useless and injurious things as tea, &c., and give what they cost to the cause, they would receive more blessings here, and a reward in heaven." In a private letter to a brother struggling with the tobacco habit Ellen White added that her "accompanying angel" told her that the weed was not to be used even for medicinal purposes, because doing so greatly dishonored God. Although she regarded tobacco and tea as physically harmful, it is significant that in her early years she was clearly much more concerned about the money squandered on such needless items than she was about their possibly injurious effects.[21]

Now that God had spoken, tobacco began disappearing from among the sabbatarian Adventists. In September, 1849, while Bates was roaming the state of Maine seeking out "the scattered sheep," he happily reported that "pipes & Tobacco are travling [sic] out of sight fast I tell you." With the Second Coming so close, it seemed to him that nothing was "to[o] dear or precious to let go in end of the cause now." A couple of months later James White gave a similarly encouraging account of progress in New York. "Tobacco and snuff are being cleared from the camp with few exceptions," he wrote following a conference at Oswego.[22]

Aside from the individual labors of Bates and the Whites, there seems to have been little antitobacco activity among the Adventists in the early 1850s. In fact, little was said about health at all until af-

---

men, kept kegs of ale and beer in their cellars." During these years his own father used both beverages. "The Significance of Our Work," *Medical Missionary,* XIV (March, 1905), 82.

21. James White, "Western Tour: Kansas Camp-Meeting," *R&H,* XXXVI (November 8, 1870), 165; EGW, *Supplement to the Christian Experience and Views of Ellen G. White* (Rochester: James White, 1854), p. 42; EGW to Brother Barnes, December 14, 1851 (B-5-1851, White Estate).

22. Joseph Bates to Brother and Sister Hastings, September 25, 1849 (White Estate); James White to Brother Howland, November 13, 1849, quoted in EGW, *Spiritual Gifts* (1860), p. 119.

ter February, 1854, when Ellen White received a second heavenly message on the subject, notably broader in scope than her first. In words that echoed Sylvester Graham she told of seeing that Sabbath-keepers were making "a god of their bellies," that instead of eating so many rich dishes they should take "more coarse food with little grease." "I saw," she said, "rich food destroyed the health of the bodies and was ruining the constitution, was destroying the mind, and was a great waste of means." It was also brought to her attention that the Sabbath-keepers were not as clean and tidy as God wanted them to be. Uncleanliness was not to be tolerated, and those persisting in their filthy ways were to "be put out of the camp."[23]

The Adventists launched their campaign against tobacco in the summer of 1855 with two lead articles in the *Review and Herald* on "the filthy, health-destroying, God-dishonoring practice of using tobacco."[24] In this way they joined the growing number of antitobacco crusaders who had begun in the 1830s to speak out against the undesirable habits of their fellow citizens. Americans had long been fond of their pipes and snuffboxes, but with the rise of the common man in the Jacksonian era they took to the unsightly but time-saving practice of chewing. The ever-practical American, it was pointed out, "can saw wood, or plow, or hoe corn, at the same time while he is chewing a good 'cud' of tobacco. He can, if need be, plead before a jury, or preach a sermon, while at the same time he holds the precious bolus in one side of his mouth."[25] Tobacco consumption increased in the late 1840s with the popularization of the cigar during the war against Mexico. Now, complained an irritated nonsmoker, from one end of the country to the other there was "one mighty *puff,-puff,-puff.*" Critics began calling attention to the dire consequences — from insanity to cancer — of so much tobacco using and

---

23. EGW, MS dated February 12, 1854 (MS-1-18,54, White Estate). An exception to the general silence on tobacco was a selected article entitled "Tobacco" that appeared in the *Review and Herald,* IV (December 13, 1853), 178.

24. "On the Use of Tobacco," *R&H,* VII (July 24, 1855), 9-10, and (August 7, 1855), 17-18; James White, "The Office," ibid., VII (July 24, 1855), 13.

25. Joel Shew, *Tobacco: Its History, Nature, and Effects on the Body and Mind* (New York: Fowler and Wells, 1850), p. v. On American tobacco habits and the antitobacco crusade, see Joseph C. Robert, *The Story of Tobacco in America* (Chapel Hill: University of North Carolina Press, 1967), pp. 99-104, 107-12.

in 1849, in conscious imitation of the temperance workers, organized the American Anti-Tobacco Society. With the outbreak of the Civil War, however, their movement came to an untimely end.[26]

A few months after the appearance of the *Review and Herald* articles, the editor noted that the subject of tobacco was "engaging the attention of many of our brethren in different places." It had certainly caught the attention of the brethren in Vermont. At a general meeting in Morristown on October 15, 1855, representatives from churches throughout the state voted resolutely to withdraw "the hand of fellowship" from any member who, after being "properly admonished," continued to use tobacco. Upon returning to their home churches, however, they discovered that their enthusiasm for reform was not shared by their fellow members. Consequently, at a statewide conference a year later they rescinded their previous action and in its place unanimously adopted a milder resolution more compatible with the practices of their constituency: "*Resolved,* That the use of Tobacco is a fleshly lust, which wars against the soul; and therefore we will labor in the spirit of meekness, patiently and perseveringly to persuade each brother and sister who indulge in the use of it, to abstain from this evil."[27]

Adventist leaders worked strenuously for years to get their members to break the tobacco habit. Ellen White even wrote personal testimonies on occasion to those shown her in vision as being in special need. The editors of the *Review and Herald* pursued an "uncompromising course" in presenting the evils of tobacco to their readers. They filled their pages with articles by prominent sabbatarian ministers like J. N. Andrews, J. H. Waggoner, and M. E. Cornell, urging the faithful to overcome "this inexcusable worldly lust." Perhaps the most persuasive argument came from the pen of

---

26. Robert, *Story of Tobacco in America,* p. 112; William A. Alcott, "Physiological Effects of Tobacco," *Water-Cure Journal,* IV (November, 1847), 316; "Anti-Tobacco Society," ibid., VII (April, 1849), 120. On the relationship between tobacco and cancer, see Shew, *Tobacco,* p. 50; and "The Smoker's Cancer," *Water-Cure Journal,* XXXIII (May, 1862), 110.

27. Editorial introduction to George Trask, "Popular Poisons," *R&H,* VII (October 16, 1855), 62; Stephen Pierce, "The Use of Tobacco: Doings of the Church in Vermont," ibid., VII (December 4, 1855), 79; Pierce, "Conference in Wolcott, Vt.," ibid., IX (March 5, 1857), 144.

James White, who pointed out the economic advantages of not using tobacco and tea. According to his calculations, if the one thousand Sabbath-keeping families all discarded those two items, ten thousand dollars would be saved annually, enough "to sustain thirty Missionaries in new fields of labor." How shameful it was, he said, that some members too poor to take the *Review and Herald* or to support the ministry nevertheless found sufficient cash to purchase tobacco and tea.[28]

By the late 1850s Adventist ministers no longer smelled of tobacco, and it was impossible for users to obtain a "card of recommendation" licensing them to preach.[29] But among the laity, who could not so easily be controlled, tobacco continued to be a problem for years. In 1858 Elder Cornell wrote of being distressed by "the thought that some among us, who are called *brethren,* after all that has been written on the subject, should still persist in using the infamous weed." Three years later Elder Isaac Sanborn complained of finding tobacco among professed Sabbath-keepers in Wisconsin. And as late as 1867 there were still some members in northern Michigan who had not yet gained the victory.[30]

With the spotlight focused on tobacco, other aspects of health reform tended to get lost in the shadows. Even some of the practices Ellen saw condemned in vision received scant attention. Coffee, which had recently replaced tea as "the American beverage," was

---

28. EGW to Victory Jones, January [?], 1861 (J-1-1861, White Estate); S. Myers, "From Bro. Myers," *R&H,* XII (October 7, 1858), 159; J. N. A[ndrews], "The Use of Tobacco a Sin Against God," ibid., VIII (April 10, 1865), 5; J. H. W[aggoner], "Tobacco," ibid., XI (November 19, 1857), 12-13; M. E. Cornell, "The Tobacco Abomination," ibid., XII (May 20, 1858), 1-2; J[ames] W[hite], "Tobacco and Tea," ibid., VIII (May 1, 1856), 24. On the economics of tobacco using, see also "Arithmetic Applied to Tobacco," ibid., XXI (April 28, 1863), 171.

29. J. N. Loughborough, "Sketches of the Past — No. 107," *Pacific Union Recorder,* X (December 15, 1910), 1-2. Loughborough tells of one candidate for a ministerial card, Gilbert Cranmer, who, upon being turned down for secretly using the weed, left the Adventists and started printing an opposition paper, *The Hope of Israel.*

30. Cornell, "The Tobacco Abomination," p. 1; Isaac Sanborn, "To the Glory of God," *R&H,* XVII (May 14, 1861), 205; George W. Amadon, "Trip to Northern Michigan," ibid., XXX (September 10, 1867), 204. See also EGW to the church at Caledonia, December [?], 1861 (C-12-1861, White Estate); and D. T. Bourdeau, "Tobacco and Tea," *R&H,* XXI (March 17, 1863), 125-26.

seldom mentioned. Tea was definitely frowned upon, but still too widely used to be made a test of fellowship. Often the conscience-smitten rationalized their actions by taking "part of a cup," having it "just colored," or making it "weak." Such laxity about a drink God had specifically forbidden naturally bothered some of the more scrupulous members. In an open letter appearing in the *Review and Herald* in 1863 Elder A. S. Hutchins took his erring brethren and sisters to task for not heeding the light the Lord had given. "Are we ashamed of the position that we as a people and organized churches have taken in regard to the use of this herb?" he asked. "If not let us *live* out our faith, when with tea-drinkers, as well as when with those who drink cold water."[31]

The dietary reforms of the 1854 vision seem to have been wholly ignored. The only serious question relating to food was whether or not, in light of the Old Testament ban against swine's flesh, Sabbath-keepers could properly eat pork, a staple of the American diet. On this issue the Whites stood firmly against the extremists who wanted the church to take a position against eating it. When the problem first arose in the early days of the sabbatarian movement, James wrote in the *Present Truth* that, although too much pork-eating could be harmful, he did "not, by any means, believe that the Bible teaches that its proper use, in the gospel dispensation, is sinful." Referring to the decision of the apostles and elders at Jerusalem not to impose certain Mosaic practices on converted Gentiles (Acts 15), he asked, "Shall we lay a greater 'burden' on the disciples than seemed good to the Holy Ghost, and the holy apostles of our Lord Jesus Christ? God forbid. Their decision, being right, settled the question with them and it should forever settle the question with us."[32]

With some believers, however, the question was far from settled. They failed to see why the church should abide by one part of the Old Testament — the seventh-day Sabbath — and not another. Thus agitation over swine's flesh continued until 1858, when a vision settled

---

31. Richard Osborn Cummings, *The American and His Food: A History of Food Habits in the United States* (rev. ed.; Chicago: University of Chicago Press, 1941), pp. 34-35; A. S. Hutchins, "Let Your Light Shine," *R&H,* XXI (January 13, 1863), 56. See also D. M. Canright, "Tea Poisoned," ibid., XXI (May 12, 1863), 187.

32. [James White], "Swine's Flesh," *Present Truth,* I (November, 1850), 87-88.

the controversy. Ellen White was shown, she said, that while it was all right for individuals to refrain from eating pork, the church should not make a test of it. "If it is the duty of the church to abstain from swine's flesh," she wrote to a couple who were urging the extreme position, "God will discover it to more than two or three."[33] Later, she answered another sister's inquiry about what course to take with the reply that "if it is your husband's wish to use swine's flesh, you should be perfectly free to use it." And to make sure the point got across, James scribbled on the back of the letter: "That you may know how we stand on this question, I would say that we have just put down a two hundred pound porker."[34]

The revival of hoop skirts in the 1850s prompted Ellen White to speak out on still another reform of the day — dress. Since childhood she had associated austere attire with true Christianity, and she wanted her followers to be known by their simplicity of dress. She herself always wore plain, durable clothing, devoid of any "unnecessary bows and ribbons." Hoops she found particularly objectionable. They were not only "ridiculous" and "disgusting" but immoral, having been devised (as she thought) by the prostitutes of Paris as "a screen to iniquity." Sabbathkeepers were to have nothing to do with this godless fashion. *"Do not put on hoops by any means,"* she admonished one minister's wife; "let us preserve the signs which distinguish us in dress, as well as articles of faith."[35]

By the early 1860s the sabbatarian Adventists numbered thirty-five hundred members scattered over the territory east of the Missouri River and north of the Confederacy. Since Christ still had not come, some of the brethren — led by James White — now turned their attention to establishing a church on earth. Resistance to such a move

---

33. EGW, "Errors in Diet," *Testimonies,* I, 205-6, from a letter originally written October 21, 1858.

34. Quoted in H. E. Carver, *Mrs. E. G. White's Claim to Divine Inspiration Examined* (2nd ed.; Marion, Iowa: Advent and Sabbath Advocate Press, 1877), pp. 19-20.

35. Elizabeth McClellan, *History of American Costume: 1607-1870* (New York: Tudor Publishing Co., 1969), p. 466; EGW, "A Question Answered," *Testimonies,* I, 251-52; EGW to Mary Loughborough, June 6, 1861, and June 17, 1861, and EGW to the Church in Roosevelt and Vicinity, August 3, 1861 (L-5-1861, L-6-1861, and R-16a-1861, White Estate).

was great, however, and as a result James grew "desperately discouraged." He and his wife had invested their lives in the Advent movement, and it was difficult for them to take a detached view of things. Ellen explained their feelings in a poignant letter to her friend Lucinda Hall:

> The cause of God is a part of us. Our experience and lives are interwoven with this cause. We have no separate existence. It has been a part of our very being. The believers in present truth have seemed like our children. When the cause of God prospers, we are happy. But when wrongs exist among them, we are unhappy and nothing can make us glad. The earth, its treasures and joys, are nothing to us. Our interest is not here. Is it then strange that my husband with his sensitive feelings should suffer in mind?[36]

The acquisition of church buildings and a publishing house made it imperative to set up some kind of legal entity. Thus the first step toward organization was taken in the fall of 1860 when the leaders met and, over the opposition of those who disliked any compromise with the world, selected a name. Some favored the "Church of God," but the majority finally settled on the less pretentious but more distinctive "Seventh-day Adventists." Three years later delegates from several states met in Battle Creek to complete the organizational process by adopting a constitution, approving general and state conferences, and choosing officers. Unanimously elected as first president of the General Conference was James White, who tactfully declined the appointment to forestall criticism that he had created the new institution for his own political purposes. In his place the delegates selected Elder John Byington, an ardent antislavery man, who had been one of the first in the church to speak out against current trends in ladies' fashions.[37]

Although the early Seventh-day Adventists found the very idea of

---

36. "Development of Organization in SDA Church," *SDA Encyclopedia*, ed. Don F. Neufeld (Washington: Review and Herald Publishing Assn., 1966), p. 935; EGW to Lucinda Hall, April 5, 1860, quoted in Paul Gordon and Ron Graybill, "Letters to Lucinda," *R&H*, CL (August 23, 1973), 6-7.

37. "Development of Organization in SDA Church," pp. 929-35; J. Byington, "Dress," *R&H*, XII (August 5, 1858), 96.

a creed anathema — *"The Bible is our creed,"* they insisted — all members were expected to subscribe to certain doctrines and practices. Among their basic beliefs were the imminent return of Christ, the seventh-day Sabbath, the divine inspiration of Ellen White's visions, the unconscious state of the dead, and the importance of October 22, 1844, as the date on which the "investigative judgment" began in heaven. In addition, good Adventists practiced baptism by immersion, foot-washing, and "systematic benevolence," whereby members were required to give "at the rate of two cents each week upon every one hundred dollars worth of property which they possess," plus weekly donations of twenty-five cents or more. In this way the church was able to support its ministers, who had previously been sustained by gifts or their own labors.[38]

After years of poverty the Whites had settled down to a relatively comfortable life in the west end of Battle Creek, where they purchased an acre-and-a-half plot and built their first home. Battle Creek at midcentury was a village of a few thousand, only a decade or two removed from the wilderness. Its fame in those days before corn flakes and Rice Krispies rested on the flour and woolen mills that occupied much of the downtown area, which still had the appearance of a frontier community. Cows, pigs, and horses roamed at will through the often muddy streets, and garbage was everywhere. Churches and saloons provided for the social needs of the villagers, whose cultural lives were enriched by an occasional lecture on abolition, women's rights, or temperance. The arrival of the railroad and telegraph in the 1840s made Battle Creek an ideal center from which the Adventists could evangelize the West.[39]

Since moving to Michigan, James had held a steady job as president of the Publishing Association and usually doubled his income (seven to ten dollars a week) selling Bibles, concordances, Bible dic-

---

38. James White, *Life incidents, in Connection with the Great Advent Movement* (Battle Creek: SDA Publishing Assn., 1868), pp. 301, 322-36; LeRoy Edwin Froom, *Movement of Destiny* (Washington: Review and Herald Publishing Assn., 1971), pp. 88-89, 138-39. Over the years systematic benevolence evolved into tithing, in which each member contributes one-tenth of his income.

39. "Ellen Gould (Harmon) White," *SDA Encyclopedia*, p. 1408; Ross H. Coller, *Battle Creek's Centennial, 1859-1959* (Battle Creek: Enquirer and News, 1959), pp. 10-65.

tionaries, and Bible atlases on the side. Ellen not only served as wife and mother to a growing family but continued to fill speaking engagements and to write her pamphlets of *Testimonies for the Church,* nine of which had appeared by 1863. Her diary for this period reveals a woman of extraordinary strength and adaptability. At home in Battle Creek she sewed, worked with the children in the garden, and even assisted her husband at the office folding papers or stitching book signatures. She loved her family, yet felt guilty for missing them so much whenever absent. On one trip to northern Michigan she "had a weeping time before the Lord." Her writing, so important to her, often had to be squeezed in while riding the train or visiting in the homes of others.[40]

On September 20, 1860, Ellen White gave birth to her fourth baby boy, John Herbert. The delivery was apparently difficult and left her with a weak back and lame legs, which confined her to the house. She used this time unselfishly to collect clothes for some needy families and once crawled up the stairs on her knees "to get these things together for the poor." Her own suffering was increased when three-month-old Herbert contracted erysipelas and, after weeks of intense pain, passed away. His heartbroken mother was so emotionally spent by this time that she could no longer cry, but fainted at the funeral. Following the burial at Oak Hill Cemetery in Battle Creek she remained disconsolate. "This is a dark, dreary world," she confided to her diary after the death of the Loughboroughs' child that same year. "The whole human family are subject to disease, sorrow, and death."[41]

The Civil War that engulfed the nation during the early 1860s seldom touched the White household directly. Although Ellen was an outspoken abolitionist sympathetic to the Union cause, she counseled the church against active participation in the conflict. As editor of the *Review and Herald,* James reported on the progress of the war but limited his personal involvement to raising bounties for

---

40. *Defense of Elder James White and Wife: Vindication of Their Moral and Christian Character* (Battle Creek: SDA Publishing Assn., 1870), pp. 9-11; EGW, 1859 Diary, quoted in Arthur L. White, *Ellen G. White: Messenger to the Remnant* (Washington: Review and Herald Publishing Assn., 1969), pp. 100-10.

41. EGW, *Spiritual Gifts* (1860), pp. 294-96; EGW to Lucinda Hall, November 2, 1860, quoted in Gordon and Graybill, "Letters to Lucinda," p. 5.

volunteers, securing conscientious objector status for Adventist draftees, and speculating on writing paper and envelopes, which netted him a quick 100 percent profit on an initial investment of twelve hundred dollars.[42]

During the winter of 1862-63 a diphtheria epidemic swept through the country, bringing renewed anxiety to Ellen White for the safety of her remaining three sons. When two of the boys actually came down with sore throats and high fevers, her alarm increased, for medical science seemed so inadequate. Then one day she read an article from the *Yates County Chronicle* (Penn Yan, New York) in which a Dr. James C. Jackson described his highly successful water treatments for curing diphtheria. Hopefully she applied the hydropathic fomentations to her sick boys and met "with perfect success."[43] At last she had stumbled onto a system of medicine that really worked. With the fervor of a convert she began sharing her faith in hydropathy, and to her death she remained one of its staunchest advocates. The following chapter traces the rise and development of the movement she so enthusiastically joined in 1863.

---

42. Roy Branson, "Ellen G. White — Racist or Champion of Equality," *R&H*, CXLVII (April 9, 1970), 3; "War Meeting," *Battle Creek Journal*, October 24, 1862; *Defense of Eld. James White and Wife*, pp. 9-11. On Adventist attitudes toward the Civil War, see Peter Brock, *Pacifism in the United States: From the Colonial Era to the First World War* (Princeton, N.J.: Princeton University Press, 1968), pp. 852-61. Brock sometimes confuses James White with a first-day Adventist preacher named J. S. White.

43. Editorial introduction to James C. Jackson, "Diphtheria, Its Causes, Treatment and Cure," *R&H*, XXI (February 17, 1863), 89. Jackson's essay was later published in pamphlet form as *Diptheria [sic]: Its Causes, Treatment and Cure* (Dansville, N.Y.: Austin, Jackson & Co., 1868).

CHAPTER THREE

The Health Reformers

"The Water-Cure revolution is a *great* revolution. It touches more interests than any revolution since the days of Jesus Christ."

James C. Jackson[1]

For all its apparent vitality, America in the early nineteenth century was a sick and dirty nation. Public sanitation was grossly inadequate, and personal hygiene, virtually nonexistent. The great majority of Americans seldom, if ever, bathed. Their eating habits, including the consumption of gargantuan amounts of meat, were enough to keep most stomachs continually upset. Fruits and green and leafy vegetables seldom appeared on the table, and the food that did appear was often saturated with butter or lard. A "common" breakfast consisted of "Hot bread, made with lard and strong alkalies, and soaked with butter; hot griddle cakes, covered with butter and syrup; meats fried in fat or baked in it; potatoes dripping with grease; ham and eggs fried in grease into a leathery indigestibility — all washed down with many cups of strong Brazil coffee." It is no wonder that one writer called dyspepsia "the great endemic of the northern states."[2]

---

1. James C. Jackson, "Considerations for Common Folks — No. 4," *Water-Cure Journal,* X (September, 1850), 97.
2. Edgar W. Martin, *The Standard of Living in 1860* (Chicago: University of Chicago Press, 1942), pp. 45-46, 74-76; Thomas L. Nichols, *Forty Years of American Life*

When sickness inevitably came, the bleedings and purgings of regular physicians or the self-dosed patent medicines only compounded the misery. Few specific remedies were known, and many drugs in common use did more harm than good. As late as 1860 the distinguished Dr. Oliver Wendell Holmes wrote that "if the whole materia medica, as now used, could be sunk to the bottom of the sea, it would be all the better for mankind, — and all the worse for the fishes."[3]

This unhappy state of affairs gave rise to a growing body of literature on preventive measures aimed at preserving life and health. Some of the most influential early writings were imported from abroad, especially from Scotland: George Cheyne's *The Natural Method of Cureing the Diseases of the Body* (1742), George Combe's *The Constitution of Man* (1828), and his brother Andrew's *The Principle of Physiology Applied to the Preservation of Health* (1834). Inspired in part by these works, American authors joined their foreign colleagues in crying out against the popular dietary and therapeutic abuses. Health journals appeared in Boston and Philadelphia, and books with titles like *Dyspepsy Forestalled & Resisted* (by Professor Edward Hitchcock of Amherst) rolled from the presses. Through all these publications ran a common theme: the importance of a proper (often meatless) diet, plenty of sunshine and fresh air, regular exercise, adequate rest, temperance, cleanliness, and sensible dress.[4]

(London: John Maxwell and Co., 1864), I, 369; "Food," *Boston Medical Intelligencer*, II (1824), 15, quoted in John B. Blake, "Health Reform," in *The Rise of Adventism: Religion and Society in Mid-Nineteenth-Century America*, ed. Edwin S. Gaustad (New York: Harper & Row, 1974), p. 46. On bathing and dietary practices in the United States, see Richard Shryock, "Sylvester Graham and the Popular Health Movement, 1830-1870," in his *Medicine in America: Historical Essays* (Baltimore: Johns Hopkins University Press, 1966), pp. 112-14; and Harold D. Eberlein, "When Society First Took a Bath," *Pennsylvania Magazine of History*, LXVII (January, 1943), 30-48.

3. Oliver Wendell Holmes, *Medical Essays, 1842-1882* (Boston, 1891), p. 203, quoted in John B. Blake, "Mary Gove Nichols, Prophetess of Health," American Philosophical Society, *Proceedings*, CVI (June, 1962), 221.

4. Robert Samuel Fletcher, *A History of Oberlin College: From Its Foundation through the Civil War* (Oberlin: Oberlin College, 1943), 1, 316-17. Chapter XXII of this work is entitled "'Physiological Reform': The Health Movement." Among the earliest health reform periodicals were the *Boston Medical Intelligencer* (1823-28), the

The Health Reformers

These first sporadic attempts at reeducating the American public gave way in the 1830s to a full-blown health crusade led by the egotistical and controversial Sylvester Graham. Like many a health reformer, Graham had suffered through years of repeated illnesses, including a severe nervous collapse at age twenty-nine. By his early thirties he had recovered sufficiently to enter the Presbyterian ministry in New Jersey, where he acquired a reputation as a powerful and successful evangelist, especially when speaking on his favorite subject of temperance. In the summer of 1830 the Pennsylvania Society for Discouraging the Use of Ardent Spirits invited Graham to move to Philadelphia and lecture under its auspices. He accepted and soon was packing large crowds into area churches to hear his scientific and moral arguments against the use of alcohol. Also preaching in Philadelphia was the Reverend William Metcalfe, author of the first American tract on vegetarianism, who had brought his English congregation to this country in 1817 and set up the vegetarian Bible Christian Church. Perhaps influenced by Metcalfe, Graham now began adding the blessings of a meatless diet to his material on temperance. By the late spring of 1831 he had broken with the Pennsylvania Society and was lecturing independently at the Franklin Institute on "the Science of Human Life," a broad spectrum of topics ranging from proper diet to control of the natural passions. His fame spread, and when "an urgent invitation" came from New York, he removed to that city and remained to lecture for an entire year.[5]

The cholera epidemic of 1832 vaulted Graham and his program of health reform into the national spotlight. Several months before the disease reached the shores of North America, he revealed to a New York audience, estimated at two thousand, an almost sure way to ward off an attack: by abstaining "from flesh-meat and flesh soups, and from all alcoholic and narcotic liquors and substances,

---

Journal of Health (Philadelphia, 1829-33), and the *Moral Reformer,* renamed the *Library of Health* in 1837 (Boston, 1835-43).

5. Mildred V. Naylor, "Sylvester Graham, 1794-1851," *Annals of Medical History,* 3rd ser., IV (May, 1942), 236-40; Stephen W. Nissenbaum, "Careful Love: Sylvester Graham and the Emergence of Victorian Sexual Theory in America, 1830-1840" (Ph.D. diss., University of Wisconsin, 1968), pp. 35, 87-88, 112, 117-19; William Metcalfe, "Address," *Water-Cure Journal,* XVIII (November, 1854), 105-6.

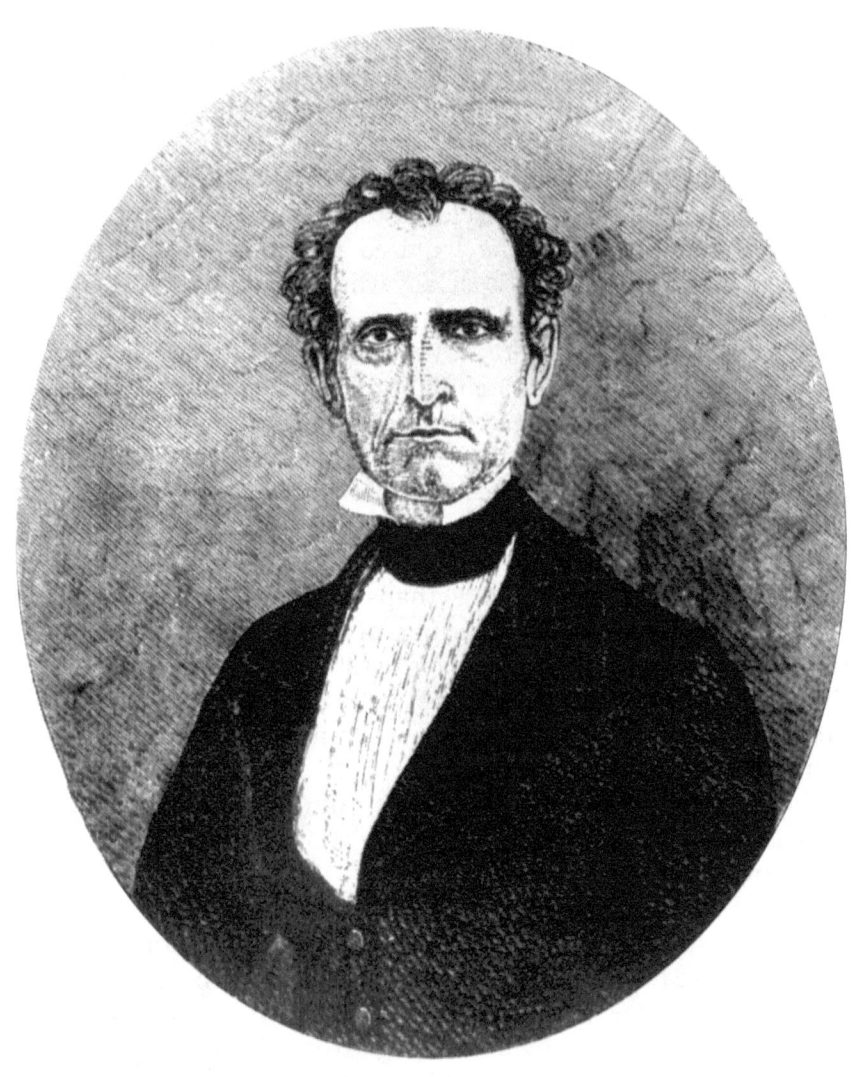

Sylvester Graham
From Graham, *Lectures on the Science of Human Life* (New York: Fowler and Wells, 1858)

and from every kind of purely stimulating substances, and [by observing] a correct general regimen in regard to sleeping, bathing, clothing, exercise, the indulgence of the natural passions, appetites, etc." When the dreaded disease finally did strike in June, he repeated his lecture on cholera to crowds of anxious listeners who had not heard him previously. After the epidemic had subsided, he happily reported "that of all who followed my prescribed regimen uniformly and consistently, not one fell a victim to that fearful disease, and very few had the slightest symptoms of an attack."[6]

During the 1830s Graham visited most of the major Eastern cities and won a widespread following among those Americans who had lost faith in the more traditional methods of preserving health. In 1839 he wrote out his oft-repeated *Lectures on the Science of Human Life,* published in Boston in two volumes. By far the most distinctive of his ideas related to diet. Borrowing liberally from the French pathologist François J. V. Broussais, whose *Treatise on Physiology* he had read in his leisure hours as a pastor, he theorized that irritation of the gastrointestinal tract, particularly the stomach, was responsible for most of man's ailments. Since the nervous system linked all the organs of the body together in "a common web of sympathy," anything that adversely affected the stomach also affected the rest of the body. Following what was too often the custom of his day, Graham insisted on his own originality and refused to acknowledge his indebtedness to Broussais or any other writer.[7]

The best way to stay healthy, advised Graham in his *Lectures,* was to avoid all stimulating and unnatural foods and to subsist "entirely on the products of the vegetable kingdom and pure water" — "the only drink that man can ever use in perfect accordance with the vital properties and laws of his nature." An ideal food, and one that came to be associated with Graham's name, was bread made from unbolted wheat flour and allowed to sit for twenty-four hours. Because of the "intimate relation between the quality of the bread and the moral character of a family," loaves from the hands of "a

---

6. Sylvester Graham, *Lectures on the Science of Human Life* (People's ed.; London: Horsell, Aldine, Chambers, 1849), p. 190; Nissenbaum, "Careful Love," pp. 119-21.

7. Nissenbaum, "Careful Love," pp. 121-33; Graham, *Lectures,* pp. ii-iii; Naylor, "Sylvester Graham," p. 238.

devoted wife and mother" were preferable to those sold in public bakeries, which were generally unfit for human consumption. Naturally, bakers did not take too kindly to this suggestion, and on one occasion, while he was lecturing in Boston, they stirred up such an unruly mob outside the hall that the Grahamites within had to disperse the protesters by dumping slaked lime out the windows on their heads.[8]

Graham regarded most dairy products as little better than meat. Butter was especially objectionable. In support of his position, he cited the recent experiments of the army surgeon William Beaumont on the unfortunate Alexis St. Martin, whose stomach had been accidentally opened for scientific observation by a shotgun blast. When butter had been introduced into Martin's stomach, it had simply floated "upon the top of the chymous mass" until most of the digesting food had passed on to the small intestine. If butter were to be used at all, said Graham, it should be "very sparingly, and never in the melted form." In its place he recommended using a moderate amount of sweet cream, which was soluble in water and thus "very far less objectionable than butter as an article of diet." Fresh milk and eggs were frowned upon but not proscribed, although the latter, being "somewhat more highly animalized than milk," were consequently more "exciting to the system." Cheese was permitted only if mild and unaged.[9]

To avoid overworking the digestive system, meals were to be taken no more frequently than every six hours and never before retiring. If this schedule could not be met, then the third meal was to be eliminated. No irritating substances were ever to appear on the table. This ban covered not only condiments and spices like pepper, mustard, cinnamon, and cloves — "all highly exciting and exhausting" — but even common salt, which was "utterly indigestible." Tea and coffee, like alcohol and tobacco, stunted growth and poisoned the system. And most pastries, with the possible exceptions of some custards and fruit and berry pies, were "among the most pernicious

8. Graham, *Lectures*, pp. 226, 232-34, 265-67; Naylor, "Sylvester Graham," p. 239.

9. Graham, *Lectures,* pp. 224-26, 243. See also William Beaumont, *Experiments and Observations on the Gastric Juice, and the Physiology of Digestion* (Plattsburgh, N.Y.: F. P. Allen, 1833).

articles of human aliment" and incomparably more harmful than simply prepared meats.[10]

In his *Lectures* Graham ranged far beyond the subject of diet to comment on just about every area of human activity, emphasizing the importance of rest, exercise, cleanliness, dress — and of never resorting to medicines. Regular hours were to be set aside for sleeping, preferably before midnight and always in a well-ventilated room. Frequent physical exercise was absolutely necessary for a healthy circulation of the blood; thus dancing, "when properly regulated," was of great medicinal value. Growing children particularly needed to exercise their bodies, and for that reason Graham opposed confining them to schoolbooks at an early age, recommending instead that they be allowed to romp outdoors like calves and colts. A sponge bath every morning upon rising was highly desirable, but better still was the "exceedingly great luxury" of standing in a tub and pouring a tumbler of water over the body. Clothing was to be both morally and physiologically unobjectionable, with no restrictive corsets, stays, or garters of any kind. Shaving the beard, Graham warned his male readers, was to be practiced only at the risk of lessening one's manly powers and shortening the life span. If, after following this regimen, a person did succumb to illness, the cardinal rule to remember was that "ALL MEDICINE, AS SUCH, IS ITSELF AN EVIL." The safest policy when sick was simply to let nature take its own beneficent course.[11]

The public outcry against Graham's strange reforms was more than matched by its outrage at his views on sex. In fact, one of his fellow reformers was convinced that "while the public odium was ostensibly directed against his anti-fine flour and anti-flesh eating doctrines, it was his anti-sexual indulgence doctrines, in reality, which excited the public hatred and rendered his name a by-word and a reproach." According to one (possibly apocryphal) story, the shock of seeing mixed bathing at the ocean one day first aroused his interest in sexual abuses and prompted him to sit down and write *A*

---

10. Graham, *Lectures*, pp. 242, 250-54, 271-75.

11. Ibid., pp. 188, 277-86. The reference to children playing outdoors is from Graham, *A Lecture to Young Men on Chastity* (10th ed.; Boston: Charles H. Pierce, 1848), p. 162.

Lecture to Young Men on Chastity, published in 1834. As Stephen Nissenbaum has pointed out, this work broke with the older moralistic literature on the subject in two ways: It was based largely on scientific rather than biblical arguments, and it focused not on the sins of adultery and fornication but on the previously neglected problems of masturbation and marital excess, which Graham defined for most people as intercourse more than once a month. In his mind, diet and sex were intimately related since stimulating foods inevitably aroused the sexual passions. Thus one of the best means of controlling these unwholesome urges was to adopt a meatless diet and forsake condiments, spices, alcohol, tea, and coffee.[12]

Despite the animosity of butchers, bakers, and corset-makers, "Bran-Bread Graham" — as one Boston paper named him — won numerous converts throughout the nation, including members of the educated and upper classes. In 1837 he began publishing a monthly called the *Graham Journal of Health and Longevity,* edited by a Boston disciple, David Cambell (or Campbell), who later engaged William Miller in a protracted debate on the interpretation of Bible prophecies. To meet the dietary needs of his growing following, he encouraged the opening of temperance boarding houses in the larger cities of the East and personally wrote a set of strict rules and regulations governing such establishments. All boarders were expected to sleep on hard beds, rise promptly at four o'clock in the morning — five during the winter months — and retire by ten each evening. Before breakfasting on ripe fruit and whole wheat or corn mush, they were to exercise for at least a half hour and attend morning prayers. Meat was permitted at dinner, but strongly discouraged. Suppers were light and simple. Pure soft water was "earnestly recommended as the exclusive drink of a Graham Boarding House," and those caught drinking alcoholic beverages, tea, coffee, or hot chocolate were thrown out. Baths were required at least once a week, three times a week in the summer. These boarding houses became a favorite haunt of many reformers, especially abolitionists. One out-of-town visitor reported that the guests in New York City were "not only

---

12. William A. Alcott, *The Physiology of Marriage* (Boston: Dinsmoor and Co., 1866), pp. 116-17; Naylor, "Sylvester Graham," p. 239; Nissenbaum, "Careful Love," pp. 6-9; Graham, *Lecture to Young Men on Chastity,* pp. 83, 144-48.

The Health Reformers

Grahamites, but Garrisonites — not only reformers in diet, but radicalists in Politics." Horace Greeley resided for some time at the New York house and married one of the women boarders.[13]

While the abolitionists flocked to the Graham boarding houses, other reformers tried to adapt the Graham system to different institutions. The revivalist Charles G. Finney and his fellow pioneers at Oberlin turned that college into a Grahamite stronghold in the 1830s, allowing the students "only plain & wholesome food" with little variety. But their experiment ended in the spring of 1841 after dissidents held a mass meeting protesting the all-vegetable fare in the dining hall. Bronson Alcott founded his utopian colony of Fruitlands on Grahamite principles, leaving his little daughter Louisa May with memories of rising at five in the morning, showering in cold water, and subsisting on Graham bread and fruit. At nearby Brook Farm there was always a popular "Graham table" for vegetarians. And many Shaker communities, whose "Millennial Laws" prohibited such health-destroying habits as taking fruit after supper and eating freshly baked bread, embraced the Graham way of life.[14]

In 1836, while lecturing in Boston, Graham met William A. Alcott, cousin of Bronson and a prominent health reformer in his own right. In contrast to the impetuous, largely self-educated Gra-

---

13. The nickname given by the *Boston Traveller* is mentioned in [William A. Alcott], "Mr. Graham," *Moral Reformer*, I (October, 1835), 322; Graham's rules and regulations are found in [Asenath Nicholson], *Nature's Own Book* (2d ed.; New York: Wilbur & Whipple, 1835), pp. 13-22; the comment on Garrisonites is in a letter from William S. Tyler to Edward Tyler, October 10, 1833 (Hitchcock Memorabilia Collection, Amherst College), quoted in Thomas H. Le Duc, "Grahamites and Garrisonites," *New York History*, XX (April, 1939), 190. On Greeley, see his *Recollections of a Busy Life* (New York: J. B. Ford and Co., 1868), pp. 103-4. Campbell's exchange with Miller appeared in the *Signs of the Times*, I (1840-41), passim.

14. Fletcher, *History of Oberlin College*, pp. 319-30; Clara Endicott Sears (ed.), *Bronson Alcott's Fruitlands* (Boston: Houghton Mifflin Co., 1915), p. 106; Alice Felt Tyler, *Freedom's Ferment: Phases of American Social History from the Colonial Period to the Outbreak of the Civil War* (New York: Harper & Row, 1962), p. 174; John Thomas Codman, *Brook Farm: Historic and Personal Memoirs* (Boston: Arean Publishing Co., 1894), pp. 120-21; Edward Deming Andrews, *The People Called Shakers: A Search for the Perfect Society* (new enlarged ed.; New York: Dover Publications, 1963), pp. 156, 194-95, 245-46.

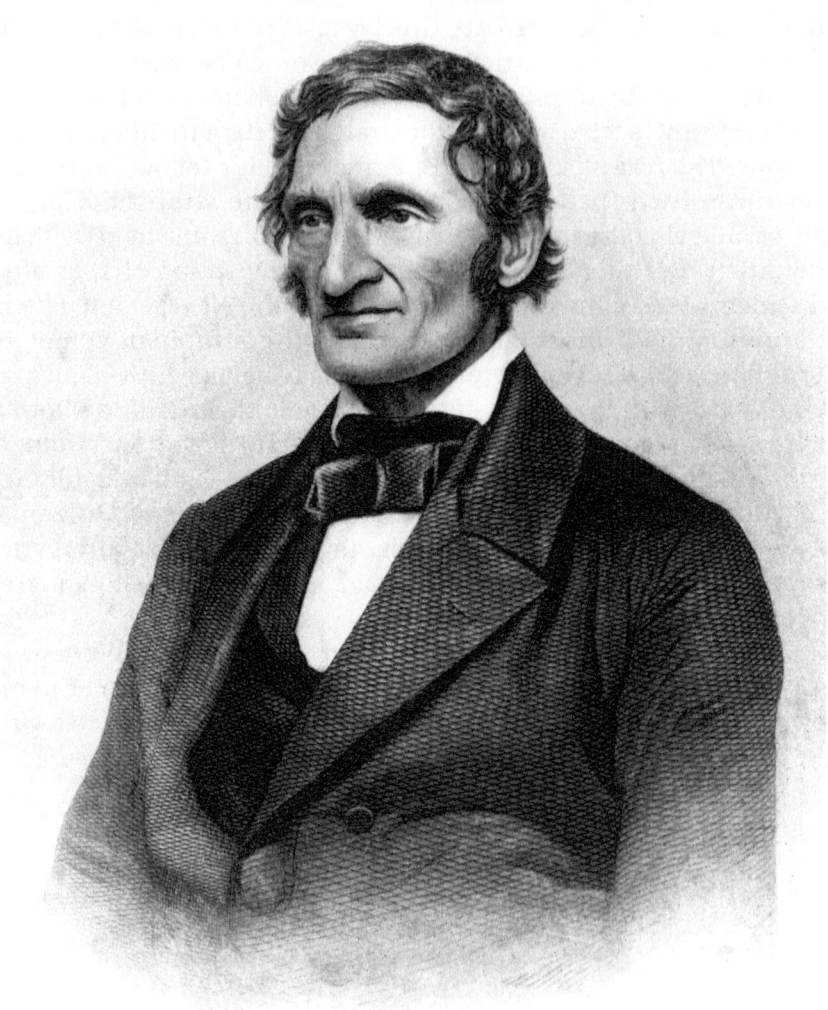

William A. Alcott
From Alcott, *Lectures on Life and Health* (Boston: Phillips, Sampson, and Co., 1853)

ham who reveled in the limelight, Alcott was a thoughtful Yale-trained physician who enjoyed teaching school most of all. A constant sufferer from pulmonary disorders, he decided in 1830 to try to regain his health by giving up all drinks but water and all animal foods except milk. When his health improved, he turned to writing manuals for the benefit of his fellow citizens and soon became one of the most widely read authors of his day. Over the years he produced no fewer than eighty-five volumes on a multitude of subjects, including most of the reforms advocated by Graham. Perhaps his most popular work was his *Young Man's Guide,* which passed through twenty-one editions between its appearance in 1833 and 1858. In 1835 he began editing the *Moral Reformer,* a journal dedicated to wiping out the evils of intemperance, gluttony, and licentiousness.[15]

Alcott shared with Graham an extreme reluctance to acknowledge any intellectual debts — especially to the flamboyant crusader for bran bread whom he at first found offensive. "Now let it be distinctly understood, once and for all," he wrote in 1837, "that . . . we have nothing to do, either directly or indirectly, with Mr. G. or his doctrines. Nay more . . . we adopted nearly all our present views as independently of Mr. G. as if he had never written on the subject." That same year, however, Alcott buried his misgivings and joined with Graham in forming the first of many health reform associations, the American Physiological Society, which aimed to promote all reforms involving "Air, Temperature, Clothing, Exercise, Sleep, Dress, Diet, and Drink." Alcott was elected president, Graham's as-

---

15. William A. Alcott, *Forty Years in the Wilderness of Pills and Powders* (Boston: John P. Jewett and Co., 1859), pp. 86, 380-83; [Alcott], "Objections to Animal Food," *Moral Reformer,* I (September, 1835), 283. On Alcott's life and writings, see James C. Wharton, "'Christian Physiology': William Alcott's Prescription for the Millennium" (unpublished paper read at the 47th Annual Meeting of the American Association for the History of Medicine, Charleston, S.C., May 2, 1974); Carl Bode, *The Anatomy of American Popular Culture, 1840-1861* (Berkeley and Los Angeles: University of California Press, 1960), pp. 119-27; E. Douglas Branch, *The Sentimental Years, 1836-1860* (New York: Hill and Wang, 1965), p. 221; and Sidney Ditzion, *Marriage, Morals and Sex in America: A History of Ideas* (New York: Bookman Associates, 1953), pp. 322-23. For a typical exposition of Alcott's views on the importance of fresh air and exercise, proper diet, dress, and cleanliness, see his *Laws of Health* (Boston: John P. Jewett and Co., 1859).

sociate David Cambell, corresponding secretary. The health reform movement now had a united front.¹⁶

Women, who joined the movement in large numbers, accounted for almost one-fourth of the American Physiological Society's membership. They were among the most effective evangelists for health reform, organizing societies from Maine to Ohio and lecturing widely on the gospel of health. As Regina Markell Morantz has recently shown, health reform held special significance for the American woman:

> In a society in which women were expected to play an increasingly complex role in the nurture of children and the organization of family life, health reform brought to the bewildered housewife not just sympathy and compassion, but a structured regimen, a way of life. In an era characterized by weakening ties between relatives and neighbors, health reform lectures, journals, and domestic tracts provided once again the friendly advice and companionship of the now remote kinswoman. Women were promised a way to end their isolation and make contact with others of their sex. At lectures, study groups and even through letters to the various journals, they shared their common experiences with other women. A deep sense of sisterhood was evidenced by the frequent use of the term. No longer must woman bear her burden alone.¹⁷

Allied with the women health reformers in the work of educating the American public were many men. Of particular importance for our story are three whose writings later had a noticeable influence on the thinking of Ellen White: Horace Mann, Dio Lewis, and

---

16. William A. Alcott, *The Library of Health, and Teacher on the Human Constitution* (Boston: George W. Light, 1837), I, 4; [Alcott], "Mr. Graham," *Moral Reformer,* I (July, 1835), 227; Hebbel E. Hoff and John F. Fulton, "The Centenary of the First American Physiological Society Founded at Boston by William A. Alcott and Sylvester Graham," Institute of the History of Medicine, *Bulletin,* V (October, 1937), 687-96, 712-14; William B. Walker, "The Health Reform Movement in the United States, 1830-1870" (Ph.D. diss., Johns Hopkins University, 1955), pp. 113, 123.

17. Hoff and Fulton, "Centenary of the First American Physiological Society," p. 696; Regina Markell Morantz, "Nineteenth-Century Health Reform and Women: An Ideology of Self-Help" (paper read at a symposium on "Medicine without Doctors," University of Wisconsin-Madison, April 14, 1975), p. 24.

The Health Reformers

Larkin B. Coles. Mann, best remembered as the champion of public schools during his tenure as secretary to the Massachusetts State Board of Education, was an eloquent spokesman for the causes of temperance and personal hygiene. Apparently inspired by William Alcott, he urged the state board in his annual report for 1842 to require the teaching of "physiology" in all common schools. By this term he meant the laws of health relating to fresh air, pure water, and proper diet. His campaign culminated in 1850 in the passage of an act by the Massachusetts General Court requiring that the principles of physiology and hygiene be taught in all public schools by properly certified teachers.[18]

Dio (Dioclesian) Lewis, a younger contemporary of Mann's, was an active temperance, health, and educational reformer, whose greatest contributions lay in the areas of physical education and gymnastics. In 1845 he enrolled in the medical department of Harvard College, only to be forced out by financial difficulties before receiving his diploma. Not one to let such a minor setback deter him, he returned to his home in New York City and went into partnership with his family doctor, a homeopath. (In 1851 the Homeopathic Hospital College in Cleveland, Ohio, awarded him an honorary M.D. degree.) He first caught the nation's eye in the 1850s as a highly successful temperance lecturer, who on one foray into Michigan managed to close down all but one of the forty-nine drinking places in the town of Battle Creek. In his lectures and writings he espoused most of the same reforms as Graham and Alcott, regarding it "an honor and privilege" to range himself with such conscientious and abused men. However, on two relatively minor issues he broke with many of the older reformers and took positions also advocated by Ellen White: He recommended the use of salt in moderation and came out strongly in favor of only two meals a day.[19]

---

18. Horace Mann, "Report for 1842," *Life and Works of Horace Mann* (Boston: Lee and Shepard, 1891), III, 129-229; Walker, "The Health Reform Movement," pp. 94-98. See also Mann's *Two Lectures on Intemperance* (Syracuse: Hall, Mills, and Co., 1852).

19. Mary F. Eastman, *The Biography of Dio Lewis, A.M., M.D.* (New York: Fowler & Wells, 1891), pp. 36-37, 67-68; Dio Lewis, *Weak Lungs, and How to Make Them Strong* (Boston: Ticknor and Fields, 1863), pp. 101, 134; Lewis, *Our Digestion; or, My Jolly Friend's Secret* (New York: Fowler & Wells, 1872), p. 147. For a recent survey of Ameri-

Larkin B. Coles, although never as prominent a reformer as Mann or Lewis, is of special interest because of his background as a Millerite preacher-physician. A native of New Hampshire, he graduated from Castleton Medical College in 1825 during that institution's heyday as New England's most popular medical school. He is reputed also to have been trained as a minister.[20] As early as 1836 he seems to have been associated with William Miller, and at the height of the Millerite movement he was actively distributing Miller's books and writing theological articles for the *Signs of the Times*. Shortly after the Great Disappointment of 1844 he settled in Boston and joined both the Boston Medical Association and the Massachusetts Medical Society as an orthodox physician in good and regular standing. His two great loves seem to have been preaching and traveling. For years he occupied a pulpit every Sabbath and traveled extensively up and down the Ohio and Mississippi valleys, once going as far from home as Galveston, Texas. He died in January, 1856, while visiting Louisville, Kentucky.[21]

---

can views on the importance of exercise, see John Rickards Betts, "American Medical Thought on Exercise as the Road to Health, 1820-1860," *Bulletin of the History of Medicine*, XLV (March-April, 1971), 138-52.

20. Frederick Clayton Waite, *The First Medical College in Vermont: Castleton, 1818-1862* (Montpelier: Vermont Historical Society, 1949), p. 204, lists Coles as a graduate of both Castleton and Newton Theological Seminary. However, a check of the records of The Newton Theological Institution by Mr. Ellis E. O'Neal, Jr., librarian of Andover Newton Theological School, turned up no mention of Coles.

21. On a letter from Emerson Andrews, July 20, 1836, Miller wrote the name "Doct Coles" (William Miller Papers, Aurora College). Admittedly, this is skimpy evidence for establishing an early relationship between the two men, but it does fit with Barnes Riznik's assertion that Coles experienced a religious change between 1830 and 1835; "Medicine in New England, 1790-1840" (report prepared by the Department of Research, Old Sturbridge Village, Massachusetts, 1962), p. 152-RRR. On a scrap of paper (ca. 1842, Miller Papers) Miller noted having sent Coles thirty-seven copies of one of his books. Typical of Coles's contributions to the *Signs of the Times* are: "On the 24th of Matthew," V (April 12, 1843), 2; "Proof from Opposers," V (April 12, 1843), 2; and "The Jews-Romans XI," V (May 17, 1843), 6-7. At the time of writing these pieces Coles was living in Lowell, Mass. Earlier, in the late 1820s, he had practiced medicine in Fitzwilliam, N.H.; John F. Norton, *The History of Fitzwilliam, New Hampshire, from 1752 to 1887* (New York: Burr Printing House, 1888), p. 429. Coles's name first appeared in the Boston Directory in 1845. On Dec. 17, 1847, he joined the Boston Medical Association; "List of Members, 1806-1910" (The Francis A. Count-

Coles's claim to a place among the health reformers rests on two books: *Philosophy of Health: Natural Principles of Health and Cure* and *The Beauties and Deformities of Tobacco-Using.* The former volume was remarkably successful, selling thirty-five thousand copies during its first five years and another nine thousand before Coles's death. When the twenty-sixth edition appeared in 1851, one medical journal joked that it seemed "as though the friends of reform not only read, but eat the books."[22] Taking as his theme the proposition that "it is as truly a sin against Heaven, to violate a law of life, as to break one of the ten commandments," he went on to develop the now-traditional arguments of the health reformers for fresh air and exercise, a vegetarian diet, the nonuse of stimulants, reform in dress, sexual purity, and drugless medicine. On this last point — drugless medicine — he failed to go far enough to suit some of the more radical reformers who wanted him to come out against medicine of any kind.[23] But his generally moderate stance won him the respect of his peers in the medical community. "Dr. Coles hails from the ranks of the vegetable eaters," noted the *Boston Medical and Surgical Journal,* "but if he really abominates beef-steaks and butter, he is modest and unobtrusive with regard to his opinion, which should be regarded as a virtue in this age of radicalism."[24]

The Beauties and Deformities of Tobacco-Using elicited praise from reformers and nonreformers alike. The *Water-Cure Journal* called it "the best looking work on the subject," while the orthodox *Boston Medical and Surgical Journal* highly recommended it as a devastating attack on "the vile weed." In Coles's opinion as a physician and minister, tobacco was doing far more damage than alcohol to

---

way Library of Medicine, Harvard University). Eleven days later he was admitted into the Massachusetts Medical Society; "Catalogue of Gentlemen Elected and Admitted into the Society, 1826-50" (Countway Library).

22. "Philosophy of Health," *Boston Medical and Surgical Journal,* XLV (November 26, 1851), 358. For an earlier comment on Coles's manuscript in this same journal, see XXXVII (November 10, 1847), 305.

23. Coles, *Philosophy of Health,* p. 216; cf. p. 8. The criticism of Coles's views on medicine is in "Literary Notices," *Water-Cure Journal,* XVI (September, 1853), 66-67.

24. "Philosophy of Health," *Boston Medical and Surgical Journal,* XXXVIII (February 2, 1848), 26. When his *Philosophy of Health* first appeared in 1848, Coles received a congratulatory message from William Alcott; this and other endorsements appear on pp. 119-20 of the 8th edition of *Philosophy of Health.*

the health and welfare of Americans, whose per capita consumption of the stuff was eight times higher than the French and three times more than the English. Epileptic fits, weak eyesight, and insanity were just a few of its many frightening physical effects. Morally it was no less insiduous, for it formed an unholy "triplet union" with rum and profanity. "RARELY CAN A PROFANE OATH BE FOUND ISSUING FROM A CLEAN MOUTH AND A PURE BREATH," he observed. Obviously the only safe course was never to take up this body- and soul-destroying habit.[25]

Coles's moralistic view of health reform, as seen in his elevation of hygienic laws to equality with the Ten Commandments, was not unique among health reformers. William Alcott, for example, also emphasized the moral obligation to preserve health. Yet the theological assumptions and expectations of the two men differed significantly. While Alcott and other Christian perfectionists looked forward to the virtual eradication of disease in a millennium of perfect health, the millenarian Coles — and later Ellen White — saw obedience to the laws of health primarily as a requirement for entry into heaven and only secondarily as a means of living a more enjoyable life on earth. The rewards in either case, however, provided ample motivation to live more hygienically.[26]

By the mid-1840s the health reformers had developed a comprehensive system for maintaining good health; what they lacked was an effective means of restoring health once it was lost. Several reformers had attended regular medical schools, but the heroic therapy they had learned — bleeding, blistering, and purging — no longer seemed worthy of confidence. The Adventist printer L. V. Masten, whose cholera had not responded to blood-letting and calomel, was expressing a popular opinion when he called such treatment *"sure death!"* Most health reformers agreed with him on the risks of regular medicine and thus chose one of the safer sectarian systems: Thomsonianism, homeopathy, or hydropathy.[27]

---

25. "Book Notices," *Water-Cure Journal*, XII (October 1851), 93; "Beauties and Deformities of Tobacco-Using," *Boston Medical and Surgical Journal*, XLVIII (March 2, 1853), 104-5; Coles, *Beauties and Deformities of Tobacco-Using*, pp. 7, 58, 64, 88.

26. See Coles, *Philosophy of Health*, pp. 214, 286; and Whorton, "'Christian Physiology.'"

27. L. V. Masten, "Experience of Bro. Masten," *R&H*, III (September 30, 1852),

The Health Reformers

Samuel Thomson, the New Hampshire farmer who founded the Thomsonian medical sect, substituted "natural" botanic remedies for the bleeding and mineral drugs of regular physicians. Early in his healing career he became convinced that the cause of all disease was cold and that the only cure was the restoration of the body's normal heat. This he accomplished by steaming, peppering, and puking his patients, with heavy reliance on lobelia, an emetic long used by Native Americans.[28]

Not one to ignore the commercial possibilities of his discovery, Thomson in 1806 began selling "Family Rights" to his practice, patented in 1813. For twenty dollars purchasers enrolled in the Friendly Botanic Society and received a sixteen-page instruction booklet, *Family Botanic Medicine,* later expanded into a more substantial *New Guide to Health.* The section on preparing medicines contained various botanical recipes, but with key ingredients left out. Agents filled in the blanks only after buyers pledged themselves to secrecy "under the penalty of forfeiting their word and honour, and all right to the use of the medicine."[29]

---

86. On the low status of the regular medical profession, see Charles E. Rosenberg, *The Cholera Years: The United States in 1832, 1849, and 1866* (Chicago: University of Chicago Press, 1962), pp. 154-60. A fourth major medical sect, eclecticism, relied exclusively on botanical remedies; for a recent discussion, see Ronald L. Numbers, "The Making of an Eclectic Physician: Joseph M. McElhinney and the Eclectic Medical Institute of Cincinnati," *Bulletin of the History of Medicine,* XLVII (March-April, 1973), 155-66.

28. Samuel Thomson, *New Guide to Health; or, Botanic Family Physician* (2nd ed.; Boston: For the author, 1825), Part 1, pp. 42-45. Alex Berman, "The Impact of the Nineteenth-Century Botanico-Medical Movement on American Pharmacy and Medicine" (Ph.D. diss., University of Wisconsin, 1954), remains the most thorough treatment of Thomsonianism; but see also Berman, "The Thomsonian Movement and Its Relation to American Pharmacy and Medicine," *Bulletin of the History of Medicine,* XXV (September-October, 1951), 405-28, and (November-December, 1951), 519-38; Madge E. Pickard and R. Carlyle Buley, *The Midwest Pioneer: His Ills, Cures, & Doctors* (New York: Henry Schuman, 1946), chap. 4, pp. 167-98; Joseph F. Kett, *The Formation of the American Medical Profession: The Role of Institutions, 1780-1860* (New Haven: Yale University Press, 1968), chap. 4, pp. 97-131; and James Harvey Young, *The Toadstool Millionaires: A Social History of Patent Medicines in America before Federal Regulation* (Princeton: Princeton University Press, 1961), chap. 4, pp. 44-57.

29. Thomson, *New Guide to Health,* Part 2, p. 4; Samuel Thomson, *Family Botanic Medicine* (Boston: T. C. Bangs, 1819).

During the 1820s and 1830s Thomsonian agents fanned out from New England through the southern and western United States urging self-reliant Americans to become their own physicians. Almost everywhere they met with success. By 1840 approximately one hundred thousand Family Rights had been sold, and Thomson estimated that about three million persons had adopted his system. In states as diverse as Ohio and Mississippi, perhaps as many as one-half of the citizens were curing themselves the Thomsonian way. And as Daniel Drake observed, the devotees of Thomsonianism were not "limited to the vulgar. Respectable and intelligent mechaniks, legislative and judicial officers, both state and federal barristers, ladies, ministers of the gospel, and even some of the medical profession 'who hold the eel of science by the tail' have become its converts and puffers."[30]

By the 1840s internal squabbles were fragmenting the Thomsonians; and as botanic strength began to wane, a new sect, homeopathy, rose to national prominence. Homeopathy was the invention of a regularly educated German physician, Samuel Hahnemann, who had grown dissatisfied with the heroics of orthodox practice. During the last decade of the eighteenth century he began constructing an alternate system based in large part upon the healing power of nature and two fundamental principles: the law of similars and the law of infinitesimals. According to the first law, diseases are cured by medicines having the property of producing in healthy persons symptoms similar to those of the disease. An individual suffering from fever, for example, would be treated with a drug known to increase the pulse rate of a person in health. Hahnemann's second law held that medicines are more efficacious the smaller the dose, even as small as dilutions of one-millionth of a gram. Though regular practitioners — or allopaths, as Hahnemann called them — ridiculed this theory, many patients flourished under homeopathic treatment, and they seldom suffered.[31]

---

30. Berman, "The Impact of the Nineteenth-Century Botanico-Medical Movement," pp. 150-52; Daniel Drake, "The People's Doctors," *Western Journal of the Medical and Physical Sciences* (1829), p. 407, quoted ibid., pp. 42-43.

31. On homeopathy, see Martin Kaufman, *Homeopathy in America: The Rise and Fall of a Medical Heresy* (Baltimore: Johns Hopkins University Press, 1971); Harris L. Coulter, *Divided Legacy: A History of the Schism in Medical Thought* (Washington:

The Health Reformers

Following its appearance in this country in 1825, homeopathy rapidly grew into a major medical sect. By the outbreak of the Civil War there were nearly twenty-five hundred homeopathic physicians, concentrated largely in New England, New York, Pennsylvania, and the Midwest, and hundreds of thousands of devoted followers. Homeopathy's appeal is not difficult to understand. Instead of the bleedings and purgings of the regulars, or the equally rigorous therapy of the Thomsonians, the homeopaths offered pleasant-tasting pills that produced no discomforting side effects. Such medication was particularly suitable for babies and small children. As the orthodox Dr. Holmes observed, homeopathy "does not offend the palate, and so spares the nursery those scenes of single combat in which infants were wont to yield at length to the pressure of the spoon and the imminence of asphyxia." Perhaps because of its suitability for children, homeopathy won the support of large numbers of American women, who constituted approximately two-thirds of its patrons and who were among its most active propagators.[32]

Both Thomsonianism and homeopathy attracted some health reformers. For example, Alva Curtis of Cincinnati combined Thomsonianism with Grahamism, and Elisha Bartlett observed that a "non-resistant, transcendentalist, and Grahamite, makes the most devoted disciple, and the stanchest [sic] advocate of homeopathy."[33] But by and large the health reformers distrusted all medicines, in large or small doses, botanical or mineral. Thus the majority of them opted for the one system of therapeutics that offered healing without drugs: hydropathy.

Hydropathy was a mélange of water treatments devised by a Silesian peasant, Vincent Priessnitz, to heal his wounds after accidentally being run over by a wagon. His therapy proved to be so suc-

---

McGrath Publishing Co., 1973), vol. 3; and Kett, *Formation of the American Medical Profession*, chap. 5, pp. 132-64.

32. Coulter, *Divided Legacy*, vol. 3, pp. 101-16; Oliver Wendell Holmes, "Some More Recent Views on Homeopathy," *Atlantic Monthly* (December, 1857), p. 187, quoted ibid., p. 114.

33. Blake, "Health Reform," p. 34; Elisha Bartlett, *An Essay on the Philosophy of Medical Science* (Philadelphia: Lea & Blanchard, 1844), p. 245. For an example of a homeopathic health reformer, see J. H. Pulte, *Homoeopathic Domestic Physician* (Cincinnati: H. W. Derby & Co., 1850).

cessful, he opened his home in Graefenberg as a "water cure" and invited his ailing neighbors to submit their bodies to a bewildering variety of baths, packs, and wet bandages. When news of his methods reached the United States in the mid-1840s, it touched off a "great American water-cure craze" that continued unabated until the outbreak of the Civil War. Part of the popularity of hydropathy undoubtedly stemmed from the inadequacies of nineteenth-century medicine, but equally significant was the fact that it harmonized perfectly with the Jacksonian spirit of the times. "The water treatment of disease may fairly be said to originate with an un-titled man," wrote one devotee. "This is the people's reform. It does not belong to M.D.'s of any school." The three persons most responsible for introducing Americans to hydropathic techniques — Joel Shew, Russell T. Trall, and Mary Gove — all had previous histories as reformers and succeeded, as Richard H. Shyrock pointed out, in superimposing "Grahamism upon hydropathy, and later, in the most catholic spirit imaginable, in [adding] every other hygienic procedure available."[34]

The first American water cures appeared in New York City about 1844 under the proprietorship of Drs. Shew and Trall, both graduates of regular medical schools. When Trall's first patients, "a set of desperate cases from Broadway Hospital," all recovered, the success

---

34. Richard H. Shyrock, "Sylvester Graham and the Popular Health Movement, 1830-1870," in *Medicine in America: Historical Essays* (Baltimore: Johns Hopkins University Press, 1966), pp. 121-22. The quotation about the "people's reform" is from James C. Jackson, "Considerations for Common Folk — No. 3," *Water-Cure Journal*, X (August, 1850), 67. On hydropathy in America, see Walker, "The Health Reform Movement," pp. 161-288; Harry B. Weiss and Howard R. Kemble, *The Great American Water-Cure Craze: A History of Hydropathy in the United States* (Trenton, N.J.: Past Times Press, 1967); and Marshall Scott Legan, "Hydropathy in America: A Nineteenth-Century Panacea," *Bulletin of the History of Medicine*, XLV (May-June, 1971), 267-80. In *Catharine Beecher: A Study in American Domesticity* (New Haven: Yale University Press, 1973), pp. 205-9, Kathryn Kish Sklar argues that the water cures treated "a predominantly female clientele." Women frequented these places, she says, because they allowed the indulgence of otherwise forbidden desires for physical sensuality" and "provided a supportive female environment and frequently employed women doctors." While it is true that many women patronized water cures, my research suggests that men found them equally attractive. And although roughly one-fifth of professional hydropaths were women (Weiss and Kemble, p. 44) — a large proportion in an age of few women doctors — the chief physicians at water cures were usually men.

of hydropathy was guaranteed. Within three or four years twenty-odd water cures were operating in nine states, largely concentrated in New York, Pennsylvania, and New Jersey, and numbering among their patrons such luminaries as Horace Greeley, Henry Wadsworth Longfellow, and James Fenimore Cooper. At first, Shew, who made two early pilgrimages to Graefenberg, simply duplicated Priessnitz's methods, but Trall soon went beyond the simple water treatments of the Austrian peasant to develop a fairly sophisticated system of "hygienic medication," embracing not only hydropathy but surgery and health reform as well. In December, 1845, Shew began publishing a *Water-Cure Journal* aimed broadly at providing the general reader with up-to-date information on "BATHING AND CLEANLINESS . . . CLOTHING . . . AIR AND VENTILATION . . . FOOD AND DRINKS . . . TOBACCO . . . TEA AND COFFEE . . . THE WATER-CURE . . ." and all other worthy reforms. Later, Trall took over the editorship and instituted such practical features as a matrimonial section where love-starved Grahamites and hydropaths could advertise for like-minded spouses.[35]

In the spring of 1846 Mary Gove arrived in New York City and opened a third water cure in competition with Shew's and Trall's. A long-time Grahamite and women's lecturer, Mrs. Gove had spent most of the previous year observing other water cures in operation before setting up her own. Through her lectures and writings she did much to popularize hydropathy in its early days. In 1851 she and her second husband, Thomas Low Nichols (M.D., New York University), decided the time was ripe to launch a water-cure school to meet the ever-increasing demand for trained hydropaths. That fall the American Hydropathic Institute admitted its first class of twenty-six students, and three months later graduated twenty of them — eleven men, nine women. After three fairly prosperous terms the Nicholses

---

35. Walker, "The Health Reform Movement," p. 193; Weiss and Kemble, *Great American Water-Cure Craze*, p. 41; "Russell T. Trall," *Herald of Health*, IV (July, 1864), 2-5; "Prospectus of the Water-Cure Journal, and Herald of Reforms," *Water-Cure Journal*, V (May, 1848), 79. Trall defines his system of "hygienic medication" in *Pathology of the Reproductive Organs; Embracing All Forms of Sexual Disorders* (Boston: B. Leverett Emerson, 1862), pp. vii-ix. For a list of famous patrons, see *The Water Cure in America*, ed. by a Water Patient (2nd ed.; New York: Wiley and Putnam, 1848), p. vii.

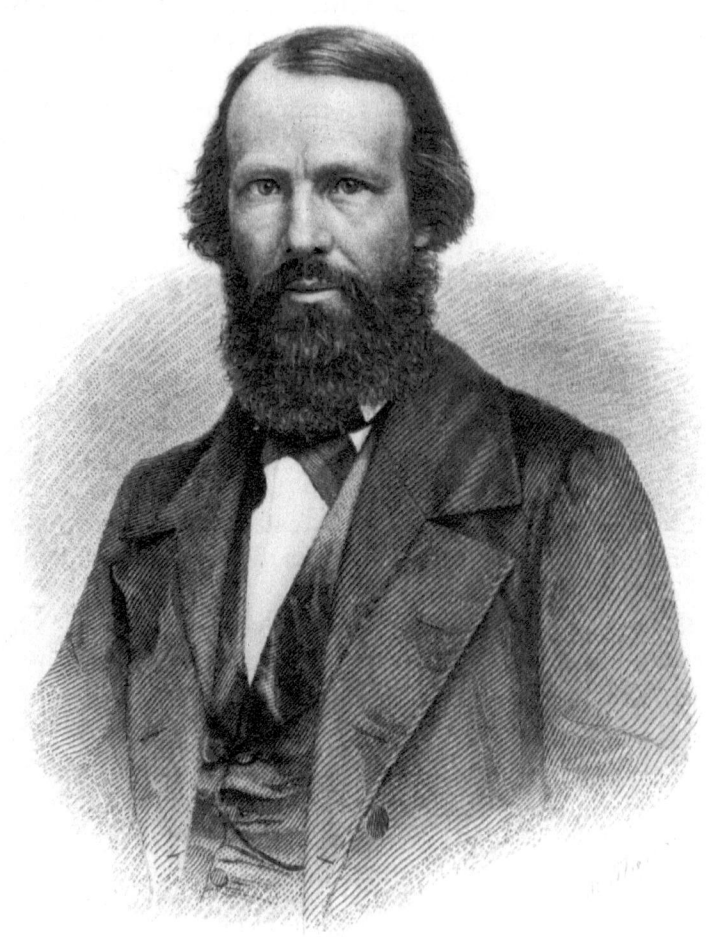

Russell T. Trall
From Trall, *Pathology of the Reproductive Organs* (Boston: B. Leverett Emerson, 1862)

suddenly lost interest in their educational venture and drifted off in the direction of free love and spiritualism, much to the dismay of their former colleagues. With the Nicholses gone, Trall wasted no time in opening his own hydropathic school in New York. His institution, christened the New York Hygeio-Therapeutic College after receiving a state charter in 1857, quickly became the water-cure center of the United States, while Trall himself, following the death of Shew in 1855 and the defection of the Nicholses, won recognition as dean of American health reformers.[36]

Listed among the original faculty of Trall's college was Lorenzo N. Fowler, lecturer on phrenology and mental science, whose presence symbolized the close union that had been forming between health reformers and phrenologists. Phrenology was the "science" of the human mind developed by two German physicians, Franz Joseph Gall and his student Johann Gaspar Spurzheim, and brought to the United States in the 1830s by Spurzheim and a Scottish convert, George Combe. According to phrenological theory, the human brain was made up of a number of different "organs" — some counted thirty-seven — each corresponding to an exotically named mental "faculty" like amativeness, acquisitiveness, or philoprogenitiveness. The organs governing man's "animal" or "domestic" propensities were located in the back and lower part of the head, while the organs of intellect and reason occupied the frontal region. Since the relative strength of any propensity could be determined by measuring the size of its matching organ, it was not difficult for the initiated to "read" a person's character by carefully examining the skull.[37]

Mistakes, however, did occur. The following incident supposedly took place when William Miller accompanied a friend to see a Boston phrenologist in March, 1842. The phrenologist, who had no idea he was examining the famous preacher's head,

---

36. Blake, "Mary Gove Nichols," pp. 219-34; Walker, "The Health Reform Movement," pp. 216-30; Weiss and Kemble, *Great American Water-Cure Craze*, pp. 33-38.

37. O. S. and L. N. Fowler, *Phrenology Proved, Illustrated, and Applied* (38th ed.; New York: Fowlers and Wells, 1848), pp. 7-51; John D. Davies, *Phrenology, Fad and Science: A 19th-Century American Crusade* (New Haven: Yale University Press, 1955), pp. 6-20; Madeleine B. Stern, *Heads & Headlines: The Phrenological Fowlers* (Norman: University of Oklahoma Press, 1971), p. 161.

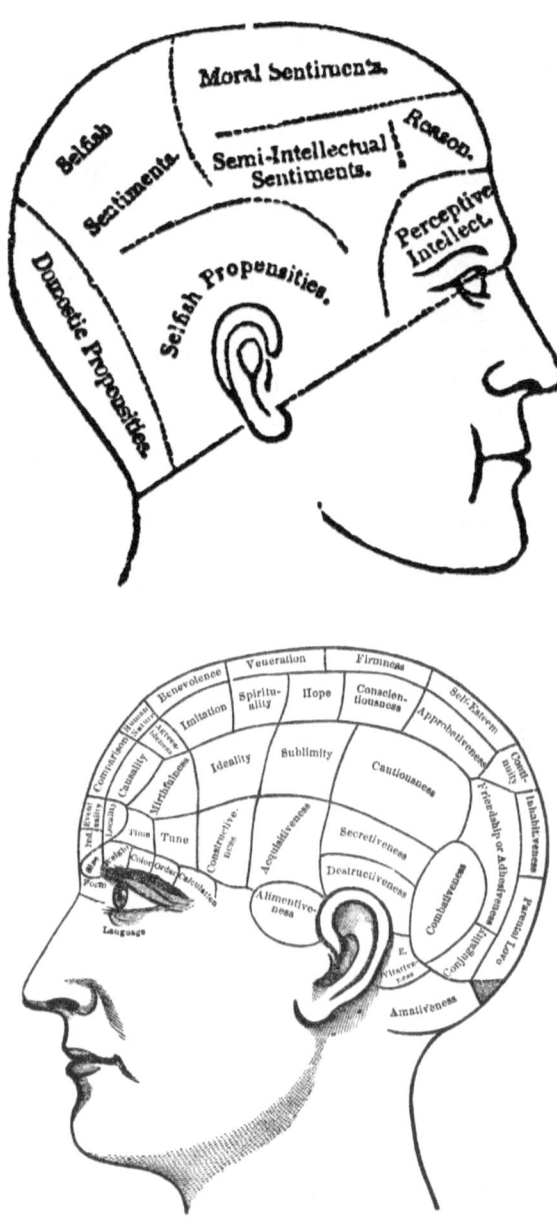

Phrenological Illustrations
From O. S. and L. N. Fowler, *New Illustrated Self-Instructor in Phrenology and Physiology* (New York: Fowler and Wells, 1859)

commenced by saying that the person under examination had a large, well-developed, and well-balanced head. While examining the moral and intellectual organs, he said to Mr. Miller's friend:

"I tell you what it is, Mr. Miller could not easily make a convert of *this man* to his hair-brained theory. He has too much good sense."

Thus he proceeded, making comparisons between the head he was examining and the head of Mr. Miller, as he fancied it would be.

"Oh, how I should like to examine Mr. Miller's head!" said he; "I would give it one squeezing."

The phrenologist, knowing that the gentleman was a particular friend of Mr. Miller, spared no pains in going out of the way to make remarks upon him. Putting his hand on the organ of marvellousness, he said: "There! I'll bet you anything that old Miller has got a bump on his head there as big as my fist"; at the same time doubling up his fist as an illustration.

The others present laughed at the perfection of the joke, and he heartily joined them, supposing they were laughing at his witticisms on Mr. Miller. . . .

He pronounced the head of the gentleman under examination the reverse, in every particular, of what he declared Mr. Miller's must be. When through, he made out his chart, and politely asked Mr. Miller his name.

Mr. Miller said it was of no consequence about putting his name upon the chart; but the phrenologist insisted.

"Very well," said Mr. M.; "you may call it Miller, if you choose."

"Miller, Miller," said he; "what is your first name?"

"They call me William Miller."

"What! the gentleman who is lecturing on the prophecies?"

"Yes, sir, the same."

At this the phrenologist settled back in his chair, the personation of astonishment and dismay, and spoke not a word while the company remained. His feelings may be more easily imagined than described.[38]

---

38. Sylvester Bliss, *Memoirs of William Miller* (Boston: Joshua V. Himes, 1853), pp. 160-61. Bliss includes Miller's phrenological scores.

The amazing popularity of phrenology during the 1840s and 1850s was in large measure the work of its two American high priests, Orson Squire Fowler and his brother Lorenzo. From their headquarters at Clinton Hall in New York City the Fowler brothers created a phrenological empire that reached into every segment of American society. Each month twenty thousand families pored over their *American Phrenological Journal,* one of the nation's most successful magazines, while thousands of others went out and purchased the multitude of guides and manuals the Fowlers annually published on all aspects of mental and physical health. As part of their effort to improve the human race, they rapidly branched out from phrenology to embrace the whole gamut of health reforms then in vogue: hydropathy, Grahamism, temperance, chastity, and even the Bloomer costume, named after a friend of Lorenzo's wife, Lydia.[39]

Through the years a close relationship developed between the leading phrenologists and health reformers. Shew and Trall became familiar figures at Clinton Hall and issued many of their books through the publishing house of Fowlers and Wells. Graham and Alcott also visited the Fowlers' phrenological palace, as did Horace Mann, who cheerfully submitted to a head reading. When the *Water-Cure Journal* almost folded in the spring of 1848, the Fowlers stepped in and promptly raised its circulation twenty-fold. In May, 1850, Clinton Hall was the setting for the organizational meeting of the American Vegetarian Society, which brought together many of the biggest names in health reform. Among the officers elected were William Alcott, president; Sylvester Graham and Joel Shew, vice-presidents; R. T. Trall, recording secretary; William Metcalfe, corresponding secretary; and Samuel R. Wells, brother-in-law and associate of the Fowlers, treasurer. Indeed, by the 1850s, as Sidney Ditzion has observed, "the vegetarians, phrenologists, water-cure doctors, and anti-tobacco, anti-corset, and temperance people" were so often crossing paths, "they began to look like participants in a single reform movement."[40]

39. Davies, *Phrenology,* pp. 60, 106-13.
40. Stern, *Heads & Headlines,* pp. 49-52, 129; T. L. Nichols, "American Vegetarian Convention," *Water-Cure Journal,* X (July, 1850), 5-6; Ditzion, *Marriage, Morals, and Sex in America,* p. 328. Although Graham was sympathetic to phrenology, he nevertheless had certain doubts about its validity; see his *Lectures,* pp. ii-iii, 89-94.

The Health Reformers

The outbreak of civil war in 1861 diverted much of the nation's attention from bran bread, baths, and Bloomers to other, more pressing, issues. From time to time die-hards attempted to revive interest in health reform — they actually founded a World's Health Association in Chicago in June, 1862 — but the movement as a whole had already crested. In the postwar years, as spectacular breakthroughs in scientific medicine drew more and more patients back to the regular fold, patronage at the water cures fell off markedly. Many went under, but a few did manage to survive until late in the century. Among the most flourishing was Dr. James Caleb Jackson's "Home on the Hillside" in Dansville, New York.[41]

James Caleb Jackson was born on March 28, 1811, in the little town of Manlius, New York, near Syracuse. Recurring poor health ended his formal education at age twelve, and his father's untimely death only a few years later left him with the onerous responsibility of managing the family farm. As he went about his daily chores, he dreamed of exchanging his dreary, bucolic life for the excitement of the public arena. Opportunity came in 1834, when he began receiving invitations from nearby towns to lecture on temperance and slavery. As his speaking engagements multiplied, time for farming vanished, and before long he was on the road full time. The rigors of the lecture circuit, however, proved to be too much for his frail constitution and forced him to take less physically demanding jobs editing antislavery papers and serving as secretary to abolitionist societies. Through his antislavery activities, he formed a warm friendship with Gerrit Smith, a New York philanthropist, who readily lent his wealth and prestige to virtually every reform that came along, from abolition and temperance to Sunday schools and Bloomers. Inevitably Smith joined the health reformers; and when Jackson's health failed so completely in 1847 that he "went home to die," Smith encouraged him to go to Dr. Silas O. Gleason's water cure in Cuba (New York) and personally raised the funds to pay his expenses there.[42]

---

41. Walker, "The Health Reform Movement," pp. 262-80; R. T. Trall, "Rambling Reminiscences — No. 12," *Water-Cure Journal*, XXXIV (August, 1862), 26.

42. William D. Conklin, *The Jackson Health Resort* (Dansville, N.Y.: Privately distributed by the author, 1971), pp. 105-7, 303; Ralph Volney Harlow, *Gerrit Smith: Philanthropist and Reformer* (New York: Henry Holt and Co., 1939), pp. 90-96. Infor-

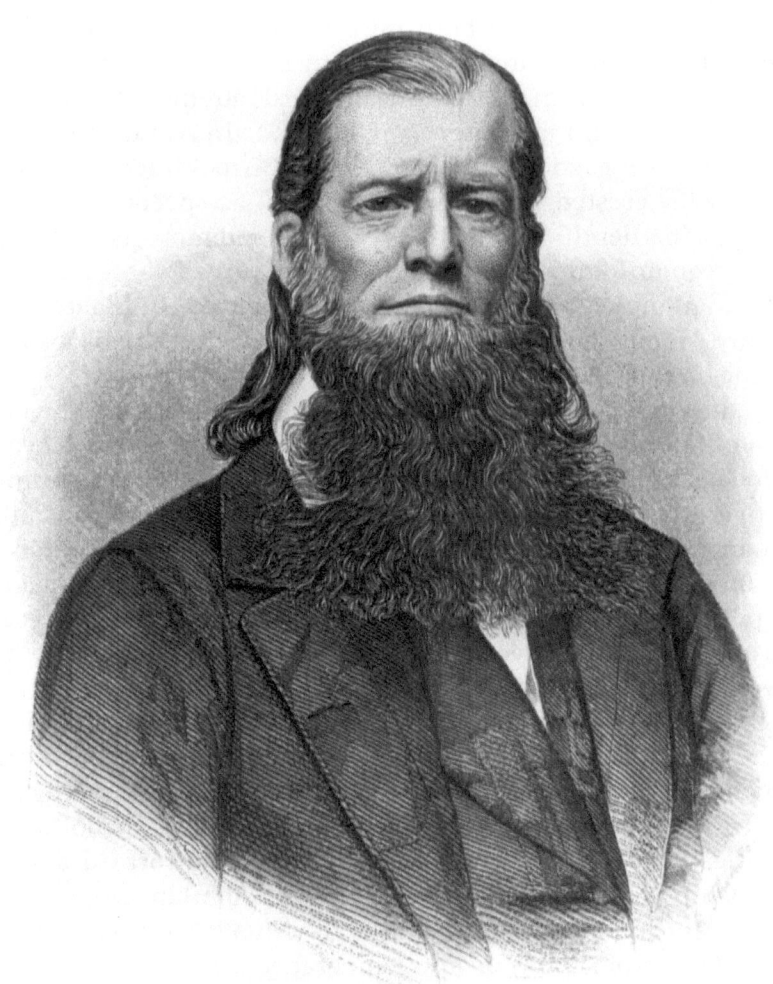

James Caleb Jackson
From Jackson, *The Sexual Organism* (Boston: B. Leverett Emerson, 1862)

The Health Reformers

Although Gleason's water treatments were often so harsh Jackson feared for his very life, his health did improve, and his interest in hydropathy grew correspondingly. By the end of his stay in Cuba, he and Gleason had agreed to go into partnership and open another water cure, Glen Haven, at the south end of Skaneateles Lake. Unfortunately, this venture turned out to be something of a disappointment, and after a few years Gleason sold his interest and moved elsewhere with all but two of the patients, leaving Jackson, the business manager, with a practically vacant building and no physician. Prospects for the future looked bleak indeed, but Jackson was not one to throw in his towels without a fight. He temporarily closed down the institution for the winter, enrolled in an eclectic medical college in Syracuse, and returned in three months, diploma in hand, to run the water cure himself.[43]

One day Dr. Harriet N. Austin, an alumna of Mary Gove Nichols's shortlived hydropathic college who was now practicing in nearby Owasco, called on Jackson for a professional consultation. She made such a favorable impression, he invited her to join the staff of Glen Haven, now doing so thriving a business that the assistance of a second physician was needed. Eventually Jackson adopted the young woman as his daughter, and together they turned Glen Haven into a thoroughly hygienic institution where only vegetarian meals were served and only reform dresses were worn. Women's clothing received their special attention, convinced as they were that current styles were doing irreparable harm to the health of American women. Inspired by the so-called Bloomer costume — actually designed by Gerrit Smith's daughter Elizabeth Smith Miller — they devised their own short dress-and-trousers combination, dubbed the "American costume." To display their handiwork and to promote its adoption elsewhere, they entertained a convention of dress reformers at Glen Haven in February, 1856, which resulted in the founding of a National Dress Reform Association.[44]

---

mation regarding Jackson's early life comes largely from his unpublished autobiographical memoir, now in private hands and quoted extensively in Conklin.

43. Conklin, *The Jackson Health Resort*, pp. 108-9.

44. Ibid., pp. 113-14; Walker, "The Health Reform Movement," p. 213; James C. Jackson, *How to Treat the Sick without Medicine* (Dansville, N.Y.: Austin, Jackson & Co., 1872), pp. 66-67. Harriet Austin also attended the 1854-55 winter session of the

In 1858 a disastrous fire swept through Glen Haven, leaving Jackson and Austin not only without a water cure but also without compensation, since their insurance company had just gone bankrupt. Undaunted, the two hydropaths somehow scraped together sufficient cash to purchase a defunct cure about fifty miles south of Rochester outside the town of Dansville, and on October 1 they proudly opened the doors of "Our Home on the Hillside" for patients. At first the local townspeople seemed less than delighted with their eccentric new neighbors who lived communally and dressed so queerly, and Jackson took precautionary measures to avoid undue hostilities. He later described the situation:

> All the women who came with us to enter into our employment wore the American Costume. A style of dress of this kind had never been seen in the town and so I issued an edict, forbidding any of our helpers to go into the village at all, until I gave the word, knowing that this would be the point around which opposition could rally and it would be impossible to keep our women from being stared at and perhaps insulted if they undertook to walk the streets.... At that day, for a woman to wear the American Costume was to so apparel herself as to lead everyone to suppose she was loose in virtue.[45]

Eventually the novelty wore off, and the health reformers and the citizens of Dansville settled down to a life of peaceful coexistence.

Our Home was not a resort for pleasure seekers. The physical facilities were comfortable, but nothing more. Long, narrow corridors wound through the rambling main building leading to small, uncurtained rooms, heated in winter by wood-burning "box stoves." Each day began promptly at six o'clock with the ritual beating of a Chinese gong and, for the hearty, a cold plunge in sometimes icy water. A half-hour after rising all residents gathered in the large parlor for

---

Eclectic Medical Institute of Cincinnati; "Eclectic Medical Institute: Eleventh Annual Announcement," *Eclectic Medical Journal*, XIV (September, 1855), 399.

45. James Caleb Jackson, autobiographical memoir, quoted in Conklin, *The Jackson Health Resort*, p. 116. In addition to espousing socialism, Jackson wanted to modify the traditional marriage and family structure; "Letter from Dr. Jackson," *Laws of Life*, X (December, 1867), 185.

"Father" Jackson's daily exhortation on the laws of life. Then it was on to the dining hall for a vegetarian breakfast around long, common tables, where seats were assigned by lot each week to ensure a properly democratic mix at mealtime. Jackson's water cure was one of the very few that served only two meals a day — breakfast at eight, dinner at two-thirty. Food, plentiful but plain, consisted principally of a variety of "Graham" dishes, vegetables, and piles of fresh fruit. Meat, butter, white-flour bread, tea and coffee were positively not allowed on the premises. A miscellany of water treatments, simple exercises, and amusements filled the remaining hours of the day. By eight-thirty all kerosene lamps were extinguished, and the weary patients tumbled into their hard beds of sea-grass and cotton mattresses on wooden slats.[46]

In the early days of Our Home specific treatments were "limited chiefly to half-baths, packs, sitz baths, plunges and dripping sheets." Under no circumstances would Jackson prescribe drugs. "In my entire practice," he once boasted, "I have never given a dose of medicine; not so much as I should have administered had I taken a homeopathic pellet of the seven-millionth dilution, and dissolving it in Lake Superior, given my patients of its waters." His medical faith rested implicitly on ten natural remedies: "First, air; second, food; third, water; fourth, sunlight; fifth, dress; sixth, exercise; seventh, sleep; eighth, rest; ninth, social influence; tenth, mental and moral forces."[47]

Through the 1850s and the following decades Jackson wrote compulsively on all facets of health reform. "This reformation has gotten my soul by a grip as strong as death," he explained, "and woe is me if I falter." For years his by-line graced virtually every issue of the *Water-Cure Journal,* and after moving to Dansville in 1858 he began publishing his own health paper, first called the *Letter Box,* then *Laws of Life.* His most popular book, *How to Treat the Sick without Medicine,* en-

---

46. This account of life at Our Home is based on personal reminiscences collected in Conklin, *The Jackson Health Resort,* pp. 31-32, 79-81, 171. On the number of meals per day at the water cures, see J. C. Jackson, "Clifton Springs and Our Home," *Laws of Life,* III (September, 1860), 137; and "Two Meals a Day," ibid., III (November, 1860), 174.

47. Conklin, *The Jackson Health Resort,* p. 81; Jackson, *How to Treat the Sick without Medicine,* pp. 25-26.

joyed widespread use among those who distrusted physicians, while his numerous little pamphlets circulated throughout the country. His favorite subject and professional specialty was sexual disorders. In eleven years he treated over *four thousand* cases of spermatorrhea alone, and grew so astute at diagnosing sexual abuses, he could spot masturbators merely by the gait of their walk or the flatness of their breasts. For those who could not afford a personal consultation with the doctor, he provided a series of cheap six-cent tracts dealing with various sexual problems, as well as a special fifty-cent "private circular" on "How to Rear Beautiful Children."[48]

Of all Jackson's writings, probably the most influential in terms of long-range effects was a modest-looking article on diphtheria published January 15, 1863, in a rural New York newspaper, the *Yates County Chronicle*. At the time of the article's appearance, a severe diphtheria epidemic was raging through much of the United States, and by a twist of fate the paper fell into the hands of an anxious mother who was nursing her two sons through an apparent attack. When the simple water treatments described by the Dansville physician proved successful, the grateful mother at once began sharing her discovery with others and thus embarked upon a lifelong career as a prophetess of health reform. Her name was Ellen G. White.[49]

---

48. J. C. Jackson, "Work! Yes, Work!" *Water-Cure Journal,* XXVII (January, 1859), 3; Jackson in an advertisement for Our Home, ibid., XXXI (May, 1861), 77; Jackson, *The Sexual Organism, and Its Healthful Management* (Boston: B. Leverett Emerson, 1862), pp. 65-67. For a sample list of Jackson's tracts see *The Letter Box,* I (December 15, 1858), 104.

49. J. C. Jackson's article was reprinted, with an editorial introduction, in the *R&H,* XXI (February 17, 1863), 89-91.

CHAPTER FOUR

Dansville Days

"... it is as truly a sin against Heaven, to violate a law of life, as to break one of the ten commandments."

L. B. Coles[1]

"It is as truly a sin to violate the laws of our being as it is to break the ten commandments."

Ellen G. White[2]

Ellen White's chance reading of Jackson's article on diphtheria in January, 1863, was by no means the first Adventist encounter with health reform. Adventist involvement actually went back to the days before the Great Disappointment of 1844 when prominent Millerites such as the Reverend Charles Fitch, Ezekiel Hale, Jr., and Dr. Larkin B. Coles publicly allied themselves with the reformers. Such an alliance was not at all unusual; as Charles E. Rosenberg has pointed out, the unorthodox in religion commonly displayed a marked affinity for heterodox medicine, which they tended to view in a moral rather than in a scientific light.[3]

    1. L. B. Coles, *Philosophy of Health: Natural Principles of Health and Cure* (rev. ed.; Boston: Ticknor, Reed, & Fields, 1853), p. 216.
    2. EGW, *Christian Temperance and Bible Hygiene* (Battle Creek: Good Health Publishing Co., 1890), p. 53.
    3. Charles E. Rosenberg, *The Cholera Years: The United States in 1832, 1849, and*

In the early 1860s Jackson's water cure in Dansville became a favorite retreat for ailing Sunday-keeping Adventists. Daniel T. Taylor, Adventist hymnist and minister, resided at Our Home for an entire year while undergoing the water treatment — "mostly hot or warm externally & internally perpetually." He in turn influenced Joshua V. Himes, formerly Miller's top assistant, to join him when the latter's health broke early in 1861. Elder and Mrs. Himes had been friends of the Jacksons for some time, but it was Joshua's remarkable cure at Our Home that finally made wholehearted health reformers out of them. Favorable notices of Jackson's books and water cure began appearing in Himes's *Voice of the Prophets,* and later, after Himes moved to Michigan and changed the name of his paper to *Voice of the West,* each issue for a while featured a "Health Department," to which Jackson was an occasional contributor.[4]

Even the sabbatarians displayed more than passing interest in the health-reform movement. Joseph Bates, as we have already noted, adopted Grahamism in 1843 and spent decades as a temperance crusader. John Loughborough took to eating Graham bread and reading the *Water-Cure Journal* in 1848, after learning about health reform from an uncle in western New York. J. P. Kellogg, of Tyrone, Michigan — father of Merritt, John Harvey, Will Keith, and thirteen other children — raised his sizable brood by the *Water-Cure Journal* and sent three of his older sons, including Merritt, to reform-minded Oberlin College. Roswell F. Cottrell, who served on the editorial committee of the *Review and Herald* after the move to

---

1866 (Chicago: University of Chicago Press, 1962), pp. 161-62. Fitch's health reform activities are mentioned in Hebbel E. Hoff and John F. Fulton, "The Centenary of the First American Physiological Society Founded at Boston by William A. Alcott and Sylvester Graham," Institute of the History of Medicine, *Bulletin,* V (October, 1937), 704. On Hale, see Francis D. Nichol, *The Midnight Cry* (Washington: Review and Herald Publishing Assn., 1944), pp. 212-14.

4. Daniel T. Taylor to Samuel F. Haven, August 7, 1861 (from a copy in the library of the Review and Herald Publishing Association, Washington, D.C.; original at the American Antiquarian Society); J. V. Himes, "My Sickness and Cure," *Voice of the Prophets,* II (January, 1861), 37-38; [Himes], "Two Important Books on Health," ibid., IV (January, 1863), 16; J. C. Jackson, "Morning Worship Talk-No. 1," *Voice of the West,* II (November 7, 1865), 176; "Good Words," *Laws of Life,* VIII (August, 1865), 122. John Himes and his wife also spent some time at Dansville; Obituary of John G. L. Himes, *Advent Herald,* XXV (July 26, 1864), 119.

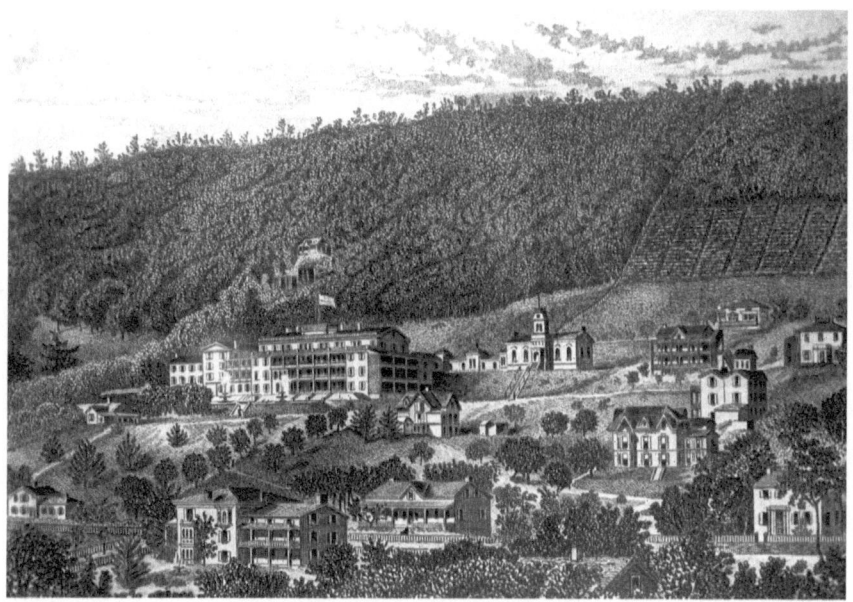

Our Home on the Hillside, Dansville, New York, as it appeared in the 1860s
Courtesy of Mr. William D. Conklin

Battle Creek, began experimenting in the late 1840s with a vegetarian diet and a daily bath.[5] All these men were closely associated with the Whites and undoubtedly spoke to them of their experiences in health reform.

And there were others. J. W. Clarke, of Green Lake County, Wisconsin, turned to vegetarianism and hydropathy in the late 1840s. William McAndrew in Michigan and an anonymous sister in Rhode

---

5. Joseph Bates, "Experience in Health Reform," *HR,* VI (July, 1871), 20-21. J. N. Loughborough, "Waymarks in the History of the Health Reform Movement," *Medical Missionary,* X (December, 1899), 6-7; John Harvey Kellogg, autobiographical memoir, October 21, 1938, and "My Search for Health," MS, January 16, 1942 (Kellogg Papers, MHC); R. F. Cottrell, "Experience in Health Reform," *HR,* VII (August, 1872), 251. See also W. C. White, "The Relationship of the White and Kellogg Families," MS. *circa* 1931 (DF 127g, White Estate). The pervasiveness of health-reform knowledge among Seventh-day Adventists is revealed by the fact that many members immediately noted the similarity between Mrs. White's views and those of Jackson and Trall; EGW, "Questions and Answers," *R&H,* XXX (October 8, 1867), 260.

Island embraced health reform in the early 1850s. Uriah Smith's sister Annie, after copy-editing the *Review and Herald* in Saratoga Springs and Rochester, spent several months at a water cure before her death in 1855. H. F. Phelps and H. C. Miller were reading water-cure publications and taking their first steps toward health reform in the early 1860s. And by early 1863 Marietta V. Cook, of Kirkville, New York, was dressing in the American costume, enjoying meals of "plain food," and corresponding with the doctors at Dansville.[6]

Despite these early signs of interest, Seventh-day Adventists as a body did not awaken to the cause of health reform until 1863, a period during which a major change in attitudes toward health occurred among the leaders of the sect. One of the first indications of a health-reform awakening was the reprinting of Dr. Jackson's "Diphtheria, Its Causes, Treatment and Cure" on the front page of the February 17 issue of the *Review and Herald,* accompanied by a note from the pen of James White recommending the hydropathic approach to medicine. On the basis of Ellen's recent experience using Jackson's treatments on her two boys, as well as on the six-year-old child of Elder Moses Hull, James had come to place "a good degree of confidence in [Jackson's] manner of treating diseases." He failed to mention that over two years earlier, while suffering from lung fever in Wisconsin, he had had another successful encounter with the water cure.[7]

---

6. J. W. Clarke, "A Vegetarian Survives Disease without Drugs," *HR,* III (April, 1869), 194-95; Wm. McAndrew to Uriah Smith, February 11, 1857, *R&H,* IX (February 26, 1857), 135; 5. N. Haskell, "What the Health Reform Has Done," *HR,* VI (July, 1871), 13; Mrs. Rebekah Smith, *Poems: With a Sketch of the Life and Experience of Annie R. Smith* (Manchester, N.H.: John B. Clarke, 1871), pp. 96-107; H. F. Phelps, "My Experience: No. 1," *HR,* II (March, 1868), 142-43; H. C. Miller, "Experience," *HR,* III (September, 1868), 52; "A Good Beginning," *Laws of Life,* VI (March, 1863), 43; "Good Words from the Readers of the Laws Received during the Month of March," ibid., VI (April, 1863), 53. See also "The People's Estimate of the 'Laws,'" ibid., VI (November, 1863), 176. In 1858 a Joseph Clarke recommended "Plain, coarse food at regular intervals, regular rest and exercise, habits of temperance in all things"; "Health," *R&H,* February 11, 1858, 106. I have been unable to prove that J. W. Clarke, Phelps, and Miller were Seventh-day Adventists, but it is likely that they were.

7. James C. Jackson, "Diphtheria, Its Causes, Treatment and Cure," *R&H,* XXI (February 17, 1863), 89-91; James White, "Western Tour," *R&H,* XVI (November 13, 1860), 204. Jackson reprinted White's endorsement in the *Laws of Life,* VI (April,

Dansville Days

The Jackson article not only described specific treatments for diphtheria, it spelled out the basic principles of health reform in tips on eating properly, dressing sensibly, and breathing lots of fresh air. We know that James White was beginning to recognize the importance of these measures, for in the February 10 *Review and Herald* he called air, water, and light "God's great remedies," preferable to "doctors and their drugs." He reported proudly that both he and his wife slept year-round with the windows wide open and took "a cold-water sponge-bath" every morning. Four pages later he inserted an article on the evils of sleeping in poorly ventilated rooms, taken from an exchange publication. The language appears to be Dr. W. W. Hall's, but the selection is not found in earlier issues of *Hall's Journal of Health*.[8]

During the month of May, James White continued to focus on hygienic living in the *Review and Herald* with a note from Dio Lewis on dress reform and two extracts from *Hall's Journal of Health,* one urging a meatless, low-fat diet during spring and summer, the other recommending two meals a day.[9] Thus by June of 1863 Seventh-day Adventists were already in possession of the main outlines of the health reform message. What they now needed to become a church of health reformers was not additional information, but a sign from God indicating his pleasure.[10]

1863), 64. How the Whites ran across Jackson's essay, first published in Penn Yan, New York, is not certain; it is possible that the newspaper clipping was sent to them by Elder John N. Andrews, an Adventist evangelist then preaching in western New York, who caught diphtheria during the 1863 epidemic and who was among the earliest sabbatarians to visit Our Home. See Diary of Mrs. Angeline Stevens Andrews, entry for February 17, 1863 (C. Burton Clark Collection).

8. [James White], "Pure Air," *R&H,* XXI (February 10, 1863), 84; "What Is in the Bedroom?" ibid., p. 88. Portions of "What Is in the Bedroom?" are similar to passages in W. W. Hall, "Unhealthy Houses," *Hall's Journal of Health,* IX (June, 1862), 144; and Hall, *Sleep; or The Hygiene of the Night* (New York: Hurd and Houghton, 1870), p. 322.

9. Dio Lewis, "Talks about Health," *R&H,* XXI (May 5, 1863), 179; W. W. Hall, "Spring Suggestions in Regard to Health," *R&H,* XXI (May 12, 1863), 185; [Hall], "Eating and Sleeping," *R&H,* XXI (May 19, 1863), 195. An earlier selection from Lewis appeared in 1862; "Talks about Health: A Word about Dress," *R&H,* XX (November 25, 1862), 203.

10. J. H. Waggoner offered a similar interpretation in 1866. The Adventist con-

Divine approval of the health crusade came on the evening of June 5, 1863, while Ellen White and a dozen friends were kneeling in prayer at the home of the Aaron Hilliards, just outside the village of Otsego, Michigan. Earlier that Friday the Whites had driven up from Battle Creek with several carriages full of Adventists to lend their support to a series of tent meetings being held in the village. At sundown the Battle Creek visitors gathered in the Hilliard home to usher in the Sabbath with prayer. Ellen, the first to speak, began by asking the Lord for strength and encouragement. Lately, neither she nor James had been well. Her familiar fainting spells were recurring once or twice a day, while excessive cares and responsibilities had brought James to the verge of a mental and physical collapse.[11]

As Ellen prayed, she slipped to her husband's side and rested her hands on his bowed shoulders. In a short time she was off in vision, receiving heaven-sent instructions on the preservation and restoration of health. She and James were directed not to assume such a heavy burden in the Adventist cause, but to share their responsibilities with others. She was to curtail her sewing and entertaining; James was to quit dwelling on "the dark, gloomy side" of life. In a less personal vein, she saw that it was a religious duty for God's people to care for their health and not violate the laws of life. The Lord wanted them "to come out against intemperance of every kind, — intemperance in working, in eating, in drinking, and in drugging." They were to be his instruments in directing the world "to God's great medicine, water, pure soft water, for diseases, for health, for cleanliness, and for luxury."[12]

For a couple of weeks following her vision Ellen White seemed reluctant to say much about its contents. Then one day while riding

---

tribution to health reform was not adding new knowledge, he said, but making it "an essential part of present truth, to be received with the blessing of God, or rejected at our peril." Waggoner, "Present Truth," *R&H,* XXVIII (August 7, 1866), 76-77.

11. William C. White, "Sketches and Memories of James and Ellen G. White," *R&H,* CXIII (November 24, 1936), 3; Martha D. Amadon, "Mrs. E. G. White in Vision," November 24, 1925 (DF 105, White Estate); EGW, MS sermon, May 21, 1904 (MS-50-1904, White Estate). The date of the event is frequently given as June 6, because it occurred after sundown on June 5.

12. Amadon, "Mrs. E. G. White in Vision"; EGW, MS relating the Vision of June 6, 1863 (MS-1-1863, White Estate).

Dansville Days

in a carriage with Horatio S. Lay, a self-styled Adventist physician from Allegan, she briefly mentioned some of the things she had seen. What he heard whetted his curiosity. When the Whites visited Allegan for a funeral a few days later, he took the opportunity to invite them and nine-year-old Willie home to dinner. After the meal he immediately began pumping Mrs. White for more details of her recent vision. As Willie recalled seventy-three years later, his mother at first demurred, saying "that she was not familiar with medical language, and that much of the matter presented to her was so different from the commonly accepted views that she feared she could not relate it so that it could be understood." Lay's persistence eventually overcame her hesitance, however, and for two hours she related what she had witnessed. According to Willie,

> She said that pain and sickness were not ordinarily, as was commonly supposed, due to a foreign influence, attacking the body, but that they were in most cases an effort of nature to overcome unnatural conditions resulting from the transgression of some of nature's laws. She said that by the use of poisonous drugs many bring upon themselves lifelong illness, and that it had been revealed to her that more deaths had resulted from drug taking than from any other cause.

At this point Lay interrupted to say that certain "wise and eminent physicians" were currently teaching exactly what she had been shown. Thus encouraged, she went on to condemn the use of all stimulants and narcotics, to caution against meat eating and to emphasize "the remedial value of water treatments, pure air, and sunshine."[13]

Ellen White's first published account of her June 5 vision, a short thirty-two-page sketch tucked into the fourth volume of *Spiritual Gifts* did not appear until fifteen months after the event. She had hoped to provide a fuller report, but other duties and poor health had made that impossible. For the past year she had labored at her desk almost constantly, often writing twelve hours a day. At

---

13. W. C. White, "Sketches and Memories," pp. 3-4; W. C. White, "The Origin of the Light on Health Reform among Seventh-day Adventists," *Medical Evangelist,* XX (December 28, 1933), 2.

times her head continually ached, and for weeks she seldom got more than two hours' sleep at night.[14]

In her essay "Health," which reads in places like L. B. Coles, she recited the established principles of health reform, attributing them to her recent vision. Willful violations of the laws of health — particularly "Intemperance in eating and drinking, and the indulgence of base passions" — caused the greatest human degeneracy. Tobacco, tea, and coffee depraved the appetite, prostrated the system, and blunted the spiritual sensibilities. Meat-eating led to untold diseases; swine's flesh alone produced "scrofula, leprosy and cancerous humors." Living in low-lying areas exposed one to fever-producing "poisonous miasma."[15]

---

14. EGW, "Writing Out the Light on Health Reform" (MS-7-1867, White Estate); EGW, *Spiritual Gifts: Important Facts of Faith, Laws of Health, and Testimonies Nos. 1-10* (Battle Creek: SDA Publishing Assn., 1864), pp. 120-51. An announcement for this fourth volume of *Spiritual Gifts* appeared in the *R&H*, XXIV (September 6, 1864), 120.

15. EGW, *Spiritual Gifts* (1864), pp. 120-51. The similarities between Ellen White and L. B. Coles can be seen in the following passages taken from EGW, *Spiritual Gifts* (1864), and Coles, *Philosophy of Health* (3rd ed.; Boston: Ticknor and Fields, 1855):

EGW, p. 128: Tobacco is a poison of the most deceitful and malignant kind, having an exciting, then a paralyzing influence upon the nerves of the body.	Coles, p. 84: [Tobacco's] first influence is felt upon the nervous system. It excites and then deadens nervous susceptibility.
EGW, p. 129: The whole system under the influence of these stimulants [tea and coffee] often becomes intoxicated. And to just that degree that the nervous system is excited by false stimulants, will be the prostration which will follow after the influence of the exciting cause has abated.	Coles, p. 79: [Tea] is a direct, diffusible, and active stimulant. Its effects are very similar to those of alcoholic drinks, except that of drunkenness.... Like alcohol, it increases, beyond its healthy and natural action, the whole animal and mental machinery; after which there comes a reaction — a corresponding languor and debility.
EGW, p. 133: I was shown that more deaths have been caused by drug-taking than from all other causes combined. If there was in the land one physician in the place of thousands, a vast amount of premature mortality would	Coles, p. 207: It has been my settled conviction, for many years, as before stated, that there is more damage than good done with medicine ... it has been, for many years, my belief that the standard of health and longevity of our

Dansville Days

Her strongest language, however, was reserved for the medical profession: "I was shown that more deaths have been caused by drug-taking than from all other causes combined. If there was in the land one physician in the place of thousands, a vast amount of premature mortality would be prevented." All drugs, vegetable as well as mineral, were proscribed. The Lord specifically and graphically forbade the use of opium, mercury, calomel, quinine, and strychnine. "A branch was presented before me bearing flat seeds," Ellen recalled. "Upon it was written, *Nux vomica, strychnine*. Beneath was written, No antidote." Of all the medical sects, only drugless hydropathy received divine sanction. Since medicines were so dangerous and had "no power to cure," the only safe course was to rely on the natural remedies recommended by the health reformers: pure soft water, sunshine, fresh air, and simple food — preferably eaten only twice a day.[16]

In the months following her June 5 vision, as Ellen White traveled about the Midwest and Northeast speaking on her favorite topic of health, curious listeners sometimes inquired if she had not previously read the *Laws of Life,* the *Water-Cure Journal,* or any of the works of Drs. Jackson and Trall. Her stock reply was that she had not and

---

be prevented. Multitudes of physicians, and multitudes of drugs, have cursed the inhabitants of the earth, and have carried thousands and tens of thousands to untimely graves.	land would now be far above its present position, if there had never been a single physician or a single drug in it. . . . Dr. Johnson says: "I declare my conscientious opinion . . . that if there were not a single physician, surgeon, apothecary, chemist, druggist, or drug, on the face of the earth, there would be less sickness and less mortality than now."

Compare also Ellen White with Coles, *The Beauties and Deformities of Tobacco-Using* (rev. ed.; Boston: Ticknor and Fields, 1855):

EGW, p. 126: [Tobacco] affects the brain and benumbs the sensibilities, so that the mind cannot clearly discern spiritual things. . . .	Coles, p. 97: [Tobacco-users] so deaden the natural sensibilities of body and mind, by using it, that they are not immediately susceptible of the impulses of the Holy Spirit, by which alone a true spirit of devotion and religious enjoyment are induced.

16. Ibid., pp. 129-30, 133-40, 142-45.

would not until she had fully written out her views, "lest it should be said that I had received my light upon the subject of health from physicians, and not from the Lord." But the embarrassing questions persisted until finally she issued a formal statement in the *Review and Herald* disclaiming any familiarity with health-reform publications prior to receiving and writing out her vision. Referring specifically to Jackson's, she said: "I did not know that such works existed until September, 1863, when in Boston, Mass., my husband saw them advertised in a periodical called the *Voice of the Prophets,* published by Eld. J. V. Himes. My husband ordered the works from Dansville and received them at Topsham, Maine. His business gave him no time to peruse them, and as I determined not to read them until I had written out my views, the books remained in their wrappers."[17]

In her anxiety to appear uninfluenced by any earthly agency — "My views were written independent of books or of the opinion of others" — Ellen White failed to mention certain pertinent facts. Not only did she ignore her reading of Jackson's article on diphtheria nearly six months before her vision, but she incorrectly gave the time when James had first learned of Jackson's other works. On August 13, 1863, one month before James supposedly had any knowledge of Dansville, Dr. Jackson wrote him apologizing for his long delay in replying to White's request for information about his books. It seems that James had written Jackson sometime in June, for in December of 1864 he stated that eighteen months earlier (June, 1863) he had sent off to Dansville "for an assortment of their works, that might cost from ten to twenty-five dollars. Then we knew not the name of a single publication offered for sale at that house. We heard from reliable sources that there was something valuable there, and resolved to put in for a share."[18]

If James's account is accurate, then Ellen was also wrong in implying that her husband first learned of the Dansville publications from an advertisement in the *Voice of the Prophets.* James said that he knew not "the name of a single publication" when he wrote Dr.

17. W. C. White, "Sketches and Memories," p. 4; EGW, "Writing Out the Light on Health Reform"; EGW, "Questions and Answers," p. 260.
18. EGW, "Writing Out the Light on Health Reform"; James C. Jackson to James White, August 13, 1863 (White Estate); J[ames] W[hite], "The Health Reform," *R&H,* XXV (December 13, 1864), 20.

Jackson; but had he read the notice in Himes's journal, he would have known at least three titles: *Consumption* and *The Sexual Organism* by Jackson, and *Pathology of the Reproductive Organs* by Trall.[19]

Two other details bear on the accuracy of Ellen White's disclaimer. She insisted that the books from Dansville remained in their wrappers after arriving in Topsham, but already by December 12 James was mailing Jackson's *Consumption* from Topsham to a friend in Brookfield, New York. And if Ellen White regularly read the *Review and Herald* that her husband edited, as surely she did, then she saw in the October 27 issue an article by Dr. Jackson on hoops, taken from the *Laws of Life*.[20]

Ellen White's conversion to health reform did much to change the eating habits of Seventh-day Adventists. The revolution began in her own household. She desperately wanted to switch all at once to the two-meal Graham system, but her stomach rebelled. Having been a self-confessed "great meat-eater," she found the substitution of unbolted wheat bread intolerable. For a few meals she could eat nothing, but at last the victory was gained when she resolutely placed her hands on her recalcitrant stomach and warned it, "You may wait

---

19. "Two Important Books on Health," *Voice of the Prophets*, IV (January, 1863), 16. If James White did see an advertisement in the *Voice of the Prophets* in September, 1863, this was undoubtedly the one. In an attempt to harmonize the statements of James and Ellen White, Ron Graybill of the White Estate has suggested "that James called her attention to the ad in *Voice of the Prophets* during their stay in Boston in September of 1863 and stated to her that he had ordered these books. She could easily have assumed that he meant that he had ordered them on that occasion — September of 1863 — when in fact he had ordered them earlier." (Ron Graybill to the author, March 11, 1975.) This explanation raises the question of why James made no effort to correct Ellen's wrong impression when the true sequence of events was so important an issue.

20. James White to Ira Abbey, December 12, 1863 (White Estate); [J. C. Jackson], "Which Will You Have, Hoops or Health?" *R&H*, XXII (October 27, 1863), 176. Although James White was editor of the *Review and Herald* in 1863, he was traveling in the East when Jackson's article appeared in October. During the second half of 1863 the *Review and Herald* carried several other articles on health reform that Ellen White probably read before writing out what she had seen in her June 5 vision: "Keep Your Teeth Clean," *R&H*, XXII (July 28, 1863); Dio Lewis, "How to Prevent Colds," *R&H*, XXII (August 4, 1863), 75; Lewis, "Eating when Sick," *R&H*, XXII (August 11, 1863), 86-87; Lewis, "Talks about Health: A Word to My Fat Friends," *R&H*, XXII (August 25, 1863), 98-99; W. T. Vail, "Eating and Sleeping," *R&H*, XXIII (December 8, 1863), 11.

until you can eat bread." Before long she actually came to enjoy the once-hated article and accorded it a central place, along with fruit and vegetables, in the White family diet. "Our plain food, eaten twice a day, is enjoyed with a keen relish," she was able to write by 1864. "We have no meat, cake, or any rich food upon our table. We use no lard, but in its place, milk, cream, and some butter. We have our food prepared with but little salt, and have dispensed with spices of all kinds. We breakfast at seven, and take our dinner at one." On this regimen, her health took a marked turn for the better. Her periodic "shocks of paralysis" ceased; her "dropsy and heart disease" abated; and her weight dropped by twenty-five unneeded pounds she had gained since her youth. For years she had never felt better.[21]

Unfortunately, not all the members of her family shared her experience. Her husband's health improved at first but then declined alarmingly in the next couple years, and during the winter of 1863-64 two of her boys came down with critical cases of pneumonia. Despite (or because of) the efforts of a physician, her eldest son, Henry, died of the disease at age sixteen and was laid to rest beside his baby brother, Herbert, in the Oak Hill Cemetery in Battle Creek. A short time after the funeral Willie, too, caught "lung fever." This time his frightened parents decided not to consult a physician, but to administer water treatments and pray for his recovery. For five anxious days he lingered near death, but then his mother had an inspired dream in which a heavenly physician assured her that Willie would not die, "for he has not the injurious influence of drugs to recover from." All he needed was cool, fresh air, said the messenger; "Stove heat destroys the vitality of the air, and weakens the lungs." By the next day Willie was feeling better and was soon fully recovered. Needless to say, these two events substantially increased Ellen White's faith in the curative power of water over that of earthly physicians.[22]

For most Adventists, acceptance of health reform meant principally three things: a vegetarian diet, two meals a day, and no drugs

---

21. EGW, *Spiritual Gifts* (1864), pp. 153-54; EGW, *Testimonies*, II, 371-72.
22. EGW, "Our Late Experience," *R&H*, XXVII (February 27, 1866), 97; EGW, *Spiritual Gifts* (1864), pp. 151-53; Dores E. Robinson, *The Story of Our Health Message* (3rd ed.; Nashville: Southern Publishing Assn., 1965), pp. 86-87; EGW, "That Spare Bed," *HR*, IX (February, 1874), 41.

or stimulants. Its progress among them was immortalized in a song, "The Health Reform," composed by Elder Roswell Cottrell:

> When men are beginning the work of reform,
> Casting off their gross idols, as ships in a storm
> Cast off the most cumbersome part of their freight,
> They feel the improvement and progress is great.
>   Oh, yes, I see it is so,
>   And the clearer it is the farther I go.
>
> First goes the tobacco, most filthy of all,
> Then drugs, pork and whisky, together must fall,
> Then coffee and spices, and sweet-meats and tea,
> And fine flour and flesh-meats and pickles must flee.
>   Oh, yes, I see it is so,
>   And the clearer it is the farther I go.
>
> Things hurtful and poisonous laying aside,
> The good and the wholesome alone must abide;
> And these with a moderate, temperate use,
> At regular seasons, avoiding abuse.
>   Oh, yes, I see it is so,
>   And the clearer it is the farther I go.
>
> A proper proportion of labor and rest,
> With good air and water, the purest and best,
> And clothing constructed to be a defense,
> Not following custom, but good common sense.
>   Oh, yes, I see it is so,
>   And the clearer it is the farther I go.
>
> Our frames disencumbered, our spirits are free,
> Our minds once beclouded now clearly can see;
> Brute passions no longer our natures control,
> But instead we act worthy a rational soul.
>   Oh, yes, I see it is so,
>   And the clearer it is the farther I go.
>
> Faith, patience and meekness, more brightly now shine
> Evincing the human allied to divine;

And religion, once viewed as a shield against wrath,
Becomes a delightsome and glorious path.
  Oh, yes, they know it is so,
  Who have chosen this light-giving pathway to go.[23]

Since so few knew anything about preparing meatless meals or giving fomentations, the *Review and Herald* undertook the task of educating the uninitiated by regularly excerpting appropriate selections from the writings of prominent reformers like Russell Trall, Dio Lewis, and L. B. Coles. Individuals who desired additional help could send in to the *Review* office in Battle Creek for cookbooks by Trall and Jackson or for special irons to make "Graham gems," a popular form of whole-wheat bread. A handful of Adventists were able to draw upon their own experiences to assist their fellow members through the transition. Martha Byington Amadon, daughter of the General Conference president, thoughtfully provided readers of the *Review and Herald* with hints on "How to Use Graham Flour," a ubiquitous substance used in making everything from bread and biscuits to puddings and cakes. By the time of the 1864 Michigan State Fair some Battle Creek sisters were so proficient at vegetarian cookery that they hauled stoves to the fairgrounds and publicly demonstrated their newly acquired skills.[24]

Right from the beginning of their health-reform days the Seventh-day Adventists, like their Sunday-keeping brethren, displayed a singular fondness for the Jackson water cure in Dansville. The person apparently most responsible for establishing this relationship was John N. Andrews, an itinerant preacher — later General Conference president and pioneer missionary — who in the early sixties was pitching his evangelistic tent in the towns and villages of western New York. It is not clear how or when he first learned of Our Home, but he possibly heard of it through Daniel T. Taylor, whom he had come to know while writing his *History of the Sabbath*, and whose

---

23. R. F. Cottrell, "'Oh, Yes, I See It Is So,'" *HR*, I (February, 1867), 105. For what it meant to be an Adventist health reformer, see the scores of testimonials in the early volumes of the *Health Reformer*.

24. M. D. Amadon, "How to Use Graham Flour," *R&H*, XXIV (November 1, 1864), 178-79; EGW, MS-27-1906, quoted in EGW, *Counsels on Diet and Foods* (Washington: Review and Herald Publishing Assn., 1938), p. 442.

brother Charles was a colleague of his in the ministry. The unpublished diary of Mrs. Andrews reveals that she and her husband were routinely using water treatments in their home by the spring of 1863 and that in January, 1864, John's co-laborers offered to send him to Our Home for a few weeks of rest and treatment. John, "loath to quit" his preaching, declined the invitation, but a few months later sent his badly crippled six-year-old son Mellie (Charles Melville) for a fifteen-week stay. After several weeks Mrs. Andrews joined her boy at Dansville, and although she at first felt "like a stranger in a strange land" amid so many dress reformers, she eventually came to respect the place and its dedicated physicians. Mellie's leg improved remarkably at the water cure, and by July he was able to return home nearly normal. Meanwhile, both his parents had become zealous health reformers, and as his father preached throughout the state, he also solicited subscriptions for the *Laws of Life* in order to earn a free copy of Trall's *Hydropathic Encyclopedia*.[25]

Possibly encouraged by the Andrewses, James and Ellen White decided in late autumn, 1864, that the time was right for a firsthand look at the Dansville facilities. They had contemplated such a visit since shortly after Ellen's June 5 vision, when James had written Jackson inquiring about a ministerial discount; but the trip had been postponed until Ellen had sketched out most of her vision, to avoid insinuations that she had come under the influence of the Dansville reformers. At last on Monday, September 5, following a weekend stopover in Rochester with the Andrewses, the Whites arrived at Our Home. Within a few days they were joined by Edson and Willie and their chaperone, Adelia Patten. Although the local press ignored the presence of the prophetess and her family, Dr. Jackson

---

25. Diary of Mrs. Angeline Stevens Andrews, October, 1859, to January, 1865 (C. Burton Clark Collection); J. N. Andrews, "My Experience in Health Reform," *HR*, IV (July, 1869), 8-10, VII (February, 1872), 44-45, VII (March, 1872), 76-77; Daniel T. Taylor, "Sabbatical Library for Sale," advertisement included with a letter to S. F. Haven, January 26, 1863 (from a copy in the library of Review and Herald Publishing Association, Washington, D.C.; original at the American Antiquarian Society). Andrews's role in introducing the Adventists to Dansville is mentioned in D. M. Canright, "Progress of Health Reform," *HR*, XIII (May, 1878), 133; and G. I. Butler to John Harvey Kellogg, March 7, 1906 (Kellogg Collection, MSU). The Andrewses may have learned about the Dansville water cure from Marietta V. Cook, a friend of theirs.

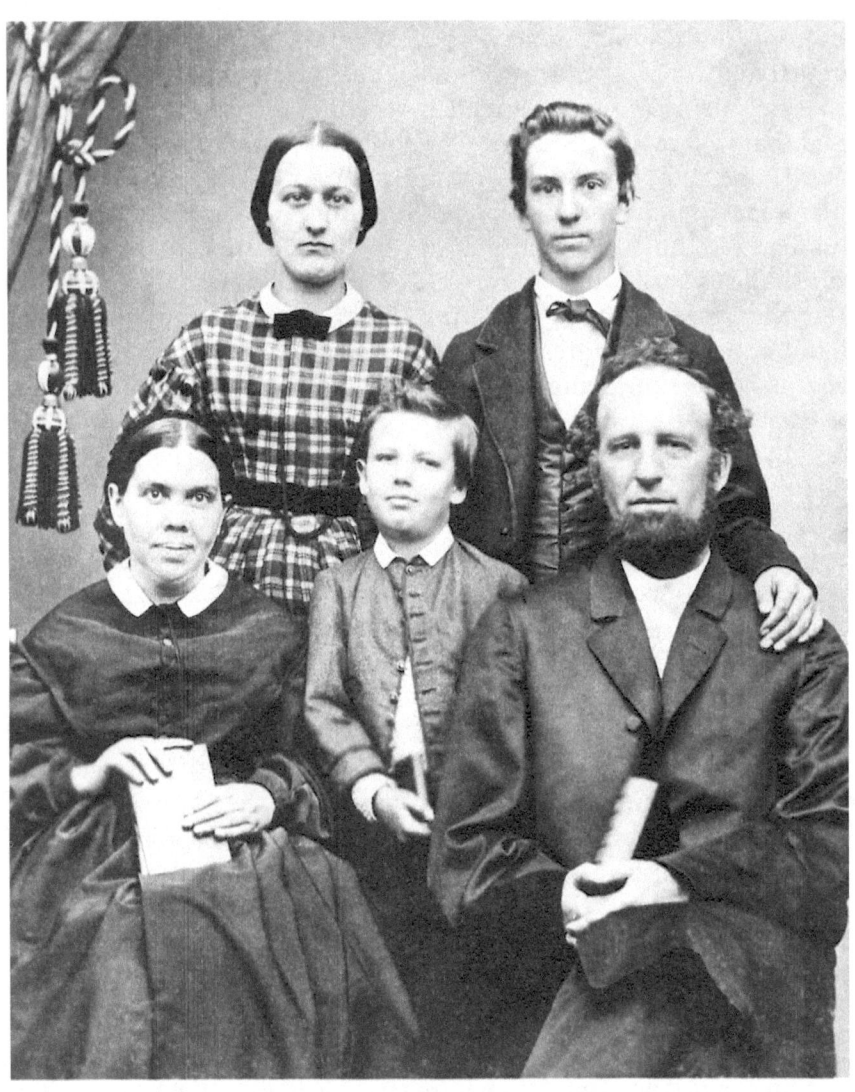

The White family and Adelia P. Patten about the time of their first visit to the Dansville water cure. Willie is between his parents; Edson is standing in the rear.
Courtesy Ellen G. White Estate, Inc.

Dansville Days

welcomed them all warmly and even invited Mrs. White to address a health-reform convention then in progress. Unlike Mrs. Andrews only a few months earlier, she had little reason to feel like a stranger, for already a colony of Adventists was forming at the water cure. Besides her family and Miss Patten, at least seven other Sabbath-keepers were there, including Dr. and Mrs. Horatio Lay, John Andrews, and Hiram Edson.[26]

For three weeks the Whites remained as guests of Our Home, gleaning all the information they could from daily observations of hydrotherapy and from Jackson's frequent lectures. Adelia Patten described the doctor's style: "he combines his theology, his medical instructions, his comical nonsense and his theatrical gestures all into his discourses. He flies about like a young man, and will come into the lecture hall with an old blue woolen cap on[,] which he takes off and puts under his arm and walks along and mounts the rostrum with all the firmness of an experienced lecturer."[27]

Fascinating to Ellen White was the "science" of phrenology, which Dr. Jackson practiced at five dollars a reading. Soon after the arrival of Edson and Willie she took them to the doctor for evaluations of their "constitutional organization, functional activity, temperament, predisposition to disease, natural aptitudes for business, fitness for connubial and maternal conditions, etc., etc." Writing to friends, she could scarcely conceal her elation with Jackson's flattering analysis: "I think Dr. Jackson gave an accurate account of the disposition and organization of our children. He pronounced Willie's head to be one of the best that has ever come under his observation. He gave a good description of Edson's character and peculiarities. I think this examination will be worth everything to Edson." Presumably she was not so pleased with the doctor's diagnosis of her condition as hysteria.[28]

---

26. Jackson to White, August 13, 1863; Diary of Mrs. Andrews; James White, "Eastern Tour," *R&H,* XXIV (November 22, 1864), 205; EGW to Edson and Willie White, June 13, 1865 (W-3-1865, White Estate). A search of the *Dansville Advertiser* and the *Herald* for 1864 and 1865 turned up no mention of the Whites. Mr. William D. Conklin, of Dansville, kindly assisted me in going through these newspapers.

27. Adelia P. Patten to Sister Lockwood, September 15, 1864 (White Estate).

28. EGW to Bro. and Sister Lockwood, September [14], 1864 (L-6-1864, White Estate); James C. Jackson, "Description of Character of Willie C. White . . . Sept. 14,

The American costume of "short" skirts over pants, worn by Dr. Harriet Austin and the other women of Our Home, also caught Ellen's fancy. The outfits did strike her as being on the mannish side, but she thought slight modifications could easily remedy that. "They have all styles of dress here," she wrote from Dansville.

> Some are very becoming, if not so short. We shall get patterns from this place, and I think we can get out a style of dress more healthful than we now wear, and yet not be bloomer or the American costume. Our dresses according to my idea, should be from four to six inches shorter than now worn, and should in no case reach lower than the top of the heel of the shoe, and could be a little shorter even than this with all modesty. I am going to get up a style of dress on my own hook which will accord perfectly with that which has been shown me [in vision]. Health demands it. Our feeble women must dispense with heavy skirts and tight waists if they value health.

"[D]on't groan now," she told her correspondent. "I am not going to extremes, but conscience and health requires a reform."[29]

The Battle Creek visitors found the food at Our Home plain even for their tastes. "We have the crackers," wrote Miss Patten; "they don't furnish 'gems' only in case of a wedding or some other extra occasion. They don't have salt. The pudding is thin and fresh squash and cabbage without salt or vinegar and oh such times. I had a little salt dish this noon and wanted to pocket the salt that was left and as none of our company had an envelope so had Bro. W[hite] tip it into his pass book."[30]

Even with an offended palate, Ellen White was so impressed with the overall program at Dansville that she began toying with the idea of setting up a similar institution in Battle Creek, "to which our

---

1864" (DF 783, White Estate). According to the testimony of a disaffected Adventist in Iowa, Mrs. White herself stated in 1865 that Jackson had "pronounced her a subject of Hysteria"; H. E. Carver, *Mrs. E. G. White's Claims to Divine Inspiration Examined* (2nd ed.; Marion, Iowa: Advent and Sabbath Advocate Press, 1877), pp. 75-76. Jackson apparently began giving "psycho-hygienic examinations of character" early in 1864; see his advertisement in *Laws of Life*, X (January, 1867), 15.

29. EGW to Bro. and Sister Lockwood, September [14], 1864.
30. Adelia P. Patten to Sister Lockwood, September 15, 1864.

Dansville Days

Sabbath keeping invalids can resort." At their own water cure the strait-laced Adventists could avoid certain problems encountered at Our Home. Dr. Jackson, she reported regretfully, allowed his patients to "have pleasureable excitement to keep their spirits up. They play cards for amusement, have a dance once a week and seem to mix these things up with religion." While such activities might be appropriate for those who had "no hope for a better life," they surely could not be condoned by Christians looking for Christ's return.[31]

Following three profitable weeks at Dansville, the Whites headed home to Battle Creek, brimming with enthusiasm for sitz baths, short skirts, and Graham mush. On the return trip they once again stopped for a brief visit with the Andrewses and indulged themselves in a little fresh fish, which James thoughtfully went out and purchased for breakfast one morning. Visions or not, vegetarianism was going to be a battle! For the next eleven months, while Sherman marched through Georgia and Grant pursued Lee in Virginia, James and Ellen campaigned throughout the Northern states proclaiming the gospel of health and salvation — at times, complained some dissident members, to the exclusion of other more pressing issues. It was difficult for these critics to understand why "nothing was shown about the duty of the brethren in view of the draft, but a vision was given showing the length at which women should wear their dresses."[32]

During these years before the Adventists had their own water cure, Ellen White could often be seen in Battle Creek going from house to house giving hydropathic treatments. In addition to this and her frequent speaking engagements, she found time to assemble six

---

31. Ibid. Ellen was not the first visitor to be disturbed by Jackson's advocacy of "worldly" amusements. The Rev. John D. Barnes, a Union chaplain who recuperated at Our Home in the summer of 1862, recalled being approached by "a delegation of long faced very serious looking men," who wanted him to sign a petition protesting the dancing and card playing. He refused, to Jackson's great delight. John D. Barnes, MS Autobiographical Memoir (Huntington Library, San Marino, California). This document was brought to my attention by Wm. Frederick Norwood.

32. Diary of Mrs. Andrews; EGW to Edson and Willie White, June 13, 1865; J. N. Loughborough, "Report from Bro. Loughborough," *R&H*, XXV (December 6, 1864), 14; [Uriah Smith], *The Visions of Mrs. E. G. White* (Battle Creek: SDA Publishing Assn., 1868), p. 85.

pamphlets on health reform, which were then bound together into a little volume called *Health; or, How to Live,* the subtitle being borrowed from a work recently issued by the house of Fowler and Wells. Each pamphlet focused on a single aspect of healthful living — diet, hydropathy, drugs, fresh air and sunlight, clothing, and exercise — and included material written both by Mrs. White and by other reformers. Most of the major names were there: Graham, Trall, Dio Lewis, Jackson, Coles, Mann, and many more. Although their selections were carefully chosen to avoid the inclusion of objectionable passages, like Coles's recommendation of bowling as an excellent form of exercise, crude phrenological analyses and sweeping statements about prenatal influences remained untouched. Ellen White's contribution, a six-part essay on "Disease and Its Causes," dealt with "Health, happiness and [the] miseries of domestic life, and the bearing which these have upon the prospects of obtaining the life to come." And to give an indication of the state of health reform among Adventists, James White told of his recent visit to Dansville.[33]

To round out the volume, twelve of Battle Creek's finest reformed cooks assembled a special collection of recipes for pies, puddings, fruits, and vegetables. Among their favorites were:

> Gems. — Into cold water stir Graham flour sufficient to make a batter about the same consistency as that used for ordinary griddle cakes. Bake in a hot oven, in the cast-iron bread pans. The pans should be heated before putting in the batter.
> Note. — This makes delicious bread. . . . If hard water is used, they are apt to be slightly tough. A small quantity of sweet milk will remedy this defect.
>
> Graham Pudding. — This is made by stirring flour into boiling water, as in making hasty pudding. It can be made in twenty

---

33. EGW, Letter 45, 1903, quoted in Arthur L. White, *Ellen G. White: Messenger to the Remnant* (Washington: Review and Publishing Assn., 1969), p. 106; EGW, *Health; or, How to Live* (Battle Creek: SDA Publishing Assn., 1865); James White, "The Health Reform," *R&H,* XXV (December 13, 1864), 20. In 1860 Fowler & Wells published a book entitled *How to Live,* by Solon Robinson. Ellen probably saw the title in Dio Lewis, *Weak Lungs, and How to Make Them Strong* (Boston: Ticknor and Fields, 1863), p. 114, a volume she was reading at the time.

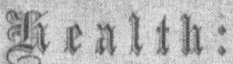

Title page of the first number of *How to Live*, Mrs. White's second volume on health reform

minutes, but is improved by boiling slowly an hour. Care is needed that it does not burn. It can be eaten when warm or cold, with milk, sugar, or sauce, as best suits the eater.

When left to cool, it should be dipped into cups or dishes to mold, as this improves the appearance of the table as well as the dish itself. Before molding, stoned dates, or nice apples thinly sliced, or fresh berries, may be added, stirring as they are dropped in. This adds to the flavor, and with many does away with the necessity for salt or some rich sauce to make it eatable. . . .

When cold, cut in slices, dip in flour, and fry as griddle-cakes. It makes a most healthful head-cheese.

In the opinion of the experts, this dish, next to Graham bread, was the most popular staple on health reform tables.[34]

According to Ellen White, the selections accompanying her essays in *How to Live* were included not to indicate her sources but solely to show the harmony of her views with what she regarded as the most enlightened medical opinion of her day. "[A]fter I had written my six articles for *How to Live*," she stated, "I then searched the various works on Hygiene and was surprised to find them so nearly in harmony with what the Lord had revealed to me. And to show this harmony . . . I determined to publish *How to Live,* in which I largely extracted from the works referred to." Even the casual reader must agree that a striking similarity does exist between Mrs. White's ideas and those commonly expressed by the health reformers. But the similarity may not be as coincidental as she implies. If we accept the testimony of John Harvey Kellogg, who as a teenager set type for *How to Live,* Ellen White was more than passingly familiar with at least Coles's *Philosophy of Health* by the time she wrote her articles. It seems that she shared with Sylvester Graham (and others) a reluctance to acknowledge her intellectual and literary debts.[35]

---

34. EGW, *How to Live,* No. 1, pp. 31-51.

35. EGW, "Questions and Answers," p. 260; John H. Kellogg, autobiographical memoir, October 21, 1938; "Interview between George W. Amadon, Eld. A. C. Bourdeau, and Dr. J. H. Kellogg, October 7, 1907," and J. H. Kellogg to E. S. Ballenger, January 15, 1929 (Ballenger-Mote Papers). In her *How to Live* essays Ellen White incorporated some ideas that had recently appeared in the *Review and Herald.* Compare, for example, her comments on the necessity of clothing the arms of babies

Although the church leaders probably never realized their goal of placing *How to Live* in every Adventist home, Mrs. White's little digest of health-reform literature sold well at $1.25 a bound copy and generally elicited a positive response. The only serious problem it encountered was the tendency of some readers to ascribe to the prophetess every notion contained in its pages. This created awkward situations at times and once moved her to protest that she did not endorse Coles's opinion, expressed in *How to Live,* that babies should be nursed only three times a day. With her blessing upon them, the various works of the health reformers began circulating freely among Adventists, and the Publishing Office in Battle Creek was soon reporting the sale of large quantities of books by Trall, Jackson, Graham, and Mann — and "tons" of pans for baking Graham bread.[36]

Despite the ground swell of reform, many Adventists continued to suffer from poor health. Physically speaking, church leadership reached its nadir in the summer of 1865 when a wave of sickness prostrated many of the leaders and brought activities at headquarters to a virtual standstill. James White and John Loughborough were both forced to their beds, causing the three-man General Conference committee to suspend meetings indefinitely. At the same time sickness prevented the Michigan state conference committee from carrying on its business and compelled Uriah Smith temporarily to relinquish his duties as editor of the *Review and Herald*.[37]

James White was the most critically ill of all. During the past year he had exhausted himself helping his wife prepare the pamphlets on *How to Live,* assisting Adventist boys drafted into the Union army, making arrangements for a general conference session in May, and attempting to put out the fires of rebellion in Iowa,

---

(No. 5, p. 68) with Dio Lewis, "Talks about Health," p. 203; or her advice on two meals a day (No. 1, pp. 55-57) with [W. W. Hall], "Eating and Sleeping," p. 195.

36. R. F. C[ottrell], "Our New Publications," *R&H,* XXVI (October 10, 1865), 148; J. N. Andrews, "How to Live," ibid., XXVI (September 12, 1865), 116; EGW, "Feeding of Infants," ibid., XXXI (April 14, 1868), 284; James White, "Health Reform — No. 4: Its Rise and Progress among Seventh-day Adventists," *HR,* V (February, 1871), 152.

37. General Conference Committee, "God's Present Dealings with His People," *R&H,* XXVII (April 17, 1866), 156; U[riah] S[mith], "Notes by the Way. No. 2," ibid., XXVI (October 3, 1865), 140.

where dissidents were splintering off to form a rival sect, the Church of God (Adventist). The strain of these additional duties severely taxed his already weakened system and literally drove him to the brink of death. Early in the morning of August 16, while he and Ellen were out walking in a neighbor's garden, a sudden "stroke of paralysis" passed through the right side of his body, leaving him practically helpless. Somehow his wife managed to get him into the house where she heard him mutter, "Pray, pray." Her prayers seemed to help a little, but still his right arm remained partially paralyzed, his nervous system shattered, and his brain "somewhat disturbed." Shock treatments with a galvanic battery were tried for a while; but this seemed like such a denial of faith in God's healing power, Ellen resolved to rely solely on the simple hydropathic techniques she had recently learned. For nearly five weeks she tenderly nursed James at home until she was too weak to continue the effort herself and could find no one else in Battle Creek willing to assume the responsibility for her husband's life. After much prayer she finally decided to take him back to Dansville and place him under the care of the skilled physicians at Our Home.[38]

Sympathetic friends and relatives waved sadly from the platform as the "Seventh-day invalid party" pulled slowly out of Battle Creek station on the morning of September 14. Accompanying the Whites on the trip to New York were Loughborough, Smith, Sister M. F. Maxson, and Dr. Horatio Lay, who had come from Dansville to escort the ailing Adventists to Our Home. After an arduous weeklong journey that included a stopover in Rochester the pathetic little band, apparently no worse for the wear, arrived at their destination, where Dr. Jackson warmly greeted them. The day after arrival the doctor examined his new patients and issued the long-awaited prognoses, which Uriah Smith reported in the *Review and Herald*. James White, clearly the most critical case, would have to remain at the water cure for six to eight months, during which time Ellen White would also take treatments. Loughborough might recover

---

38. "Sickness of Bro. White," *R&H*, XXVI (August 22, 1865), 96; H. S. Lay, "Eld. White and Wife, and Eld. Loughborough," ibid., XXVI (October 31, 1865), 172; EGW, "Our Late Experience," pp. 89-91; EGW, "Recreation for Christians," *Testimonies*, I, 518; EGW, *Life Sketches of Ellen G. White* (Mountain View, Calif.: Pacific Press, 1915), pp. 167-68.

Dansville Days

in five or six months. "But the Editor of the *Review,* unfortunately for its readers, is to be let off in five or six weeks."³⁹

The Whites soon settled into the Dansville routine. Small rooms were found close by the institution where Ellen could set up housekeeping and nursing operations. Daily she made the beds and tidied the rooms, not only for her husband and herself, but also for the other Battle Creek ministers who occupied an adjoining room. She insisted on spending as little time indoors as possible. When not taking water treatments, she and James strolled about the grounds basking in the sunlight and fresh autumn air. Three times each day they met with their brethren — including Elder D. T. Bourdeau from Vermont — for special seasons of prayer in James's behalf. Nights were the worst. Constant pain made sleep almost impossible for James, and Ellen sacrificed hours of her own much-needed rest rubbing his shoulders and arms to provide temporary relief. Often prayer proved to be the only effective therapy in bringing sleep to the weary preacher.⁴⁰

Understandably, the Whites were somewhat embarrassed by their present state of health, especially in view of their outspoken praise of health reform over the past couple of years. Certainly their own lives were not very effective witnesses to the power of abstemious living. Ellen feared that her husband's "professed friends" would secretly rejoice in his affliction and chalk it up to sin in his life. To assist in meeting possible criticism, she wrote home to her children in Battle Creek asking them to send "the health journal in which [Sylvester] Graham gives his apology for being sick." As far as the Whites were concerned, James's illness had not resulted from personal sin but from prolonged and unceasing labor for the Lord.⁴¹

Early in October James's colleagues on the General Conference committee called on Seventh-day Adventists everywhere to set aside

---

39. *R&H,* XXVI (September 19, 1865), 128; Smith, "Notes by the Way," p. 140.

40. EGW, "Our Late Experience," *R&H,* XXVII (February 20, 1866), 89-91, (February 27, 1866), 97-99; EGW to Edson White, October 19, 1865 (W-7-1865, White Estate); EGW, "The Sickness and Recovery of Elder James White," circa 1867 (MS-1-1867); D. T. Bourdeau, "At Home Again," *R&H,* XXVI (November 14, 1865), 192.

41. EGW, "Our Late Experience," p. 89; EGW to Edson and Willie White, September 22, 1865 (W-6-1865, White Estate). For James White's apology, see "Report from Bro. White," *R&H,* XXIX (January 22, 1867), 74.

Sabbath, the fourteenth, as a day of fasting and prayer for their stricken leader. At Dansville the Whites retreated a short distance from Our Home to a beautiful grove, where they spent the afternoon united in prayer with Elders Loughborough, Bourdeau, and Smith. The experience filled James with renewed hope, and the following day he appeared to be on the road to recovery. By mid-November, however, he had again slipped to a critical condition, and friends despaired for his very life. When he grew so weak he could no longer walk the short distance up the hill to the dining hall, John Loughborough kindly volunteered to bring baskets of food to the Whites' room.[42]

By this time Ellen was beginning to show signs of strain and left Dansville for a few days to be with her two boys, who had recently arrived in Rochester from Michigan. But even away from the water cure she could not get her mind off her suffering husband or the physicians caring for him. Her first night in Rochester she dreamed of being back at Dansville "exalting God and our Saviour as the great Physician and the Deliverer of His afflicted, suffering children." Apparently friction was already developing between her and the staff of Our Home, for in this dream, she told James, "Dr. Jackson was near me, afraid that his patients would hear me, and wished to lay his hand upon me and hinder me, but he was awed and dared not move; he seemed held by the power of God. I awoke very happy." In a less dramatic tone she also reported that her diet was about the same as at Dansville — "Mornings I eat mush, gems, and uncooked apples. At dinner baked potatoes, raw apples, and gems" — and that she was confident James would "astonish the whole [medical] fraternity by a speedy recovery to health."[43]

Mrs. White remained in Rochester only briefly before returning to her husband's side. On her thirty-eighth birthday, November 26, she celebrated with a dinner of "Graham mush, hard Graham crackers, applesauce, sugar, and a cup of milk." The next day she and

---

42. "Bro. White's Sickness," *R&H*, XXVI (October 3, 1865), 144; U[riah] S[mith], "Notes by the Way. No. 3," ibid., XXVI (October 24, 1865), 164; J. N. Loughborough, "Note," ibid., XXVI (October 31, 1865), 176; EGW, "Our Late Experience," p. 97.

43. EGW to James White, November 22 and 24, 1865 (W-9-1865, W-10-1865, White Estate); Adelia P. Van Horn, "A Word from Dansville, N. Y.," *R&H*, XXVI (November 21, 1865), 200.

Dansville Days

James met with Loughborough for an emotional season of prayer. "For more than one hour we could only rejoice and triumph in God," she later wrote. "We shouted the high praise of God." This "heavenly refreshing" had a cheering effect on James, but only temporarily.[44]

Shortly after this experience Ellen White became impressed with the advantages of removing James to Battle Creek, where he could recover in the more congenial atmosphere of his own home. Besides, several aspects of Dansville life were causing her deep concern. First, the inactivity prescribed for James was obviously not working. What he needed, she thought, was "exercise and moderate, useful labor." Second, James's mind was being "confused" by the religious teachings of Dr. Jackson, which did not conform with what Ellen had "received from higher and unerring authority." Third, the amusements encouraged by the management, especially dancing and card-playing, seemed out of harmony with true Christianity. Although Jackson always exempted his Adventist patients from such activities, Ellen still felt uneasy around such blatant manifestations of worldliness. One day when she was mistakenly approached in the bathroom for a donation to pay the fiddler at the dances, she declared to the doubtless startled solicitor that as a "follower of Jesus" she could not contribute and then proceeded to give an impromptu lecture on Christian principles to the ladies in the room.[45]

By early December Ellen's own strength was rapidly slipping away; and when James suffered through a particularly bad night on the fourth, she abruptly decided the time had come to leave. The doctors were notified, trunks were packed, and early the next morn-

---

44. EGW, "Our Late Experience," p. 97.

45. Ibid., pp. 90, 97-98; EGW, "The Sickness and Recovery of Elder James White"; EGW to Brother Aldrich, August 20, 1867 (A-8-1867, White Estate). On amusements at Dansville, see also Smith, "Notes by the Way. No. 3," p. 164. Clara Barton, founder of the American Red Cross, described the dances at Our Home in a letter to Jere Learned, July 15, 1876: "There is an amusement society, and one of its features is a beautiful dance once a week from 5 till 8 P.M. Piano and violin music — no round dances — but cotillions and all dances which are not injurious, and the prettiest and most elegant dancers in the hall are from among the help." Quoted in William D. Conklin, *The Jackson Health Resort* (Dansville, N.Y.: Privately distributed by the author, 1971), p. 184.

ing in driving sleet she departed for Rochester with a bundled-up James. For three weeks the Whites stayed in that city, enjoying the hospitality of Adventist friends. At James's request, other believers were summoned from surrounding churches to come to Rochester and join with the family in prayer for his recovery.[46]

While praying on Christmas evening, Ellen White was "wrapped in a vision of God's glory." To her immense relief, she saw that her husband would eventually recover. She also received a message of lasting importance: Seventh-day Adventists should open their own home for the sick, so that they would no longer have "to go to popular water-cure institutions for the recovery of health, where there is not sympathy for our faith." Adventists were to "have an institution of their own, under their own control, for the benefit of the diseased and suffering among us, who wish to have health and strength that they may glorify God in their bodies and spirits which are his." Although she appreciated "the kind attention and respect" she had received from the staff at Our Home, she wanted no more sad treks to Dansville, where "the sophistry of the devil" prevailed.[47]

New Year's Day the Whites boarded the train in Rochester and departed for home and friends in Michigan. Aided by his wife and sustained by Graham mush and gems, James survived the difficult trip to Battle Creek and arrived in good spirits. He was now fifty pounds below his normal weight, but fresh air, moderate exercise, and Ellen's gentle prodding soon had him up and about again. Still, his mental and physical health remained below par; so in the spring of 1867 he and Ellen purchased a small farm in Greenville, Michigan, where she could more effectively implement her philosophy of

---

46. EGW, "Our Late Experience," pp. 97-98; EGW, "The Sickness and Recovery of Elder James White"; EGW, *Life Sketches* (1915), pp. 170-71.

47. EGW, "Our Late Experience," pp. 91, 98; EGW, "The Health Reform," *Testimonies,* I, 485-93; EGW, "Health and Religion," ibid., I, 565. Ellen White's Christmas vision in Rochester was truly seminal. In addition to revealing the prospects for James White's recovery and the need for an Adventist water cure, it prompted testimonies on subjects as diverse as the taking of usury, erroneous political views, Sabbath observance, the Adventist cause in Maine, the duties of parents, the business interests of ministers, and the spiritual condition of several brethren and sisters. See *Comprehensive Index to the Writings of Ellen G. White* (Mountain View, Calif.: Pacific Press, 1963), III, 2980.

useful labor for the sick. Although she was fairly successful in getting James to do simple chores about the garden, he rebelled at the prospect of bringing in the hay, hoping instead to rely on the good will of nearby friends. Ellen, however, outwitted him by getting to the neighbors first and persuading them not to help her husband when he came calling on them. Thus by hook or by crook she made sure James obtained the exercise she thought he needed.[48]

According to James, his sickness led Ellen to ease up for a while in her written and oral pronouncements on health reform. Nevertheless, personal hygiene remained one of her "favorite themes," and one she regarded as being as "closely connected with present truth as the arm is connected with the body."[49] Meanwhile, during James's recuperation, exciting developments were under way in Battle Creek. There, in response to Mrs. White's Christmas vision, church leaders were laying plans to open the Western Health Reform Institute, a water cure modeled after Our Home and the first link in what was to become a worldwide chain of Seventh-day Adventist medical institutions.

---

48. EGW, "Our Late Experience," pp. 98-99; "Bro. White at Home," *R&H*, XXVII (January 9, 1866), 48; D. E. Robinson, *The Story of Our Health Message* (Nashville: Southern Publishing Assn., 1955), pp. 161-66.

49. James White, "Western Tour: Kansas Camp-Meeting," *R&H*, XXXVI (November 8, 1870), 165; James White, "Report from Bro. White," ibid., XXVIII (June 19, 1866), 20; EGW to Brother Aldrich, August 20, 1867.

CHAPTER FIVE

The Western Health Reform Institute

"More deaths have been caused by drug-taking than from all other causes combined. If there was in the land one physician in the place of thousands, a vast amount of premature mortality would be prevented."

Ellen G. White[1]

"Were I sick, I would just as soon call in a lawyer as a physician from among general practitioners. I would not touch their nostrums, to which they give Latin names. I am determined to know, in straight English, the name of everything that I introduce into my system."

Ellen G. White[2]

September 5, 1866, marked the fulfillment of one of Ellen White's fondest hopes: the grand opening of the Western Health Reform Institute in Battle Creek. Since her first visit to Dansville in the fall of 1864, she had dreamed of founding an Adventist water cure where Sabbath-keeping invalids could receive treatments in an atmo-

---

1. EGW, *Health; or, How to Live* (Battle Creek: SDA Publishing Assn., 1865), no. 3, p. 59.
2. EGW, "Health Reform Principles" (MS-86-1897), in *Selected Messages from the Writings of Ellen G. White* (Washington: Review and Herald Publishing Assn., 1958), II, 290.

The Western Health Reform Institute

sphere compatible with their distinctive faith. Her disillusionment with Our Home during James's illness and the subsequent Christmas vision of 1865 convinced her that the time had finally arrived to take positive action. Vigorous support came from the denomination's leaders, especially the numerous Dansville alumni, who shared her enthusiasm for an Adventist medical center. Uriah Smith, the influential editor of the *Review and Herald,* regarded his few weeks at Our Home as one of the most valuable experiences of his life and saw the establishment of a similiar institution in Battle Creek as "a present necessity," both for treating the sick and for educating the church in the principles of health reform. Thus while politicians in Washington quarreled bitterly over the best method of healing a divided and scarred nation, the Adventists of Battle Creek dedicated themselves to curing mankind with water.[3]

At the annual General Conference session in May, 1866, attended by church representatives from throughout the country, Ellen White announced the Lord's instruction to establish an Adventist water cure. The response was immediate and favorable. In the absence of the recuperating James White, John Loughborough, president of the Michigan conference, assumed overall responsibility for the fund-raising drive and took personal charge of the campaign in the West. John Andrews, another Dansville man, directed operations in the East, while the remaining ministers at the conference volunteered to serve as agents, selling stock in the proposed institute at twenty-five dollars a share. As soon as sufficient funds were on hand, arrangements were made to purchase an eight-acre site on the outskirts of town. Although existing buildings on the property could accommodate up to fifty patients, it was necessary to build an additional two-story structure to house a "packing room, bath room, dressing room, and a room to contain a tank of sufficient capacity to hold two hundred barrels of water."[4]

---

3. EGW to Bro. and Sister Lockwood, September [14], 1864 (L-6-1864, White Estate); [Uriah Smith], "The Health-Reform Institute," *R&H,* XXVIII (July 10, 1866), 48. The *Review and Herald* was outspokenly critical of President Andrew Johnson, whom they openly called "a rebel and traitor." See *R&H,* XXVII (February 27, 1866), 104.

4. D. E. Robinson, *The Story of Our Health Message* (3rd ed.; Nashville: Southern Publishing Assn., 1965), pp. 144-52; "The Western Health-Reform Institute," *R&H,*

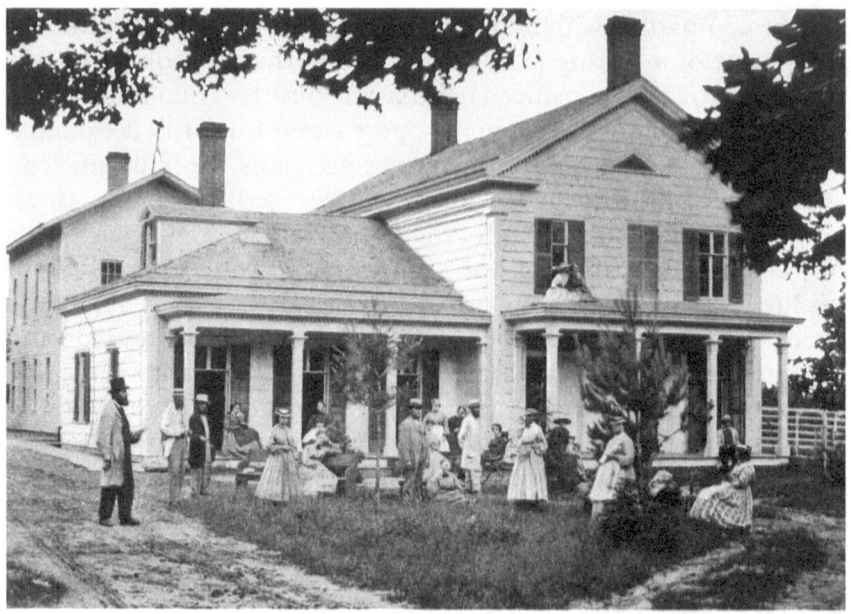

The original Western Health Reform Institute in Battle Creek

The plans to pour large sums of money into a water cure led some members to question the judgment of the brethren in Battle Creek. For years Mrs. White had been warning against heavy investments in this world, and the establishment of a big, permanent medical facility struck the critics as nothing less than "a denial of our faith in the speedy coming of Christ." To squash such sentiments, both Elders Loughborough and D. T. Bourdeau (still another former patient of Our Home) took to the pages of the *Review and Herald* to point out that the Health Reform Institute, far from being a denial of faith, would be the means of "bringing thousands to a knowledge of present truth." The institute, Loughborough predicted, "will fill its place in this cause, from the fact that scores who come to it to be healed of temporal maladies, who learn the lesson of self-denial to gain health, may also, by being brought into a place

---

XXVIII (June 19, 1866), 24; J. N. Loughborough, "Report from Bro. Loughborough," ibid., XXVIII (September 11, 1866), 117.

where they become acquainted with the character and ways of our people, see a beauty in the religion of the Bible, and be led into the Lord's service."[5]

Circulars describing the Western Health Reform Institute went out to all Adventist churches and potential stockholders and appeared in the *Review and Herald* as well. "In the treatment of the sick at this Institution," read the announcement,

> *no drugs whatever, will be administered,* but only such means employed as NATURE can best use in her recuperative work, such as Water, Air, Light, Heat, Food, Sleep, Rest, Recreation, &c. Our tables will be furnished with a strictly healthful diet, consisting of Vegetables, Grains, and Fruits, which are found in great abundance and variety in this State. And it will be the aim of the Faculty, that all who spend any length of time at this Institute shall go to their homes instructed as to the right mode of living, and the best methods of home treatment.

In language typical of American nostrum vendors, prospective patients were glibly assured that "WHATEVER MAY BE THE NATURE OF THEIR DISEASE, IF CURABLE, THEY CAN BE CURED HERE." All bills were to be paid in advance, and individuals unable to visit the institute in person could receive a prescription by letter for five dollars, the same fee charged for a personal examination.[6]

Chief physician at the institute, and one of the few Adventists with medical experience of any kind, was thirty-eight-year-old Horatio S. Lay, a man "thoroughly conversant with the latest and most approved Hygienic Methods of Treating Disease." As a youth Lay had apprenticed himself to a local doctor in Pennsylvania and acquired the fundamentals of the trade. In 1849, feeling sufficiently knowledgeable to assume the title of doctor, he moved to Allegan, Michigan, a small town northwest of Battle Creek, and began practicing as an allopathic physician. About 1856 he joined the Seventh-

---

5. D. T. Bourdeau, "The Health Reform," *R&H,* XXVIII (June 12, 1866), 12; Loughborough, "Report," p. 84.

6. "The Western Health-Reform Institute," *R&H,* XXVIII (June 19, 1866), 24; "The Western Health Reform Institute," ibid., XXVIII (August 7, 1866), 78. See Loughborough, "Report," p. 117, for a reply to complaints of excessive prices.

day Adventists, and a few years later became interested in the health-reform movement. Following Ellen White's 1863 vision on health, it was Lay who first drew her out on the subject and who informed her of the remarkable similarity between her revelation and the teachings of the health reformers.[7]

Shortly after his conversations with Mrs. White, Lay took his consumptive wife to the Dansville water cure, a move the prophetess saw in vision as being providentially arranged to train him for future work as a health reformer. At Dansville he quickly won the respect of the hydropaths. He was invited to join the staff of Our Home and in 1865 was elected a vice-president of the National Health Reform Association (along with Joshua V. Himes). During this time he toyed with the idea of "of going to N. York City to Dr. Trall's college and attend lectures, obtain a diploma and come out a regular [sic] M.D.," but he never went. In fact, it was not until 1877, long after he had severed his ties with Battle Creek, that he finally attended school and received an authentic medical degree from the Detroit Medical College.[8]

The Western Health Reform Institute was a booming success. Within months of its opening patients from all over the country filled its rooms to overflowing. But prosperity also bred problems: the need for additional space and trained personnel. During the first years of the institute Lay seems to have been the only member of "the Faculty" with significant medical experience, and even he had never seen the inside of a medical school. Several others on his staff called themselves doctors, but the term was loosely used in those days. The institute's lady physician, Phoebe Lamson, had spent some time at Dansville with her ailing father and may have picked up a rudimentary knowledge of hydropathic medicine. To

---

7. Ibid.; I. D. Van Horn, "Another Standard Bearer Fallen," ibid., LXXVII (March 13, 1900), 176; W. C. White, "The Origin of the Light on Health Reform among Seventh-day Adventists," *Medical Evangelist,* XX (December 28, 1933), 2.

8. EGW to Dr. and Mrs. Lay, May 6, 1867 (L-6-1867, White Estate); EGW to Bro. and Sister Lockwood, September [14], 1864; J. H. Kellogg, "Christian Help Work," *General Conference Daily Bulletin,* I (March 8, 1897), 309; "Constitution of the N.H.R. Association," *Laws of Life,* VIII (August, 1865), 126; C. B. Burr (ed.), *Medical History of Michigan* (Minneapolis: Bruce Publishing Co., 1930), I, 641. Lay's graduation from the Detroit Medical College (now the Wayne State University of Medicine) is verified in a letter to the author from Mary E. McNamara, March 14, 1973.

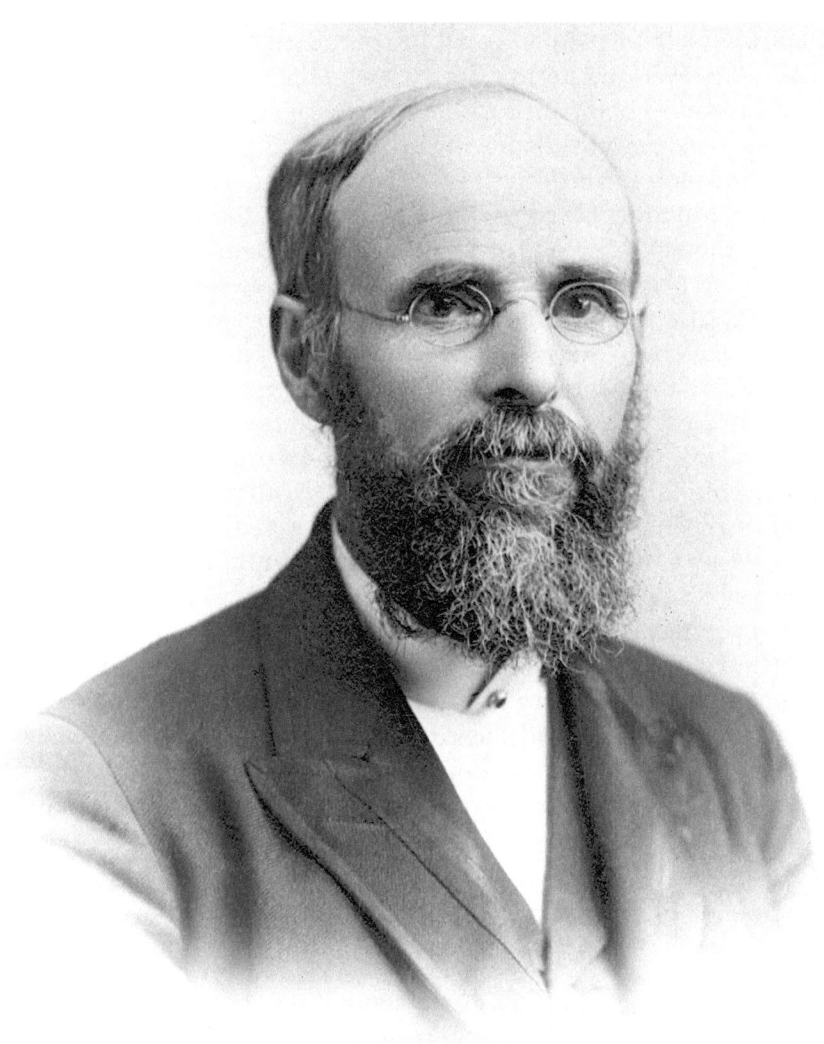

Horatio S. Lay

qualify herself more fully "to act her part in the Institution," she obtained Ellen White's permission to spend the winter 1867-68 term at Trall's Hygeio-Therapeutic College in New Jersey and returned a few months later proudly displaying an "M.D." after her name.[9]

In addition to his duties at the Health Reform Institute, Lay took on the editorship of a new monthly journal, the *Health Reformer*. During the summer of 1865, while still at Dansville, he had furnished the *Review and Herald* with a series of essays on "Health," outlining the main tenets of the reform movement. The church leaders liked his work so well that they voted at the next general conference session to have him write a second series on the same topic. But before any of his articles appeared, they ambitiously decided instead to have Lay edit "a first class Health Journal, interesting in its variety, valuable in its instructions, and second to none in either literary or mechanical execution." According to the prospectus, the journal was to be nondenominational in orientation and dedicated to curing diseases "by the use of Nature's own remedies, Air, Light, Heat, Exercise, Food, Sleep, Recreation, &c."[10]

The first issue of the *Reformer* came off the press in August, 1866, carrying the motto "Our Physician, Nature: Obey and Live." Though distinctly second class in literary quality, it was an attractive publication by nineteenth-century standards. Because of the dearth of medical writers in the church, most articles were from the pens of

---

9. "Items for the Month," *HR*, I (February, 1867), 112; Diary of Mrs. Angeline S. Andrews, entry for January 2, 1865 (C. Burton Clark Collection); EGW to Edson White, November 9, 1867 (W-14-1867, White Estate); R. T. Trall, "Visit to Battle Creek, Mich.," *HR*, III (July, 1868), 14. The original institute staff seems to have been composed of three "doctors": Lay, Lamson, and John F. Byington, son of the first General Conference president. William Russell joined the staff in the fall of 1867; and in the next few years J. H. Ginley and Mary A. Chamberlain also connected with the institute. Except for the two women, who briefly attended Trall's hydropathic college (Mrs. Chamberlain at some time in her life also graduated from the homeopathy course at the University of Michigan), none of these individuals seems to have had formal medical training. For obituaries of Byington, Chamberlain, and Ginley, see *R&H*, XL (June 25, 1872), 5; ibid., LXXVII (April 17, 1900), 256; and ibid., LXXXI (February 4, 1904), 23.

10. "Fourth Annual Session of General Conference," *R&H*, XXVIII (May 22, 1866), 196; "Prospectus of the Health Reformer," ibid., XXVIII (June 5, 1866), 8. For Lay's "Health" series, see ibid., XXVI (July 4, 1865), 37; (July 25, 1865), 61; (August 15, 1865), 85; (September 12, 1865), 117.

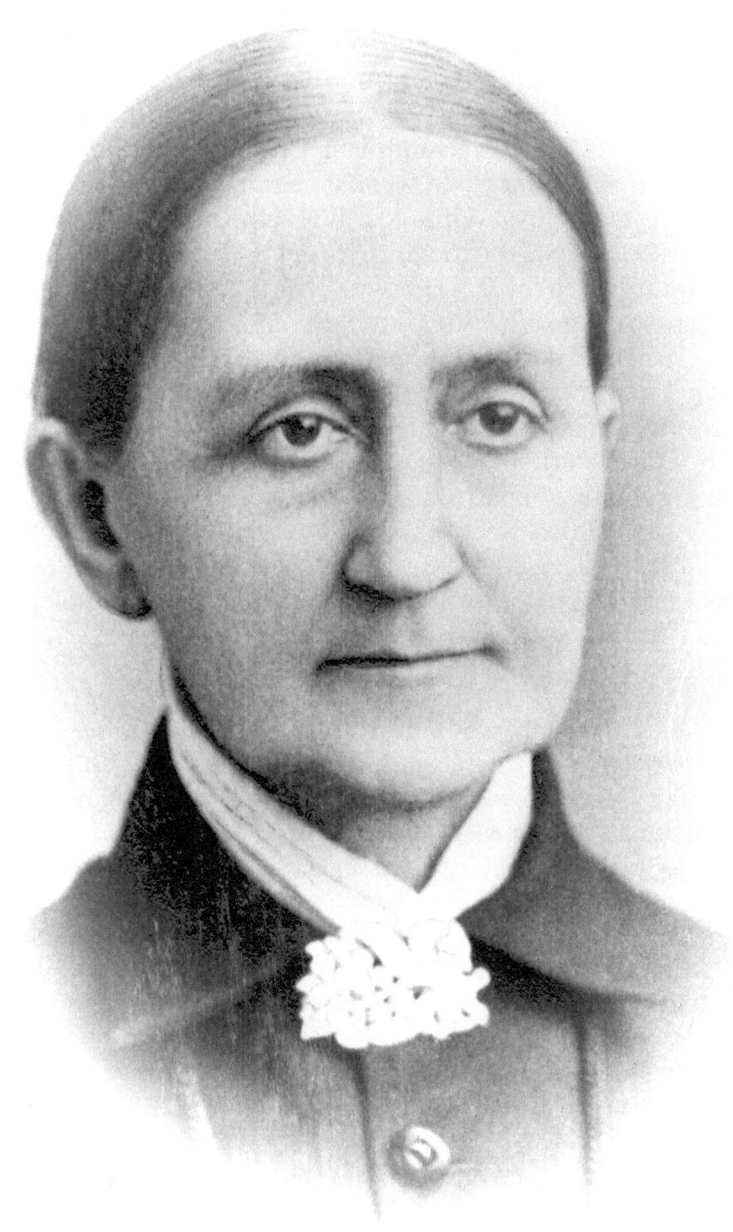

Phoebe Lamson

ministers like Loughborough, Andrews, and Bourdeau. Even Ellen White contributed a composition, "Duty to Know Ourselves," based on L. B. Coles's theme that to break one of the laws of life is "as great a sin in the sight of Heaven as to break the ten commandments." To avoid charges of religious sectarianism, the editors of the *Reformer* printed little by or about the Adventist seer in the first several volumes. Nevertheless, Mrs. White had high hopes for the magazine. "The *Health Reformer* is the medium through which rays of light are to shine upon the people," she wrote in an 1867 testimony. "It should be the very best health journal in our country."[11]

Among the most readable features of the *Reformer* were the "Question Department," where readers' queries on home treatment were answered, and numerous testimonials to the curative powers of health reform. Although the medical men in Battle Creek were prone to complain of apathy among the membership as a whole, glowing reports of how two meals a day and no butter had restored health and strength filled the pages of the *Reformer*. Typical was the progressive reform of Brother Isaac Sanborn, president of the Illinois-Wisconsin conference, who for years had suffered painfully from "inflammatory rheumatism":

> I concluded I would leave off the use of meat, which I did by leaving pork first: then beef, then condiments, fish, and mince pies. Then I adopted the two meals a day, had breakfast at seven A.M., and dinner at half past one P.M.; used no drug medicines of any kind, lived on Graham bread, fruit and vegetables, using no butter, but a little cream in place of butter. I drink nothing with my meals, and I relish and enjoy my meals as I never have before; and the result is, I am entirely well of the rheumatism, which I used to have so bad by spells that I could not walk a step for days; and although I travel through all kinds of weather, and speak often in crowded assemblies, in ill-ventilated schoolhouses, and am exposed in various ways, yet I have not had a bad cold for more than two years.[12]

---

11. EGW, "Duty to Know Ourselves," *HR*, I (August, 1866), 2-3; EGW, "The Health Reformer," *Testimonies,* I, 552.

12. J. F. Byington, "The Health Institute," *R&H*, XXIX (January 1, 1867), 43; G. W. Amadon, "My Experiences in Health Reform," *HR*, III (February, 1869), 149; Isaac Sanborn, "My Experience," ibid., I (January, 1867), 84.

The Western Health Reform Institute

Throughout its early history the *Reformer* exuded antipathy toward regular medicine, leaving no doubt of the medically sectarian loyalties of its Battle Creek promoters. This hostility reflected not only a genuine distrust of orthodox physicians but also deep-seated feelings of inferiority. "Some people seem to think that nobody can talk on Health but an M.D., and nobody on Theology but a D.D.," wrote the self-conscious and degreeless editor. "But how ever much there is in a name, or in a title, everybody will admit that all knowledge of health should not be left with the doctors, nor all theology with the ministers." J. F. Byington, Lay's associate at the institute, became almost vitriolic in denouncing the "old school," calling its therapy a "terrible humbug" and its practitioners "too bigoted and self-conceited to learn." Even the Whites were not much kinder. Ellen charged "popular physicians" with deliberately keeping their patients in ignorance and ill-health for monetary reasons, while James ridiculed "the superstitious confidence of the people in doctors' doses." Ironically, these bitter attacks on the regular medical profession came at the very period when that school was finally abandoning its long-practiced customs of bloodletting and calomel-dosing.[13]

For several months the future of the fledgling Battle Creek health institutions looked bright indeed. But it was not long before ominous storm clouds rolled in, casting shadows not only on the institute and the *Reformer,* but on Ellen White herself. The first episode began innocently in January, 1867, with an announcement by Dr. Lay that the institute was already filled to capacity and would soon be turning away incoming patients for lack of room. "What shall be done?" he inquired of readers in the *Review and Herald.* His own answer was to erect at once an additional *"large"* building capable of housing "at least one hundred more patients than we now have." The estimated cost was twenty-five thousand

---

13. [H. S. Lay], "Items for the Month," *HR,* I (September, 1866), 32; J. F. Byington, "The Greatest Humbug of the Age," ibid., III (May, 1869), 209; E[llen] G. W[hite], "Florence Nightingale," ibid., VI (July, 1871), 27; J[ames] W[hite], "The Health Reformer," ibid., V (January, 1871), 142. For a recent discussion of reforms in regular medicine, see William G. Rothstein, *American Physicians in the 19th Century: From Sects to Science* (Baltimore: Johns Hopkins University Press, 1972), p. 181.

dollars — a figure seven times the General Conference budget for that year.[14]

Before the month was out, Uriah Smith had thrown the weight of the *Review and Herald* behind the project, and interest in Lay's proposal was running high in Adventist circles. The immediate problem, as the institute's backers saw it, was how to gain a public endorsement from Mrs. White. One solution came from John Loughborough, who had just returned from a trip with Ellen and had heard her give a "good testimony" regarding the institute and its superintendent. Why not, he suggested, ask her to write out this message for *Testimony No. 11*, then going to press. This plan met with general approval, and Smith was nominated to carry out the assignment.[15]

On February 5 Smith sent a letter to Mrs. White urging her to sanction additional investments in the institute. He reminded her that a widely distributed circular had promised a statement in her next *Testimony* relative to the medical work in Battle Creek and pointed out that such a communication would be expected:

> ... a great many are waiting before doing anything to help the Institute, till they see the Testimony and now if it goes out without anything on these points, they will not understand it, and it will operate greatly against the prosperity of the Institution. The present is a most important time in this enterprise, and it is essential that no influence should be lost, which can be brought to bear in its favor.

In closing he offered to hold up the printing of the last pages of *Testimony No. 11* until she could rush her manuscript to him. Then, as if he had not already prompted her enough, the brash young Smith went on to add a postscript suggesting that she particularly emphasize the connection between the health work and "the cause of present truth." We think, he said, this relationship "should be made plainly to appear."[16]

---

14. H. S. Lay, "What Shall Be Done?" *R&H,* XXIX (January 8, 1867), 54. On the GC budget, see *R&H,* XXVII (May 22, 1866), 196; and *R&H,* XXIX (January 1, 1867), 48.

15. [Uriah Smith], "The Health Reform Institute," ibid., XXIX (January 29, 1867), 90; Uriah Smith to EGW, February 5, 1867 (White Estate).

16. Ibid.

Thus prodded, Ellen White hurriedly wrote out the desired testimony. First, following Smith's suggestion, she commented on the intimate relationship between theology and health: "The health reform, I was shown, is a part of the third angel's message [that is, Seventh-day Adventism], and is just as closely connected with it as are the arm and hand with the human body." Then, after describing the Battle Creek water cure, she stated that God had shown her in vision that the institute was "a worthy enterprise for God's people to engage in, — one in which they can invest means to his glory and the advancement of his cause." Institutions like that in Battle Creek could play a vital role in directing "unbelievers" to Adventism, for by "becoming acquainted with our people and our real faith, their prejudice will be overcome, and they will be favorably impressed." Here was "a good opportunity," she advised, for those with financial security "to use their means for the benefit of suffering humanity, and also for the advancement of the truth."[17]

Given this divine blessing — and the fact that investments were rumored to be returning an annual dividend of 10 percent — institute stock enjoyed healthy sales throughout the spring and summer months. By mid-August the basement and first floor of the new building were completed, and lumber was on hand for the remaining three stories. But the money had run out. While construction was temporarily halted, the directors of the institute appealed once again to the church membership, urging them to recall Mrs. White's counsel in *Testimony No. 11* and buy more shares in the institution.[18]

Though the directors undoubtedly did not know it, Mrs. White was at that time preparing to back away from her previous endorsement of the expansion plans. Her private correspondence reveals that by August she was having qualms that the institute might be growing too rapidly for a man of Lay's limited abilities. "Dr. Lay is not qualified to carry on so large a business as you are laying out for him," she cautioned one of the institute's directors. "Dr. Lay has done well to move out in this great work, but he can bear no heavier burdens." In addition to Lay's limitations, she and her husband

---

17. EGW, "The Health Reform," *Testimonies*, I, 485-95.
18. "Meeting of the Health Reform Institute," *R&H*, XXIX (May 28, 1867), 279; E. S. Walker, "$15,000 Wanted Immediately," ibid., XXX (August 27, 1867), 168-69.

feared that the institute's supporters were moving too fast too soon, given the available money and personnel. Some poor Adventists, she pointed out, were taking unsound financial risks, putting "from one-fifth to one-third of all they possess into the Institute." In response to these and other problems, by mid-September she had prepared *Testimony No. 12* modifying her earlier statements in *Testimony No. 11*. Now, she said, the Lord had shown her that the institute should be "small at its commencement, and cautiously increased, as good physicians and helpers could be procured and means raised." She pointed out, correctly, "that out of many hygienic institutions started in the United States within the last twenty-five years, but few maintain even a visible existence at the present time."[19]

This virtual repudiation of what the church considered to be a divinely inspired testimony demanded an explanation. Uncharitable critics later hinted that James had been behind the change, but Ellen placed the blame squarely on the shoulders of Uriah Smith and his associates. Smith's importunate letter of February 5 had caused her mental suffering "beyond description," she explained. "Under these circumstances I yielded my judgment to that of others, and wrote what appeared in No. 11 in regard to the Health Institute, being unable then to give all I had seen. In this I did wrong." Still, she refused to withdraw "one sentence" from what she had written in *Testimony No. 11*, admitting only that she had acted prematurely. Her lament that the entire affair had been "one of the heaviest trials" of her life surely evoked only sympathy. Yet her admitted wavering under pressure raised long-lasting questions about her susceptibility to human influences.[20]

Testimony No. 12 apparently caught the institute's directors by surprise. The secretary, E. S. Walker, immediately wrote James White protesting that "it would require a great amount of labor and be attended with considerable expense to undo what we have al-

---

19. EGW to Brother Aldrich, August 20, 1867 (A-8-1867, White Estate); EGW, "The Health Institute," *Testimonies*, I, 558-60.

20. Ibid., I, 559-64; D. M. Canright, *Life of Mrs. E. G. White, Seventh-day Adventist Prophet: Her False Claims Refuted* (Nashville: B. C. Goodpasture, 1953), pp. 77-78. Canright errs in implying that Mrs. White wrote *Testimony No. 12* to justify her husband's tearing down of the sanitarium building.

ready done." The directors, he said, thought it best to proceed as soon as possible with putting a roof over the new building and then to complete the interior as funds became available. To do this, they needed the Whites' public approval. On behalf of the directors he promised a reform in the management of the water cure, so that the Whites could once again "feel to work for the Institute as [they] did at its commencement."[21]

But James White did not back down. Instead, a very strange thing happened — "a real hocus pocus," remembered one old-timer. At White's insistence, and apparently with the concurrence of at least two directors, the entire structure was torn down stone by stone until not a trace remained where shortly before there had stood the proud beginning of a new sanitarium. Some placed the loss at eleven thousand dollars, but a portion of this sum was undoubtedly recovered through the sale of salvageable materials. The complex motives behind this seemingly irrational act will never be fully known. Years after the event, John Harvey Kellogg discussed the incident with White and concluded that the building had been razed "for no other reason than because James White was not consulted" at the time of its planning. By then the aging elder had come to regret his impetuous decision and confided to the young doctor that "if I had known how much power and strength there was in this thing, I never would have torn that thing down."[22]

At no time during this unpleasant episode did Ellen White allude in print to her husband's erratic behavior. Although privately con-

---

21. E. S. Walker to James White, September 24, 1867 (White Estate). In this letter the institute directors offer to buy some property from the Whites for six thousand dollars at 7 percent interest if James White will agree "to cooperate with us in raising means to pay for your place and to erect and inclose the new building at as early a day as possible."

22. "Interview between Geo. W. Amadon, Eld. A. C. Bourdeau, and Dr. J. H. Kellogg, October 7, 1907," p. 88 (Ballenger-Mote Papers). The "old-timer" mentioned was Amadon. James White may not have been consulted about plans for the new building, and he was absent the morning General Conference delegates voted to enlarge the institute; but he did attend the 1867 General Conference session and certainly was aware of plans for a new building before construction began. James White, "The Conference," *R&H*, XXIX (May 28, 1867), 282; "Business Proceedings of the Fifth Annual Session of the General Conference of Seventh-day Adventists," ibid., pp. 283-84.

cerned for his mental health during this period of his life, she publicly defended him as a man chosen of God and given "special qualifications, natural ability, and an experience to lead out his people in the advance work." James himself, instead of apologizing for throwing away the institute's money, condescendingly appealed to the church to forgive the men in Battle Creek "who have moved rashly, and have committed errors in the past for want of experience." The "large building is given up for the present, and the material is being sold," he announced matter-of-factly in the *Review and Herald* a month after his election in May, 1868, to the institute's board of directors. Then, after complaining of the large debt recently incurred, he audaciously went on to request thirteen thousand dollars for a modest two-story building and two cottages, a figure just two thousand dollars shy of what it would have cost to finish the original structure. "Send in your pledges, brethren, at once, and the money as soon as possible," he urged. "It is a SAFE INVESTMENT."[23]

To Ellen White, the extravagant plans for physical expansion were only the tip of the iceberg threatening the institute. Much more disturbing were the ubiquitous signs of worldliness: patients and staff enjoying Dansville-style amusements, physicians demanding higher wages than ministers, and workers calling each other "Mister" and "Miss" rather than "Brother" and "Sister." (Until the 1880s some Adventists refused even to use the common, but pagan, days of the week, substituting instead First-day, Second-day, etc.)[24]

The institute directors considered amusements, "when conducted within proper limits, as an important part of the treatment of disease." Their celebration of the first Thanksgiving at the water cure included songs, charades, pantomime, nonalcoholic toasts, and attempts at poetry:

Hoops on barrels, tubs, and pails,
   Are articles indispensable;
But hoops as they puff out woman's dress,

---

23. EGW to Edson and Emma White, November 15, 1871 (W-15-1871, White Estate); EGW, "The Work at Battle Creek," *Testimonies,* III, 89; James White, "The Health Institute," *R&H,* XXXI (June 16, 1868), 408-9.

24. EGW, "The Health Institute," *Testimonies,* I, 633-43. For the persistent use of First-day, etc., see the masthead of the *Review and Herald*.

The Western Health Reform Institute

Making the dear women seem so much less,
Are most reprehensible.

Such activities upset Mrs. White, especially since the Western Health Reform Institute had been established precisely to get away from such unchristian practices. And the topic became personally embarrassing when reports began circulating that Ellen White herself had taken to occasional game playing. Is it true, inquired some Adventist elders, "that you have taken an interest in the amusements which have been practiced at the Health Institute at Battle Creek, that you play checkers, and carry a checker-board with you as you visit the brethren from place to place?" Absolutely not, she replied in the *Review and Herald*. Since her conversion at the age of twelve she had forsaken all such frivolities as checkers, chess, backgammon, and fox-and-geese. "I have spoken in favor of recreation, but have ever stood in great doubt of the amusements introduced at the Institute at Battle Creek, and have stated my objections to the physicians and directors, and others, in conversation with them, and by numerous letters."[25]

By the fall of 1867 Ellen White was so disgusted with the health institute she regarded it as "a curse" to the church, a place where sincere Christians became infidels and believers lost faith in her testimonies. But later that year a spiritual revival swept through the Adventist community in Battle Creek and rekindled her enthusiasm for the water cure. The following spring she pledged renewed support, and James became a director. Her blessing and her husband's business acumen were not sufficient, however, to keep the institute solvent. By the autumn of 1869 only eight paying patrons remained. A surplus of charity patients and other factors had contributed to this situation, but so had Mrs. White's harsh criticisms that had tarnished the institute's reputation among Adventists. She naturally saw it differently and later blamed the institute's decline entirely on the managers, especially Dr. Lay, whom she had come to regard as too proud and self-centered for his position. The directors at their

---

25. J. N. Andrews, "Amusements," *HR*, I (December, 1866), 80; O. F. Conklin, "Thanksgiving at the Health-Reform Institute," ibid., pp. 74-75; EGW, "The Health Institute," *Testimonies*, I, 633-43; EGW, "Questions and Answers," *R&H*, XXX (October 8, 1867), 261.

1869 annual meeting meekly acknowledged their guilt and absolved the Whites of any culpability. Within a year Dr. J. H. Ginley had replaced the unfortunate Dr. Lay as superintendent, and businessmen had taken the place of the ministers on the board of directors.[26]

At the height of the institute controversy Merritt Kellogg paid the Whites a surprise visit. The former Oberlin student, now in his mid-thirties, was on his way back to California after attending the winter term at Trall's Hygeio-Therapeutic College and picking up an M.D. degree. The Whites, ever suspicious of close contacts with outsiders, fully expected that someone so "fresh from Dr. Trall's school" would be polluted with extreme and objectionable views. They were "happily disappointed," however, to discover that Kellogg was free from all such fanaticism. And they were delighted when he explained the remarkable harmony between what the Lord had revealed to Ellen White and what Trall taught his students. Here was just the man, thought James, to go around to the churches and revive flagging interest in health reform.[27]

At first the unknown Kellogg merely accompanied the Whites on their speaking tours, presenting the scientific side of the reform question. But at the May General Conference session, through the influence of Elder White, the church officers asked Kellogg to remain in the East as a full-time health lecturer, speaking to local churches upon request. Kellogg agreed to this arrangement, but after only three series of talks in small Michigan towns, no more invitations came in. Disheartened, he wrote Mrs. White complaining of this strange "dumbness" on the part of the churches "after so much has been shown in vision concerning the importance of this health

---

26. EGW, "The Health Institute," *Testimonies,* I, 634; EGW, "The Health Institute," ibid., III, 165-85; EGW to Dr. and Mrs. Lay, February 13, 1870 (L-30-1870, White Estate); "Second Annual Meeting of the Health Reform Institute," *R&H,* XXXI (May 26, 1868), 258; "The Health Reform Institute," *R&H,* XXXIII (May 25, 1869), 175; "Health Institute," *R&H,* XXXV (May 3, 1870), 160; Gerald Carson, *Cornflake Crusade* (New York: Rinehart & Co., 1957), p. 82. This was not a happy time for the Whites. Criticism of their conduct reached such proportions that in 1870 the church felt it necessary to publish a 112-page *Defense of Eld. James White and Wife: Vindication of Their Moral and Christian Character* (Battle Creek: SDA Publishing Assn., 1870), countering charges of misusing funds, illicit sex, and other "shameful slanders."

27. James White, "Report of Meetings," *R&H,* XXXI (April 28, 1868), 312.

movement." He felt the Whites had already said more than enough in his behalf, and he refused "to beg the privilege of lecturing." When still no calls came, the discouraged man returned to his home in California and joined an evangelistic campaign.[28] Kellogg's few months in Michigan did produce one significant result: a union between the Battle Creek reformers and Dr. Trall, the foremost American hydropath. Undoubtedly inspired by Kellogg's favorable account of Trall's teachings, the Whites arranged to bring the prominent health reformer to Battle Creek for a course of lectures at the close of the annual general conference meetings. After an opening address to the conference delegates on Sunday evening, May 17, Trall spoke twice a day for four days to somewhat smaller crowds that included many Adventist ministers in town for the conference. Thursday afternoon was reserved for a private meeting with women only and was attended by hundreds of ladies attired in the reformed "short" dress. This display of the costume, the greatest Trall had ever seen, he credited to the influence of Mrs. White, who "not only advocates the dress-reform, but practices it."[29]

The only account we have of Trall's relationship with Ellen during this visit is curious indeed. Years after the event John Loughborough (a sometimes unreliable witness) wrote that although Ellen had refused to attend Trall's public lectures she had invited him on daily carriage rides during which "it was understood that he was to listen to her ideas of hygiene, disease and its causes, the effects of

---

28. James White, "Report from Bro. White," ibid., XXXI (May 5, 1868), 328; J. N. Andrews, "Business Proceedings of the Sixth Annual Session of the General Conference of Seventh-day Adventists," ibid., XXXI (May 26, 1868), 356; M. G. Kellogg to EGW, July 16, 1868 (White Estate); "Acknowledgment," *R&H*, XXXII (August 18, 1868), 137. In the 1870s Merritt Kellogg authored at least two books on health reform: *The Bath: Its Use and Application* (Battle Creek: Office of Health Reformer, 1873), and *The Hygienic Family Physician: A Complete Guide for the Preservation of Health, and the Treatment of the Sick without Medicine* (Battle Creek: Office of the Health Reformer, 1874).

29. J. N. Andrews and Others, "Lectures by Dr. Trall," *R&H*, XXXI (May 26, 1868), 360; R. T. Trall, "Visit to Battle Creek, Mich.," p. 14; [R. T. Trall], "Dress Reform Convention," *HR*, IV (September, 1869), 57. Dr. Jackson had been invited to lecture in Battle Creek in March of 1866, but a death at Dansville forced a cancellation; "Lectures at Battle Creek," *Laws of Life*, IX (March, 1866), 43; and "Going to Battle Creek," ibid., IX (April, 1866), 58.

medicines, etc." After the second day's conversation Trall reportedly asked her where she had studied medicine and was told she had received all her information from God in vision. "He assured her that her ideas were all in the strictest harmony with physiology and hygiene, and that on many of the subjects she went deeper than he ever had." By their last session together the amazed doctor is supposed to have remarked that his hostess could just as well have given the lectures on health as he. At least this is what Loughborough claimed to have heard from John Andrews, who rode along with the Whites and Trall through the streets of Battle Creek.[30]

The rapport thus established between the Whites and Trall resulted in the doctor's being asked to become a regular contributor to the *Reformer*. The addition of a distinguished name — "admitted by all to stand at the head of the health reform in this country, so far as human science is concerned" — was calculated to pump new life into an unexciting publication and was part of an overall plan of James White's for revamping the journal. Beginning with the first issue of the third volume (July, 1868), the number of pages was increased, a disgraced Lay was replaced by an "Editorial Committee of Twelve," and Trall's "Special Department" was inaugurated. For his part, Trall cooperated by folding his monthly *Gospel of Health* and turning over its subscription list to the *Reformer,* with the assurance to his readers that it would "be managed by those who are, head and heart, in full sympathy with the true principles of the great health reformation." With this merger Battle Creek for the first time assumed national importance in the health-reform movement.[31]

The new arrangement, begun with such high hopes, proved to be less than ideal. Numerous readers, it soon turned out, resented Trall's strictures against the use of salt, milk, and sugar. And to make matters worse, the managing editor of the *Reformer,* known by insiders to use these articles of food himself, backed Trall editorially and thus prompted the pioneer reformer to speak out stronger than he otherwise would have done. The Whites, who personally re-

---

30. J. N. Loughborough, *The Great Second Advent Movement: Its Rise and Progress* (Washington: Review and Herald Publishing Assn., 1905), pp. 364-65.

31. James White, "The Health Reformer," *R&H,* XXXII (July 28, 1868), 96; R. T. Trall, "Change of Programme," *HR,* III (July, 1868), 14.

spected Trall's opinions on diet, first detected signs of discontent while on a speaking tour through some Western states. There they found that many Westerners regarded the *Reformer* as "radical and fanatical" and had no interest at all in becoming subscribers. Upon returning to Battle Creek the dismayed Whites learned that letters were pouring in from disgruntled readers canceling their subscriptions. Clearly, the journal was "going away from the people, and leaving them behind."[32]

No doubt encouraged by Ellen, James assumed the helm of the *Reformer* himself and pledged to steer a course away from all extremes. Trall, however, stayed. His department alone was, in the elder's opinion, "worth twice the subscription price of the *Reformer*." During his illness in the mid-1860s James White had given up milk, salt, and sugar, and he believed "the time not far distant" when Trall's position on the use of these items would "be looked upon by all sound health reformers with more favor than they are at the present time." To placate disgruntled subscribers, and to give the journal an air of doctrinal orthodoxy, James had Ellen begin a second "Special Department" in the March, 1871, issue, at the same time warning readers not to "feel disturbed on seeing some things in these departments which do not agree with their ideas of matters and things." Even without the sections by his wife and Dr. Trall, there were "pages enough where all can read tenfold their money's worth." With Ellen's monthly department, regular articles by James, and advertisements for son Willie's "Hygienic Institute Nursery," the new *Reformer* at times took on the appearance of a White family production.[33]

Whatever his personal problems, James White was an effective promoter. Within two years he had raised subscriptions to the *Reformer* from three thousand to eleven thousand, and by 1875 an official report showed it to have "by far the largest circulation of any

---

32. EGW, "An Appeal for Burden-Bearers," *Testimonies*, III, 19-21. The managing editor, William C. Gage, later served as a temperance mayor of Battle Creek.

33. [James White], "The Health Reformer," *HR*, V (June, 1871), 286; [James White], "Close of the Volume," ibid., VII (December, 1872), 370; James White, "Health Reform — No. 5: Its Rise and Progress among Seventh-day Adventists," ibid., V (March, 1871), 190; [James White], "The Health Reformer," ibid., V (March, 1871), 172; "Hygienic Institute Nursery," ibid., V (June, 1871), 298; EGW, "Our Late Experience," *R&H*, XXVII (February 27, 1866), 97.

journal of its kind in the world." The previous year both special departments, having served their purpose, were discontinued. The fact that Trall left the *Reformer* at the height of its success, and apparently with the Whites' blessing, gives the lie to later charges by Dr. John Harvey Kellogg that Trall was responsible for the magazine's earlier difficulties.[34]

By the early 1870s the financial outlook of the institute and the *Reformer* appeared fairly bright; yet a dire shortage of Adventist physicians continued to threaten the medical work. Before there could be any significant expansion, it was obviously necessary, said James White, to "Hustle young men off to some doctor mill."[35] As far as Adventist needs were concerned, the best "mill" was Trall's Hygieo-Therapeutic College in Florence Heights, New Jersey, where the medical course was not only hydropathic but quick.

Although Trall's school may have been one of the weakest in America, it had many competitors. As Dr. Thomas L. Nichols remarked in 1864, Americans did everything in a hurry, including the training of their physicians:

> Nominally it is required that the student shall read three years, under some regular physician, during which time he must have attended two courses of medical lectures. If, however, he pay his fees, exhibit a certificate as to the time he has studied, or pretended to study, and pass a hasty examination, made by professors who are very anxious that he should pass, he gets a diploma of *Medicinae Doctor.* He has full authority to bleed and blister, set broken bones and cut off limbs.

Most states did not require a diploma, or even a license, to practice medicine; but with medical degrees so accessible, there was little reason for any aspiring doctor to go without one.[36]

---

34. [James White], "Close of the Volume," p. 370; [J. H. Kellogg], "Hygieo-Therapy and Its Founder," *Good Health,* XVII (March, 1882), 92.

35. James White to G. I. Butler, July 13, 1874 (White Estate).

36. Thomas L. Nichols, *Forty Years of American Life* (London: John Maxwell and Co., 1864), I, 363-64. See also William Frederick Norwood, *Medical Education in the United States before the Civil War* (Philadelphia: University of Pennsylvania Press, 1944), pp. 396-406.

Thus in the fall of 1872 James White arranged with Merritt Kellogg, of the class of '68, to return to Florence Heights with four carefully chosen Battle Creek students: John Harvey Kellogg, a protégé of the Whites and Merritt's younger half-brother; Jennie Trembley, an editorial assistant with the *Reformer;* and the two White boys, Edson and Willie. For several years Ellen White had dreamed of Edson's becoming a physician, but he had turned out to be such a poor health reformer she had finally given up on him in despair. "To place you in a prominent position to prove you where a failure would be so apparent," she wrote of his medical ambitions, "would disgrace us and yourself also and discourage you." Nevertheless, when the opportunity came in 1872 for him to try his hand at doctoring, she gave her consent — provided that he rely principally on his own resources.[37]

The most promising of the four, and the one on whom the Whites were counting the most, was John Kellogg, the precocious son of J. P. Kellogg, an early Adventist health reformer. When John was only about twelve years old, James White had brought him to the Review and Herald Press to learn printing. In just a few years the lad had worked himself up from errand boy to typesetter and occasional editor — and had read all the books and journals on health reform that he could get his hands on. Aiming to become a teacher, he had enrolled at age twenty in the Michigan State Normal College in Ypsilanti. During his second term there word reached him of the Whites' decision to sponsor him at Trall's medical school.[38]

The Hygieo-Therapeutic College proved to be just what James White had ordered: a doctor mill. Standards and staff alike were woefully inadequate. On opening day, when Trall found his faculty short two teachers (he had three on hand, including himself), he improvised by pressing Merritt into service as instructor in anatomy and John as lecturer on chemistry. The arrangement worked reasonably

---

37. M. G. Kellogg, memoir dictated to Clara K. Butler, October 21, 1916 (Kellogg Papers, MHC). On Edson's medical aspirations, see the following letters in the White Estate: EGW to Edson White, December 29, 1867 (W-21-1867); EGW to Edson White, June 10, 1869 (W-6-1869); EGW to Edson and Emma White, n.d. (W-14-1872); and EGW to Edson and Willie White, February 6, 1873 (W-6-1873).

38. Richard W. Schwarz, "John Harvey Kellogg: American Health Reformer" (Ph.D. diss., University of Michigan, 1964), pp. 17-22, 113-14.

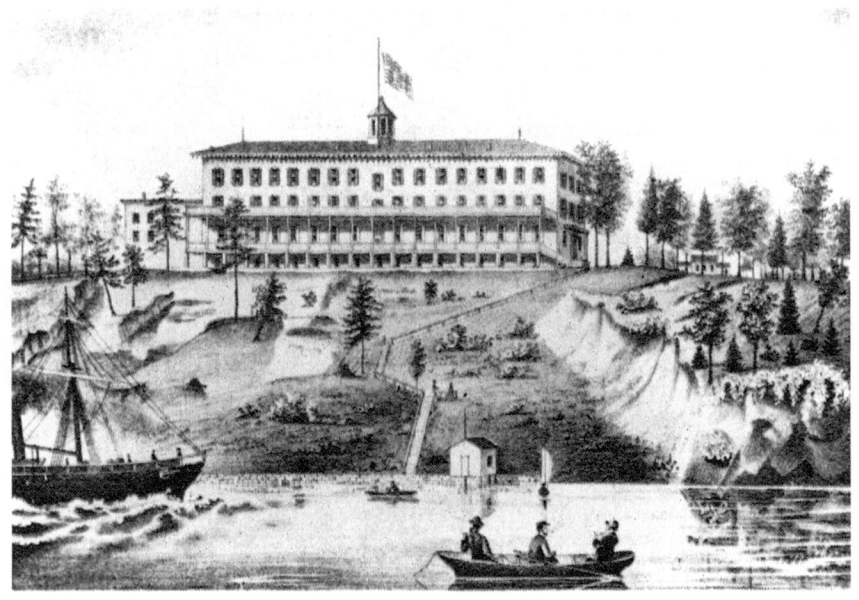

**Trall's Hygeian Home and Hygeio-Therapeutic College
at Florence Heights, New Jersey**
From J. D. Scott, *Historical Atlas of Burlington County, New Jersey* (Philadelphia, 1876),
in Harry B. Weiss and Howard R. Kemble, *The Great American Water-Cure Craze*
(Trenton, N.J.: Past Times Press, 1967)

well until John innocently wandered onto the forbidden field of *organic* chemistry — a science Trall insisted did not exist — and was subsequently relieved of his duties. Throughout the term the Kellogg and White brothers shared a room but apparently not a love for medicine. According to Merritt, Edson and Willie seldom cracked a book and always went to bed as early as possible. They did, however, attend lectures and were thus able to spy on Trall for their mother, who was curious to know if the doctor picked her writings to pieces or questioned them in any way. Despite the fact that he never examined his students, and that some were not legally old enough to practice medicine, Trall awarded them each a handsome diploma and sent them out to ply their trade on an unsuspecting world.[39]

39. M. G. Kellogg, memoir dictated to Clara K. Butler, October 12, 1916; EGW to Edson and Willie White, February 6, 1873; [J. H. Kellogg], "Hygeio-Therapy and Its

The Western Health Reform Institute

Since most of the Battle Creek students went into fields other than medicine, few patients in this instance suffered from Trall's lax standards. John Kellogg, the only one of the four to make a full-time career of medicine, wisely went on to study for two additional years at orthodox and reputable institutions: the College of Medicine and Surgery of the University of Michigan (1873-75) and the Bellevue Hospital Medical School in New York City (1874-75). Although his decision to attend Bellevue initially went against the "urgent advice" of James White, who "had the impression that so long as nature had to do the healing work anyway, it was quite unnecessary for the doctor to worry about so much minute detail," he eventually won the elder's moral and financial backing. Upon receiving his degree, five-foot, four-inch John proudly wrote Willie White that he now felt "more than fifty pounds bigger since getting a certain piece of sheepskin about two feet square. It's a *bonafide* sheep, too, by the way, none of your bogus paper concerns like the hygieotherapeutic document."[40]

Young Kellogg had a right to be proud, for he had pulled himself up from his sectarian roots to become the first Seventh-day Adventist worthy of the title "doctor." In the spring of 1875 he returned to Battle Creek and joined the staff of the Western Health Reform Institute. Being politically astute — and perhaps grateful — he at once allied himself with the Whites in their efforts to maintain control of an expanding church organization. That winter he joined Uriah Smith and Sidney Brownsberger, principal of the Adventist's Battle Creek College, in pledging to assist the Whites in bringing "discipline and order" to the work in Battle Creek. The alliance paid off handsomely the following year when the group secured his appointment, at age twenty-four, to the superintendency of the health institute, replacing Dr. William Russell, who left with over one-fourth of

---

Founder," p. 92. The entire M. G. Kellogg memoir is reproduced in Ronald L. Numbers, "Health Reform on the Delaware," *New Jersey History*, XCII (Spring, 1974), 5-12.

40. J. H. Kellogg, "My Search for Health," MS dated January 16, 1942 (Kellogg Papers, MHC); J. H. Kellogg to Willie White, March 3, 1875, and April 12, 1875 (White Estate); Richard W. Schwarz, *John Harvey Kellogg, M.D.* (Nashville: Southern Publishing Assn., 1970), p. 60. A friend of Kellogg's at Bellevue, and the only other health reformer, was Jim Jackson, son of the founder of Our Home; see Kellogg, "My Search for Health," p. 9; and Kellogg to Willie White, March 3, 1875.

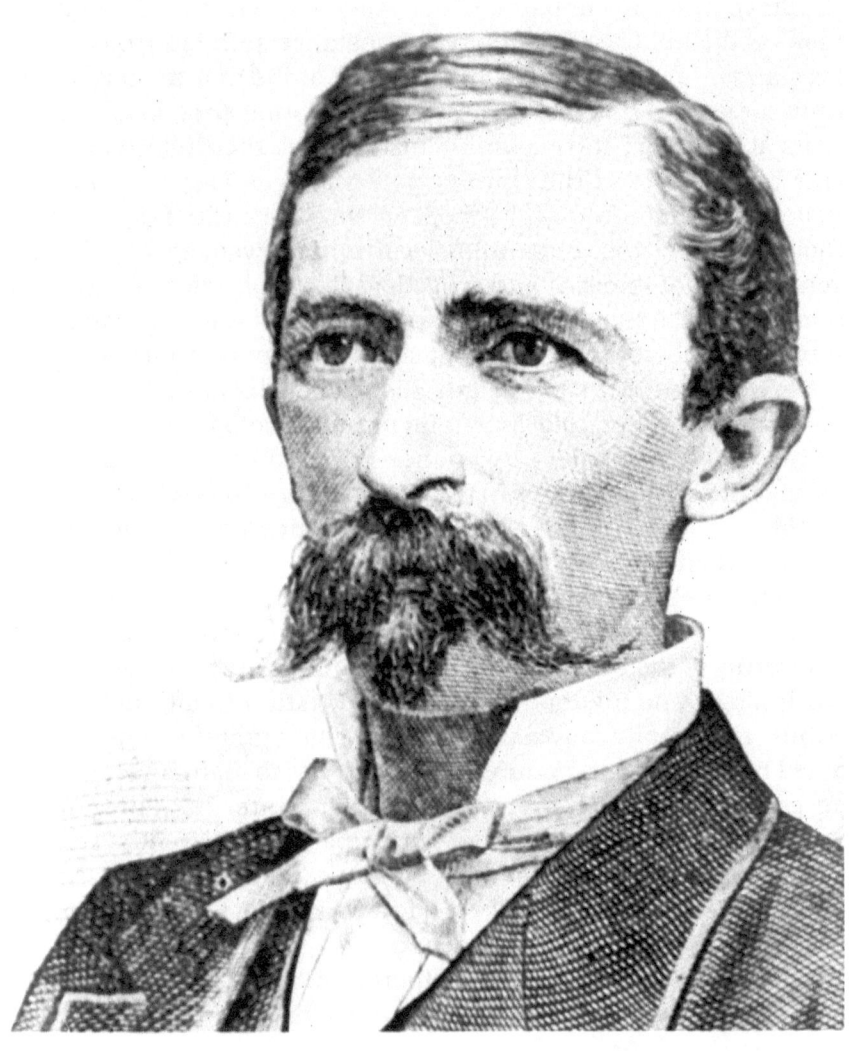

Young John Harvey Kellogg shortly after he assumed the superintendency of the Western Health Reform Institute
From Kellogg, *Plain Facts for Old and Young* (Burlington, Iowa: I. F. Segner, 1882)

the patients to run a water cure in Ann Arbor. For the next four years Kellogg thrived as James White's "fair-haired boy," but he eventually came to resent the elder's dictatorial ways.[41]

Kellogg's fondest wish was to turn the poorly equipped Battle Creek water cure into a scientifically respectable institution where a wide variety of medical and surgical techniques would be used. In this task he found a ready and powerful ally in Ellen White, who was beginning to resent having "worldlings sneeringly [assert] that those who believe present truth are weak-minded, deficient in education, without position or influence." A first-rate medical center would prove her detractors wrong and bring fame and honor to Seventh-day Adventists. In several respects the time seemed propitious for such a move. A handful of Adventist young people were coming out of recognized medical schools, patients were flocking to the institute, and the old debts were finally off the books. So when Kellogg approached the prophetess with plans for a large multistoried sanitarium, he met a warm response. And when Ellen had a dream sanctioning the erection of a large building, it was all James needed to volunteer to raise the necessary funds. "Now that we have men of ability, refinement, and sterling sense, educated at the best medical schools on the continent," he wrote glowingly in the *Review and Herald,* "we are ready to build."[42]

By the spring of 1878 an imposing new Medical and Surgical Sanitarium stood on the old institute grounds. But the Whites were not pleased. Construction costs had once again plunged the church heavily into debt and disturbed the tranquillity of Elder and Mrs. White. She had originally called for a first-class medical institution, but now that the building was finished, it reminded her of "a grand hotel rather than an institution for the treatment of the sick." Out went a testimony reprimanding the prodigal sanitarium managers for their "extravagant outlay" in "aiming at the world's standards," and for other misdeeds. Although Kellogg felt some of the charges leveled against him were grossly unfair, he attributed the outburst

41. Schwarz, "John Harvey Kellogg: American Health Reformer," pp. 174-77.

42. [J. H. Kellogg], "The Health Institute," *HR,* X (June, 1875), 192; EGW, *Testimony for the Physicians and Helpers of the Sanitarium* (n.d. [1880 ?]), p. 8; J. H. Kellogg, autobiographical memoir, October 21, 1938 (Kellogg Papers, MHC); J[ames] W[hite], "Home Again," *R&H,* XLIX (May 24, 1877), 164.

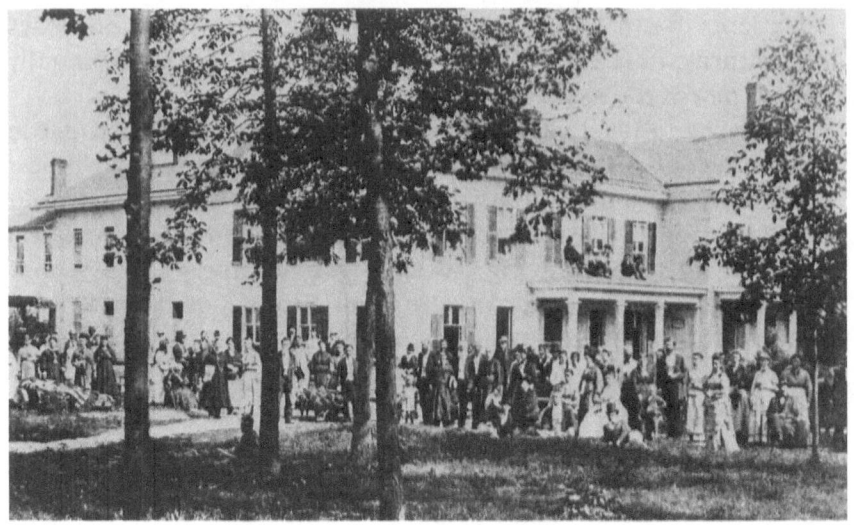

The new Western Health Reform Institute in the mid-1870s. Note Mrs. White (in her reform dress) and Elder White standing to the right of the trees.
Courtesy Ellen G. White Estate, Inc.

more to the machinations of James than to Ellen herself. In the fall of 1880 he retaliated by uniting with two of James White's rivals, Elders S. N. Haskell and G. I. Butler, to force the aging leader off the sanitarium board and to elect Haskell chairman in his place. Within a year James White lay dying in Battle Creek as a reconciled Dr. Kellogg labored in vain to save the patriarch's life.[43]

Through the following years Kellogg struggled to escape his sectarian past by identifying with the "rational medicine" of such distinguished practitioners as Jacob Bigelow and Oliver Wendell Holmes. The "rational" physician, said Kellogg, adopts "all of hygieo-therapy and all the good of every other system known or possible," not just the water cure. His ties to hydropathy were too strong to sever entirely, however; and in the mid-1880s local physicians, led

43. "Interview between Geo. W. Amadon, Eld. A. C. Bourdeau, and Dr. J. H. Kellogg," pp. 88-89; EGW, *Testimony for the Physicians and Helpers of the Sanitarium*, pp. 52-55; Schwarz, "John Harvey Kellogg: American Health Reformer," p. 177. When this testimony was reprinted for general circulation, Kellogg's name and several criticisms were deleted; see EGW, *Testimonies*, IV, 571-74.

by a former student and associate, Dr. Will Fairfield, tried (unsuccessfully) to oust him from the county medical society for sectarianism. Kellogg's vindication came sometime later when Dr. Henry Hurd, medical director of the Johns Hopkins University Hospital, publicly lauded him for "having converted into a scientific institution an establishment founded on a vision." But even after he had become a national figure, and his sanitarium world famous, Kellogg never forgot that the institution's "real founder and chief promoter" was Ellen White.[44]

44. J. H. Kellogg, "The American Medical Missionary College," *Medical Missionary*, V (October, 1895), 291; [J. H. Kellogg], "Hygeio-Therapy and Its Founder," p. 93; J. H. Kellogg to EGW, December 19, 1885, December 6, 1886, and October 30, 1904 (White Estate). Hurd is quoted in J. H. Kellogg, autobiographical memoir, October 21, 1938, p. 5.

CHAPTER SIX

Short Skirts and Sex

"God would not have his people adopt the so-called reform dress."

Ellen G. White (1863)[1]

"God would now have his people adopt the reform dress...."

Ellen G. White (1867)[2]

Ellen White took great interest in the affairs of the Western Health Reform Institute, but she did not allow the water cure to monopolize her attention. In the decades following her 1863 vision and the subsequent visits to Dansville she spoke out frequently and forcefully on the other facets of health reform: dress, sex, and diet. Of all the causes she urged on her followers, perhaps none was more personally frustrating than her ten-year effort to put the Adventist sisters into "short" skirts and pants. The need for dress reform was self-evident. Fashionable layers of long skirts and petticoats, weighing as much as fifteen pounds, swept floors and streets, while vise-like corsets tortured midriffs into exaggerated hourglass shapes, resulting in frequent fainting and internal damage. And to make

---

1. EGW, "The Cause in the East," *Testimonies,* I, 421.
2. EGW, "The Reform Dress," ibid., I, 525. Ellen White was referring here to her own reform dress as opposed to the "so-called reform dress" of Harriet Austin and others.

American women even more uncomfortable and immobile, the steel-wired hoop skirt staged a revival in the mid-1850s.³

About 1850 Elizabeth Smith Miller quietly launched a revolt to free women from their "clothes-prison." Encouraged by her reform-minded father, Gerrit Smith, she broke with fashion and donned a short skirt over pantaloons. Her unusual attire attracted little attention until she visited her cousin Elizabeth Cady Stanton in Seneca Falls, New York, and caught the eye of Amelia Bloomer, editor of a women's temperance magazine, the *Lily*. When the *Lily* began advocating Libby Miller's outfit, the national press dubbed it the "Bloomer." Seneca Falls in the 1850s was a hotbed of feminist activity, and the women's righters eagerly adopted the Bloomer as their distinctive uniform. Among the Bloomerites were such leading feminists as Sarah and Angelina Grimké, Lucy Stone, and Susan B. Anthony.⁴

Health reformers, who had long condemned the evils of tight corsets and dragging skirts, shared the feminists' enthusiasm for the Bloomer. It became especially popular at water cures, where cumbersome long dresses were definitely out of style. Almost inevitably, Gerrit Smith's protégé James Caleb Jackson supported the reform, promoting the short skirt first at Glen Haven and then at Our Home. Not being completely satisfied with the original style, he and his associate Harriet N. Austin slightly modified the Bloomer and renamed it the "American costume." Although the casual observer could scarcely distinguish their design from Mrs. Miller's, Jackson heatedly insisted that it was no more like the Bloomer than "an elephant is like a rhinoceros."⁵

---

    3. Andrew Sinclair, *The Emancipation of the American Woman* (New York: Harper and Row, 1966), pp. 102-4; Elizabeth McClellan, *History of American Costume: 1607-1870* (New York: Tudor Publishing Co., 1969), p. 466.

    4. Sinclair, *Emancipation of the American Woman,* p. 105; Elizabeth Cady Stanton and Others, *History of Woman Suffrage* (New York: Fowler & Wells, 1881), I, 127-28, 544; Alma Lutz, *Created Equal: A Biography of Elizabeth Cady Stanton, 1815-1902* (New York: John Day Co., 1940), pp. 63-64, Elizabeth Smith Miller's own account of the origin of the "Bloomer" appears in Aileen S. Kraditor (ed.), *Up from the Pedestal: Selected Writings in the History of American Feminism* (Chicago: Quadrangle Books, 1968), pp. 123-24.

    5. James C. Jackson, *How to Treat the Sick without Medicine* (Dansville, N.Y.: Aus-

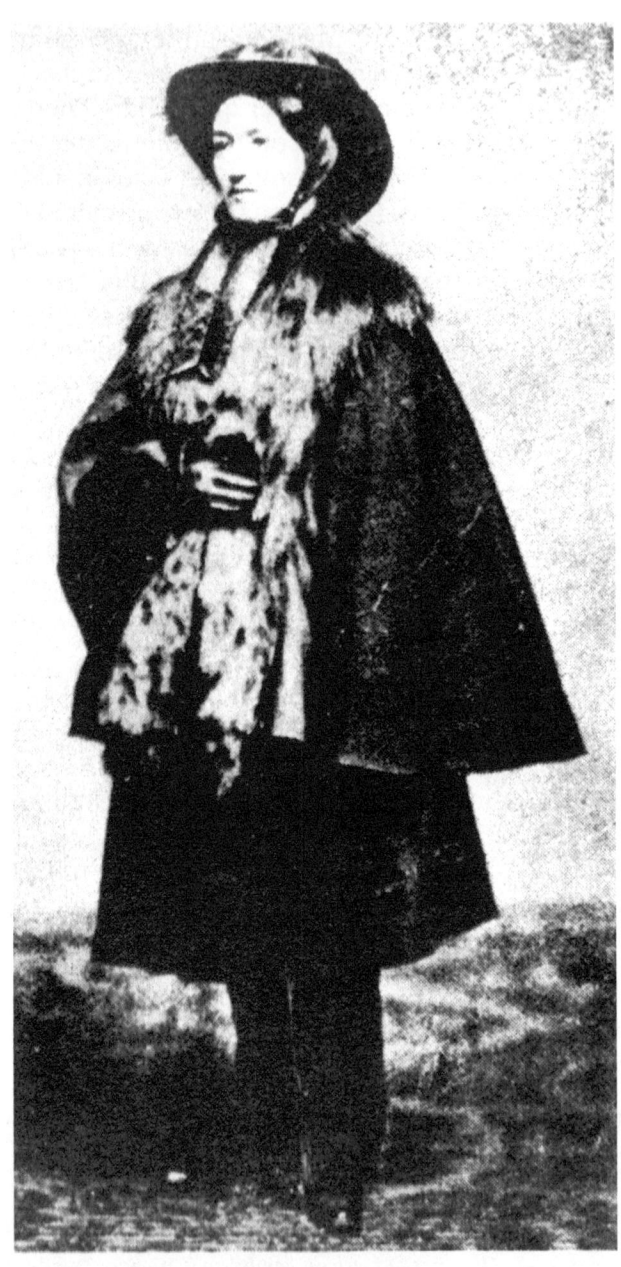

Elizabeth Smith Miller in the costume she designed
From Carrie A. Hall, *From Hoopskirts to Nudity* (Caldwell, Idaho: Caxton Printers, Ltd., 1938)

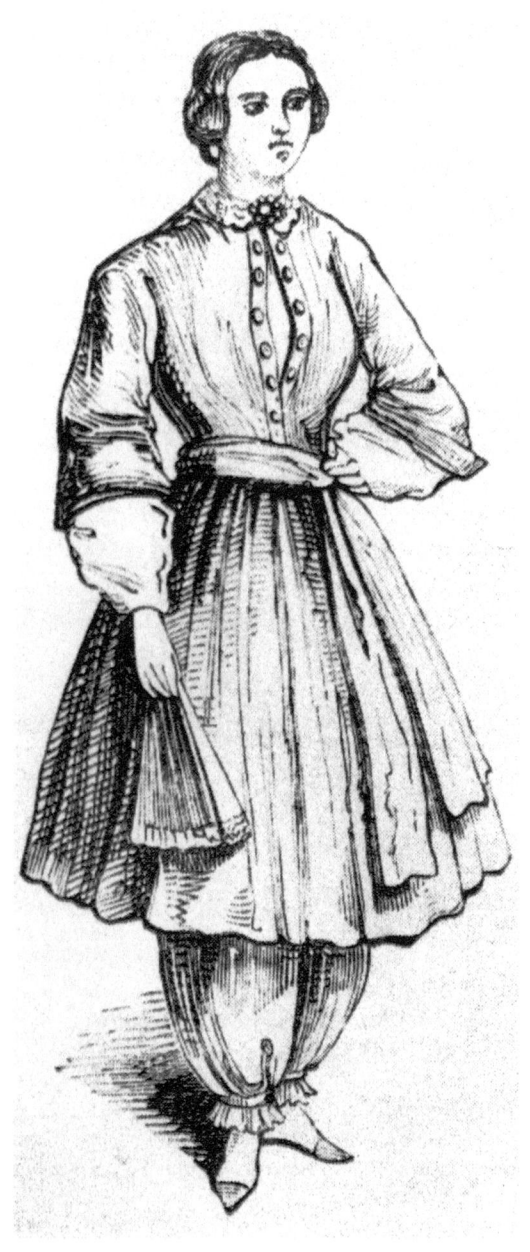

Amelia Bloomer, who lent her name to Mrs. Miller's invention
From Carrie A. Hall, *From Hoopskirts to Nudity* (Caldwell, Idaho: Caxton Printers, Ltd., 1938)

Despite the advantages of comfort and mobility it gave its wearers, the Bloomer and its variations met with universal ridicule and abuse. A hostile press characterized Bloomerites as "strong minded" and associated them with "free love" and "easy divorce." On one occasion Ellen Beard Harman, Trall's associate, was even arrested for wearing pants on the streets of New York City. To avoid such unpleasantries, both Libby Miller and Elizabeth Stanton experimented with skirts at various lengths below the knee, and Mrs. Stanton once went so far as to discard the controversial trousers. This latter act elicited a strong rebuke from Susan Anthony, who feared that it would "only be said the Bloomers have doffed their Pants the better to display their legs." Discouraged, the feminists one by one abandoned their reform. "We put the dress on for greater freedom," explained Mrs. Stanton, "but what is physical freedom compared with mental bondage?" By the 1860s the costume was no longer capturing headlines, but its influence could still be seen among hard-working housewives in the West and at places like Our Home on the Hillside, the Dansville water cure twice visited by Ellen White.[6]

Since her girlhood days Ellen had been a plain dresser — no bows, no ribbons, no rings. Among the strict Christians with whom she associated, outward adornment was not only a sure sign of a corrupt heart but a sinful waste of means as well. Thus for her, modesty

---

tin, Jackson & Co., 1872), pp. 66-67. On the American costume, see also William D. Conklin, *The Jackson Health Resort* (Dansville, N.Y.: Privately distributed by the author, 1971), pp. 137, 191-93. On the distinction between the Bloomer and the American costume, see Harriet N. Austin, "Various Things," *Laws of Life*, IX (August, 1866), 115. In 1852 Mrs. M. Angeline Merritt suggested naming the reform dress "the American dress"; see her *Dress Reform, Practically and Physiologically Considered* (Buffalo: Jewett, Thomas and Co., 1852), p. 134.

6. Stanton and Others, *History of Woman Suffrage*, I, 470; "Patrick vs. 'The Am. Costume,'" *Herald of Health*, V (June, 1865), 155; Kraditor, *Up from the Pedestal*, p. 124; Lutz, *Created Equal*, p. 86; Robert E. Riegel, "Women's Clothes and Women's Rights," *American Quarterly*, XV (Fall, 1963), 394. Susan Anthony is quoted in Sinclair, *Emancipation of the American Woman*, p. 106. Elizabeth Stanton's comment is found in Eleanor Flexner, *Century of Struggle: The Woman's Rights Movement in the United States* (New York: Atheneum, 1970), p. 84. On dress reform in the West, see "Dress Reform Pic-Nic," *HR*, IV (November, 1869), 84; and Mrs. S. W. Dodds, "Dress Reform and Health Reform in Kansas," *HR*, IV (February, 1870), 157-58.

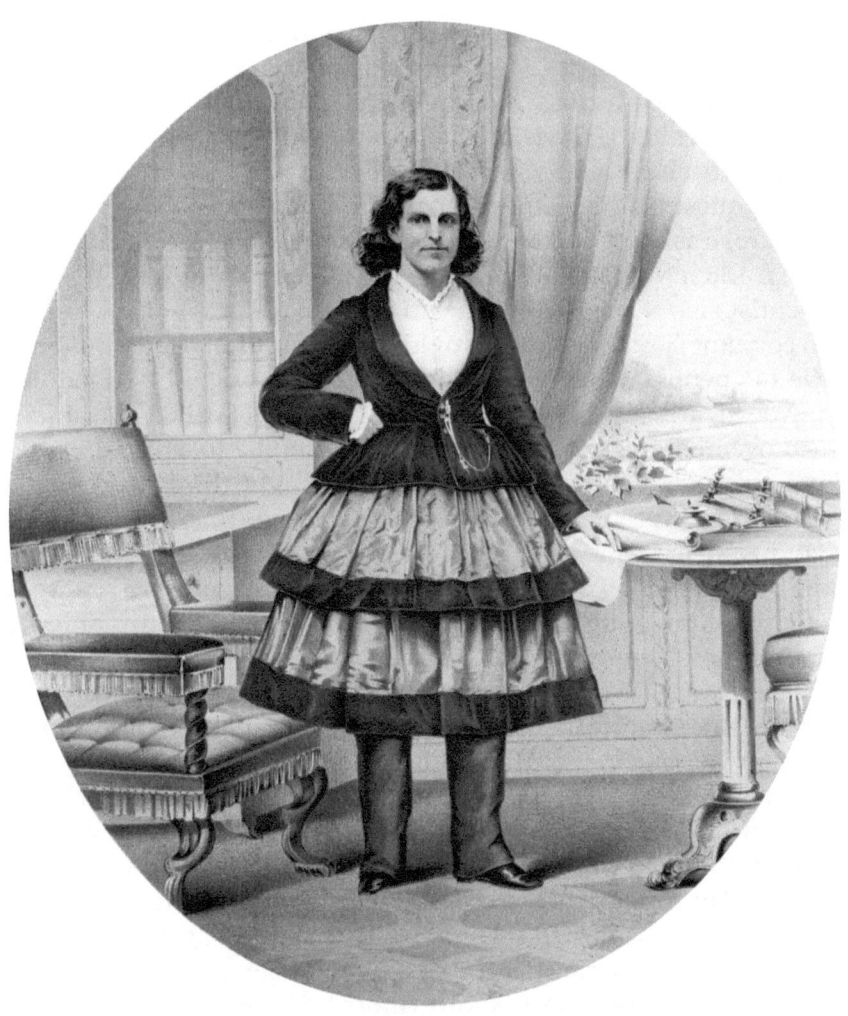

Harriet N. Austin in the American Costume
Courtesy of the Dansville Area Historical Society

in dress was not originally a matter of health but of religion. When she damned the "disgusting" hoop skirt in the early 1860s, her reason for doing so was that God would have a "peculiar" people. It was not until after her 1863 vision that she began associating the subject of dress with health.[7]

The question of whether Adventists should embrace the reform dress arose as soon as Ellen White began preaching her health message in 1863. No doubt inspired by the divine call for reform, a few Adventist sisters pressed for the immediate adoption of the American costume. But Mrs. White would have none of it. "God would not have his people adopt the so-called reform dress," she stated unequivocally in *Testimony No. 10*. "Those who feel called out to join the movement in favor of women's rights and the so-called dress reform, might as well sever all connection with the third angel's message." In her recent vision God had shown her that the American costume specifically violated the biblical injunction in Deuteronomy 22:5 against women wearing "that which pertaineth unto a man." Besides being mannish, the outfit induced "a spirit of levity and boldness" unbefitting a Christian.[8]

There was also a more personal reason for Ellen White's opposition to the American costume: she feared identification with Bloomer-wearing spiritualists. Since the 1848 experiments of Kate and Margaret Fox with the rappings of "Mr. Splitfoot," spirit communication had become an American sensation. Because of Mrs. White's ability to communicate with the supernatural world, early Seventh-day Adventists were often "branded as Spiritualists." Eli Curtis, a Millerite turned spiritualist, had upset the young prophetess by failing to discriminate between her divine revelations and the diabolical work of "the Dixboro Ghost." She was afraid that the adoption of the American costume would only add to such confu-

---

7. EGW, *Spiritual Gifts: My Christian Experience, Views and Labors* (Battle Creek: James White, 1860), pp. 13-14; EGW, "A Question Answered," *Testimonies*, I, 251-52; EGW to Mary Loughborough, June 6, 1861 (L-5-1861, White Estate). Mrs. White shortly thereafter condemned the view that "oddity and carelessness in dress" were virtuous; EGW, "Power of Example," *Testimonies*, I, 275.

8. EGW, "The Cause in the East," pp. 420-21; EGW, "Extremes in Dress," *Testimonies*, I, 424-25. Marietta V. Cook was wearing and promoting the American costume by early 1863; see "A Good Beginning," *Laws of Life*, VI (March, 1863), 43.

sion and destroy whatever influence the Adventists had. To avoid this possibility, she recommended that Adventist women simply wear their dresses "so as to clear the filth of the streets an inch or two." In this way they would appear neither "odd or singular."⁹

Within a year or so of writing these words Ellen White paid her first visit to Dansville and began having second thoughts about the reform dress. Up close it did not appear nearly as inappropriate as she had imagined. Harriet Austin's masculine appearance repulsed her; but, she wrote friends, some of the dresses were "very becoming, if not so short." Using patterns from Dansville, she planned to devise a dress "from four to six inches shorter than now worn" that would "accord perfectly" with what she had seen in vision. Of necessity it would have to be distinct from the previously condemned American costume. "We shall imitate or follow no fashion we have ever yet seen," she promised. "We shall institute a fashion which will be both economical and healthy."¹⁰

In the last of her *How to Live* pamphlets, probably completed soon after returning from Our Home, Ellen White provided the first public indication of her weakening opposition to the reform dress. Addressing her sisters in the church, she made her case for joining the dress reformers. "Christians should not take pains to make themselves gazing-stocks by dressing differently from the world," she told them. "But if in accordance with their faith and duty in respect to their dressing modestly and healthfully, they find them-

---

9. EGW, "The Cause in the East," p. 421; EGW, "Extremes in Dress," pp. 424-25; EGW, "Eli Curtis," *R&H,* I (April 7, 1851), 64. On spiritualism in America, see R. Laurence Moore, "Spiritualism and Science: Reflections on the First Decade of the Spirit Rappings," *American Quarterly,* XXIV (October, 1972), 474-500; and Moore, "Spiritualism," in *The Rise of Adventism: Religion and Society in Mid-Nineteenth-Century America,* ed. Edwin S. Gaustad (New York: Harper & Row, 1974), pp. 79-103.

10. EGW to Bro. and Sister Lockwood, September [14], 1864 (L-6-1864, White Estate). James White expressed serious doubts about the American costume shortly after arriving at Dansville, but by the time he departed he reportedly told his hosts: "If we cannot produce a better style of dress reform than that worn here, you may expect to see my wife dressed in your style." James White to Mrs. Myrta E. Steward, September 6, 1864 (White Estate); H. E. Carver, *Mrs. E. G. White's Claims to Divine Inspiration Examined* (2nd ed.; Marion, Iowa: Advent and Sabbath Advocate Press, 1877), p. 17.

selves out of fashion, they should not change their dress in order to be like the world." The pressing issue was what course to take, for the extremely short skirts of some reformers seemed scarcely less objectionable than the notorious whalebones and heavy dresses of fashionable ladies. Her solution was to lengthen the skirt of the American costume. "The dress should reach somewhat below the top of the boot; but should be short enough to clear the filth of the sidewalk and street, without being raised by the hand." No specific length was given, but alert readers were not slow in pointing out that "the top of the boot" was a good deal higher than "an inch or two" from the street.[11]

Verbally accepting the reform dress was one thing; actually putting it on was something else again. Month after month Ellen postponed the dreadful moment, praying for the perfect occasion. Her opportunity came in September, 1865, when she accompanied her ailing husband for a second visit to Our Home. There, mingling with others in short skirts and pants, she would not attract any undesirable attention. During the stopover in Rochester, shortly before arriving in Dansville, she put the finishing touches on her new wardrobe. Anxious not to appear singular in any way, she wrote home asking her children to send a dozen steel-rimmed buttons. "I need them up and down my short dress," she explained. "That is the way they all have them." Presumably her Dansville debut took place without incident; yet for over a year she remained self-conscious whenever appearing in the eye-catching garb. Under no circumstances would she wear it "at meetings, in the crowded streets of villages and cities, and when visiting distant relatives."[12]

Mrs. White no doubt would have pursued this halfhearted course indefinitely had not the eruption of an internecine conflict forced her hand. The controversy broke out when physicians at the newly opened Western Health Reform Institute, acting in harmony with the counsel in *How to Live,* urged incoming patients to dress in

---

11. EGW, *Health; or, How to Live* (Battle Creek: SDA Publishing Assn., 1865), No. 6, pp. 57-64. In the fifth pamphlet of the series Ellen had discussed proper clothing for children, largely repeating what Dio Lewis and others had earlier said. *How to Live* was published in June, 1865.

12. EGW to Edson and Willie White, September 18, 1865 (W-5-1865, White Estate); EGW, "Questions and Answers," *R&H,* XXX (October 8, 1867), 260-61.

the manner revealed by God. This policy, identifying Adventism with the disreputable short skirt, aroused the ire of some Battle Creek brethren and their fashion-conscious wives. Had not Mrs. White in *Testimony No. 10* pointedly condemned the reform dress? they asked. As the debate heated, it became clear that the authority of Ellen White's visions was at stake. Openly siding with the physicians, she lamented that among her critics, whom she characterized as possessing "a strange spirit of blind and bitter opposition," were "some who professed to be among the firmest friends of the testimonies." When news of the dissension spread beyond the confines of Battle Creek in the fall and winter of 1866, a flood of letters descended on Ellen White, demanding an explanation of the apparent contradiction between *Testimony No. 10* and *How to Live*. Which instruction was the church to follow: the 1863 admonition not to adopt the reform dress, or the later advice to wear a lengthened American costume?[13]

Deserted by friends and besieged by enemies, Mrs. White in late December withdrew with her ailing husband to the less hostile territory of northern Michigan. Here in the small town of Wright they remained six weeks attempting to recoup their lost health and influence. At first even the Adventists in Wright suspected there "was not full harmony in Mrs. White's testimony, especially on dress." But, reported James, "as she was present to speak for herself she was able to show a perfect harmony in her testimonies, and the church seems to be thoroughly aroused and prepared to receive the truth [on dress reform]." Her first two weekends in Wright Ellen cautiously kept on her "long dress" while she explained the benefits of the short skirt and pants. Then, after all prejudice had disappeared, she slipped into her reform dress. The response from the sisters was heartening, and for several years thereafter she consistently wore the divisive short skirt.[14]

During her sojourn at Wright, Ellen White wrote out a new testimony (No. 11), which she hoped would set the record straight and end the unpleasant controversy that had engulfed her. Petulantly

---

13. Ibid., p. 261.
14. James White, "Report from Bro. White," *R&H,* XXIX (January 15, 1867), 66-67; EGW, "Questions and Answers," p. 261.

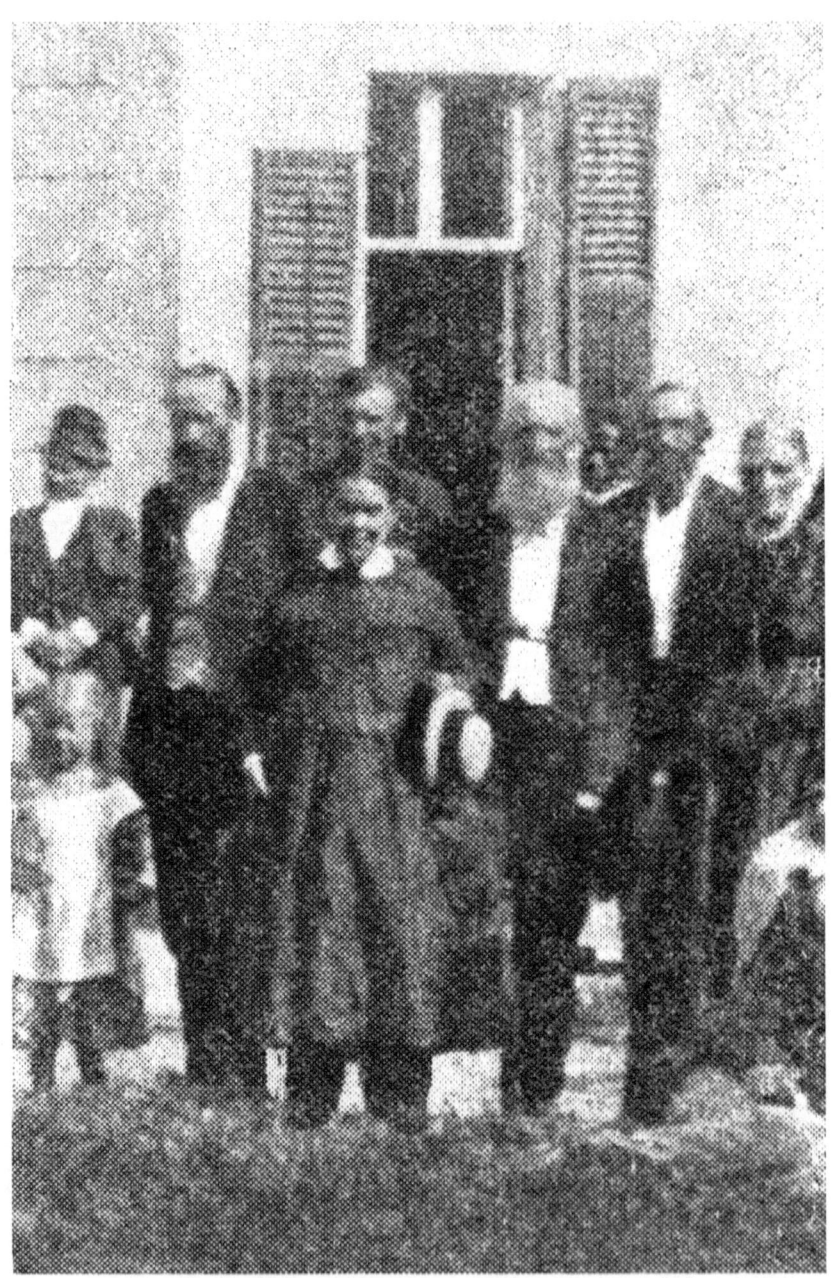

Ellen White in her short skirt and pants, about 1874

Short Skirts and Sex

she attributed the confusion surrounding her views on dress to "those who do not wish to believe what I have written" and thus fail to see the accord between *Testimony No. 10* and *How to Live*. "I must contend," she wrote, "that I am the best judge of the things which have been presented before me in vision; and none need fear that I shall by my life contradict my own testimony, or that I shall fail to notice any real contradiction in the views given me." Her two statements on dress could not possibly disagree, she asserted, for they were both based on the same vision. Therefore, "if there is any difference, it is simply in the form of expression." Her allusion to "the top of the boot" seemed to be the most troublesome. But since she had obviously been referring to those commonly worn by women — not men's high-topped boots — she professed to see no basis for misunderstanding.[15]

Elsewhere, she recalled in detail what she had seen four years earlier on the evening of June 5:

> ... three companies of females passed before me, with their dresses as follows with respect to length:
>
> The first were of fashionable length, burdening the limbs, impeding the step, and sweeping the street and gathering its filth; the evil results of which I have fully stated. This class who were slaves to fashion, appeared feeble and languid.
>
> The dress of the second class which passed before me was in many respects as it should be. The limbs were well clad. They were free from the burdens which the tyrant, Fashion, had imposed upon the first class; but had gone to the extreme in the short dress as to disgust and prejudice good people, and destroy in a great measure their own influence. This is the style and influence of the "American Costume," taught and worn by many at "Our Home," Dansville, N.Y. It does not reach to the knee. I need not say that this style of dress was shown to me to be too short.
>
> A third class passed before me with cheerful countenances, and free, elastic step. Their dress was the length I have described as proper, modest and healthful. It cleared the filth of the street and side-walk a few inches under all circumstances, such as ascending and descending steps, &c.

---

15. EGW, "Reform in Dress," *Testimonies*, I, 456-66.

Since she had not seen a lady's boot, and since the angel with her had not quoted a particular length, she went on, "I was left to describe the length of the proper dress in my own language the best I could, which I have done by stating that the bottom of the dress should reach near the top of a lady's boot, which would be necessary in order to clear the filth of the streets under the circumstances before named."[16]

Essential to Ellen White's defense was the alleged shortness of the American costume. Having previously denounced it as displeasing to God, she now found it desirable to put as much distance as possible between her own design and that associated with Dansville. To get this message across, she insisted that the American costume did "not reach to the knee," that it fell "about half-way from the hip to the knee," or that Dr. Harriet Austin wore her skirts about "six inches" above the knee. In contrast, her own dresses cleared the floor by only about nine inches and thus clearly represented a distinct style.[17]

There is evidence, however, that her zeal to appear independent of any Dansville influence led her to exaggerate the differences between Dr. Austin and herself. In her writings on dress reform Dansville's lady physician consistently advocated wearing the skirt of the American costume "a little below the knee" — not six inches above — and contemporary photographs show that this is in fact the length she wore her dresses (see photo, p. 189). Her friend Charlotte A. Joy, first president of the National Dress Reform Association, likewise advised wearing the skirt "just below the knee." When asked once about the accuracy of the Whites' description of her dress, Dr. Austin replied that "it was not the first time she had heard of Eld. White and wife making misstatements about her dress, but that she had always worn, and in her descriptions and advice to others had recommended a dress which covers the knee in walking, and which reaches six or eight inches below the knee in sitting; and that neither Eld. nor Mrs. White ever saw her in a dress which in standing or walking did not cover the bend of the knee." Some years after

---

16. EGW, "Questions and Answers," p. 260.
17. Ibid.; EGW, "Reform in Dress," p. 465; Carver, *Mrs. E. G. White's Claims to Divine Inspiration Examined,* p. 15.

the controversy over his wife's testimonies had simmered down, James White, in a moment of candor, granted that Ellen's vaunted innovation had consisted principally of lowering the skirt of the American costume a few inches: "The style of dress introduced by Mrs. W. and adopted by our sisters, with very few exceptions, is about the same as the American Costume of Our Home, with this difference, the skirt of the American Costume reaches hardly to the bend of the knee, while that introduced by Mrs. W., reaches within nine or ten inches of the floor."[18]

Following the publication of *Testimony No. 11* early in 1867, Ellen White devoted considerable energy to establishing uniformity in dress among Adventist women. Since her 1863 warning that "God would not have his people adopt the so-called reform dress," her views had changed significantly. It was currently her opinion that "God would now have his people adopt the reform dress," but not the "deformed" outfits some of the sisters were putting on in the name of reform. Above all, a standard length needed to be set. "I would earnestly recommend uniformity in length," she wrote in *Testimony No. 12* (1867), "and would say that nine inches as nearly accords with my views of the matter as I am able to express it in inches." Only a few months earlier, while still in northern Michigan, she had finally settled on that figure. When the question of a proper length had arisen, someone had brought out a ruler, measured a number of reform dresses, and simply taken the average. "Having seen the rule applied to the distance from the floor of several dresses, and having become fully satisfied that nine inches comes the nearest to the samples shown me," she explained, "I have given this number of inches in No. 12, as the proper length in regard to which uniformity is very desirable." Why the dress had seemed to be only "an inch or two" from the street immediately following her

---

18. Harriet N. Austin, "Dress Reform," *Water-Cure Journal,* XIX (April, 1855), 80; Harriet N. Austin, "The Reform Dress," ibid., XXIII (January, 1857), 3; Harriet N. Austin, "What Is the American Costume?" *Laws of Life,* X (August, 1867), 121; Charlotte A. Joy, "Suggestions to Women Who Are Interested in the Dress Reform," *Water-Cure Journal,* XXI, (May, 1856), 114; James White, "Health Reform — No. 7: Its Rise and Progress among Seventh-day Adventists," *HR,* V (May 1871), 253. Harriet Austin's comments on the Whites are based on a letter to H. E. Carver, March 26, 1868; Carver, *Mrs. E. G. White's Claims to Divine Inspiration Examined,* p. 15.

1863 vision, she did not explain, except to say that "the length was not given me in inches."[19]

To assist the sisters in dressing alike, Ellen White began peddling approved patterns as she traveled from church to church. Those unable to make the purchase directly could order them through the mail, as suggested in the following advertisement for "Reformed Dress Patterns" appended to the back of one of her *Testimony* pamphlets:

> I will furnish patterns of the pants and sack, to all who wish them; free to those not able to pay; to others for not less than 25 cents a set. The paper costs me 6 cents a pattern. Address me at Greenville, Montcalm Co., Mich. I shall take them with me wherever I travel, until all are supplied.

Assisting — or competing with — her in the pattern business was Dr. Phoebe Lamson of the Western Health Reform Institute, who advertised her design in the *Health Reformer* at fifty cents a set.[20]

As an additional means of bringing about the desired uniformity, Mrs. White prepared a small tract listing the dos and don'ts of dress reform. Gracing the front page was an engraving of a model sister neatly attired in her short skirt and pants. Just because a skirt fell eight or nine inches from the floor did not mean it was a reform dress, Ellen wrote. To qualify fully, it should "be cut by an approved pattern" and meet certain other criteria. Bright, figured materials, reflecting "vanity and shallow pride," were to be shunned. Mixed colors, "such as white sleeves and pants with a dark dress," were likewise in bad taste. As for accessories, hats and caps were to be preferred over shawls and bonnets. The high point of Ellen White's

---

19. EGW, "The Reform Dress," *Testimonies*, I, 521; EGW, "Questions and Answers," p. 260. For a somewhat different account of how the nine-inch length was selected, see J. H. Waggoner, "The Dress Reform," *HR*, II (March, 1868), 130.

20. EGW, "The Reform Dress," p. 522; EGW, "Reformed Dress Patterns." *Testimony for the Church, No. 13* (Battle Creek: SDA Publishing Assn., 1867), p. 79; "Items for the Month," *HR*, II (February, 1868), 128. The *Health Reformer* also carried reform patterns for such articles as a "flannel undergarment," a "garment combining chemise and drawers, arranged with buttons so as to support the skirts and stockings from the shoulders," and "dress drawers with leggins." "Dress Reform Patterns," *HR*, X (July, 1875), 224.

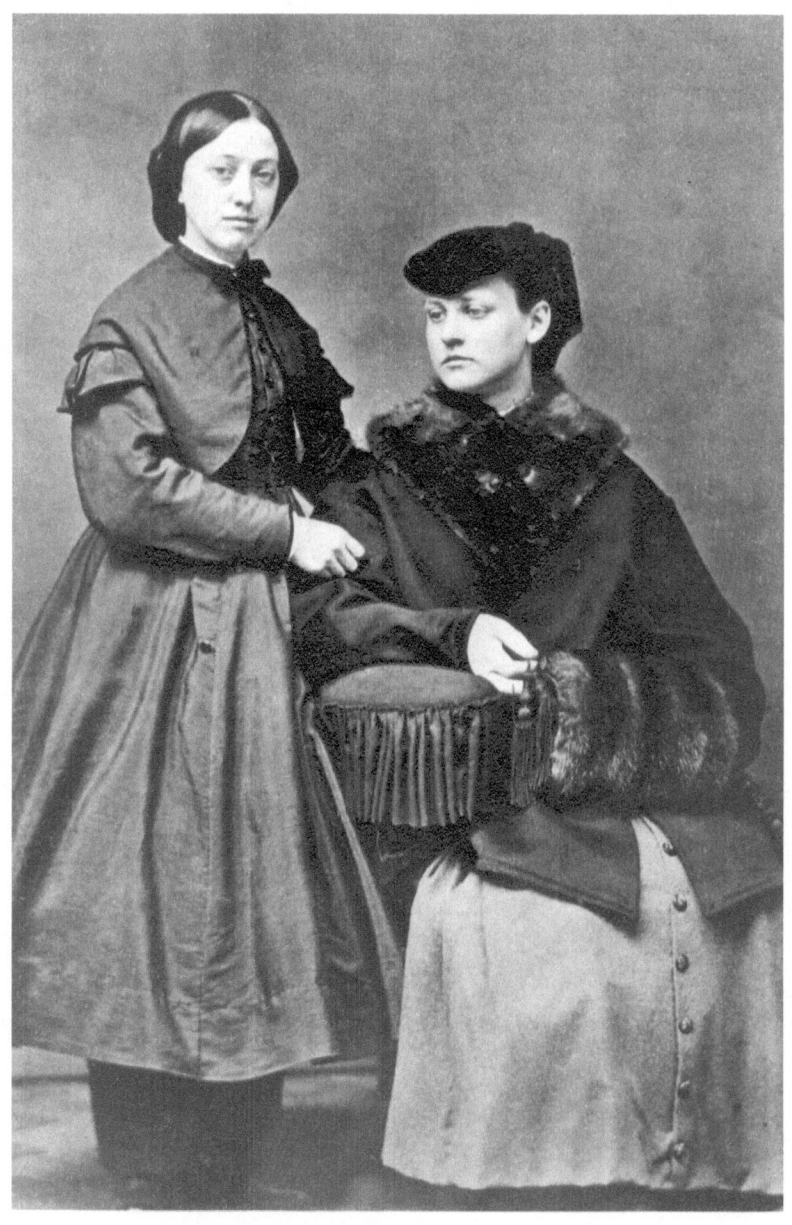

**Two young Adventist sisters,
Hannah Sawyer and Josie Chamberlain, in their reform dresses**
Courtesy of the Ellen G. White Estate

short-skirt crusade came in 1869 when the General Conference at its annual session officially endorsed the dress standards laid down in this little tract.[21]

Despite the nominal backing of the church leadership and her own tireless efforts on its behalf, the reform dress — or "woman-disfigurer," as her niece called it — never won the affection of the rank and file. Some of the Adventist brothers did seem to like it on their wives and daughters, but the women who had to wear it found the experience truly humbling. "The world is cold and distant," wrote one discouraged sister; "my neighbors seem to me sometimes to be afraid of me. (My husband says it is because I wear the short dress).... I cannot mingle with them in their social parties.... My folks do not like to have me go out much. They feel ashamed of my dress. What shall I do?"[22]

In 1873 Ellen White complained bitterly that, notwithstanding her many testimonies, the dress reform continued to be "treated by some with great indifference, and by others with contempt." The pants, especially, were a source of great embarrassment, even for those who generally favored the short skirt. But Mrs. White never quite understood this attitude. How, she wondered, could one who

---

21. EGW, *The Dress Reform: An Appeal to the People in Its Behalf* (Battle Creek: SDA Publishing Assn., 1868), pp. 14-15; "Business Proceedings of the Seventh Annual Session of the General Conference of S. D. Adventists," *R&H*, XXXIII (May 25, 1869), 173. *The Dress Reform* was reprinted in *HR*, III (August, 1868), 21-23, and (September, 1868), 41-43. Mrs. White's pamphlet is very similar in places to M. Angeline Merritt's little book *Dress Reform;* compare, for example, Ellen White on "the popular style of woman's dress" (pp. 4-5) with Mrs. Merritt's section on the inconvenience of the popular style (pp. 79-86).

22. Mary Clough to Lucinda Hall, April 21, 1876, and Mrs. A. L. Cowdrey to Emma [?], 1869 (Lucinda Hall Collection, White Estate). For reactions to the reform dress, see D. M. Canright, "Report from Bro. Canright," *R&H*, XXX (June 18, 1867), 9; L. L. Howard, "A Good Move," *R&H*, XXX (August 13, 1867), 141; C. O. Tayler, "The Reform Dress," *R&H*, XXX (September 3, 1867), 188; L. I. Belnap, "From Sister Belnap," *R&H*, XXXI (December 31, 1867), 42-43; M. J. Cottrell, "In Answer to Our Prayers," *R&H*, XXXI (February 25, 1868), 166-67. By the summer of 1872 many Adventist sisters were wearing the reform dress only to church, and support for the costume was rapidly disappearing; Ira Abbey to Lucinda Hall, September 4, 1872 (Lucinda Hall Collection). One church leader somewhat annoyed by the "everlasting Short Dress question" was Elder G. I. Butler; see Butler to James White, July 21, 1868, and an undated letter circa 1872 (White Estate).

THE DRESS REFORM.

AN APPEAL TO THE PEOPLE IN ITS BEHALF.

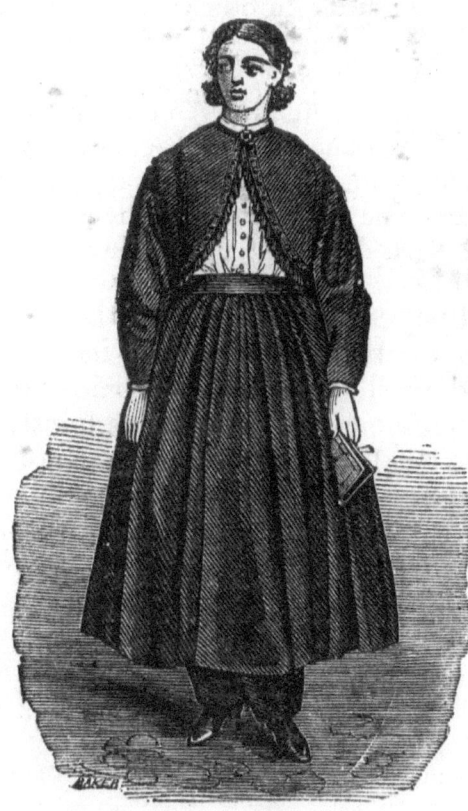

We are not Spiritualists. We are Christian women, believing all that the Scriptures say concerning man's creation, his fall, his sufferings and woes on account of continued transgression, of his hope of redemption thro' Christ, and of his duty to glorify God in his body and spirit which are his, in order to be saved. We do not wear the style of dress here represented to be odd,—that we may attract notice. We do not differ from the common style of woman's dress for any

Mrs. White's model reform dress
From Ellen G. White, *The Dress Reform* (Battle Creek: SDA Publishing Assn., 1868)

did not even blush at the "immodest exposure" of a lady's naked ankle honestly profess shock at the sight of "limbs thoroughly dressed with warm pants"?[23]

Other factors also contributed to the growing (or continuing) unpopularity of the short skirt and pants. Fanatical "extremists," for whom "this reform seemed to constitute the sum and substance of their religion," brought disrepute upon themselves and the dress by constantly pressing the issue on their less-reform-minded sisters. Lovers of the world tried to lighten "the cross" by adding superfluous trimmings or by deviating in other ways from the approved pattern. Then, with Dr. Kellogg's rise to power, the medical work passed into the hands of one who had never felt anything but chagrin at seeing the reform dress. Finally, even Ellen White, who regarded dress as a "minor" part of health reform, grew weary of the incessant bickering and longed for peace at almost any price. "Perhaps no question has ever come up among us," she noted ironically, "which has caused such development of character as has dress reform."[24]

January 3, 1875, effectively marked the end of Ellen White's ten-year struggle to impose radical dress reform upon the Adventist church. On that date God mercifully removed her burden to continue wearing and promoting the short skirt and pants. In vision she saw that the dress reform had become "an injury to the cause of truth." Rather than a blessing, it "had been made a reproach, and, in some cases, even a disgrace." The testimony calling for its adoption was now "to become silent." Journeying to California, Mrs. White discreetly left her pants behind. The ordeal was over.[25]

Freed at last from the much-despised reform costume, Adventist sisters returned to wearing apparel of their own design. But it was not long before evidences of "pride in dress" reappeared, mak-

---

23. EGW, "The Health Institute," *Testimonies,* III, 171; EGW, "The Reform Dress," *HR,* VII (May, 1872), 154-56.

24. EGW, "Simplicity in Dress," *Testimonies,* IV, 636-39; J. H. Kellogg to EGW, September 2 and October 7, 1882 (White Estate); EGW, "Questions and Answers," p. 261. Although the dress embarrassed him, Kellogg did concede that it had merit; see [Kellogg], "Dress Reform: Number Three," *HR,* XI (March, 1876), 66.

25. EGW, "Simplicity in Dress," pp. 637-39; F. E. Belden to E. S. Ballenger, February 13, 1933 (Ballenger-Mote Papers). Belden was Mrs. White's nephew.

ing it necessary for Ellen White once again to lay down rigid dress standards. This time she offered a "less objectionable style":

> It is free from needless trimmings, free from the looped-up, tied-back over-skirts. It consists of a plain sacque or loose-fitting basque, and skirt, the latter short enough to avoid the mud and filth of the streets. The material should be free from large plaids and figures, and plain in color.

"Will my sisters accept this style of dress, and refuse to imitate the fashions that are devised by Satan, and continually changing?" she inquired pleadingly. She was no longer in a mood for compromise. "All exhibitions of pride in dress," she declared, should lead to disciplinary action by the church, for continuing manifestations of such pride constituted prima facie evidence of an unconverted heart.[26]

Late in the century, when certain members tried to reintroduce the long-discarded reform dress, Ellen White wanted nothing to do with it. The Lord was not in the movement, she said. The controversies of the past were to be left behind. No "singular forms of dress" were to embarrass God's cause. "[D]o not again introduce the short dress and pants," she admonished one correspondent, "unless you have the word of the Lord for it." By now the fires of reform that had once burned so brightly within her were slowly flickering out. There would be no more patterns, no more hard-and-fast rules. Mellowed by age and experience, she advised simply to let the "sisters dress plainly, as many do, having the dress of good material, durable, modest, appropriate for this age, and let not the dress question fill the mind."[27]

Although the short skirt and pants attracted by far the most attention, dress reform for Ellen White "comprised more than shortening the dress and clothing the limbs. It included every article of dress upon the person." Through the years she offered her sage advice on every conceivable item. "Superfluous tucks, ruffles, and ornaments of any kind," for example, were positive indications "of a weak head and a proud heart." Cosmetics injured health and endangered life itself. Breast-paddings inhibited natural growth and dried

---

26. EGW, "Simplicity in Dress," pp. 640-48.
27. EGW to J. H. Haughey, July 4, 1897 (11-19-1897, White Estate).

up the supply of milk in the breasts. Once she served on a committee to select "a proper style and manufacture of hats," an appropriate assignment in view of her childhood labor as a hatmaker.[28]

Hair styles — both men's and women's — were a favorite subject of health reformers. Ellen White herself said little or nothing about the wearing of beards, but presumably she supported the action of the General Conference in 1866 condemning brethren for shaving and coloring their beards and for wearing only mustaches and goatees, which betokened "the air of the fop." A man's face was to appear either clean shaven or with full beard, "as nature designed it." As the *Health Reformer* pointed out, a man's facial hair did more than merely improve his personal appearance. "The hair of the moustache not only absorbs the moisture and the miasma of fogs, but it strains the air from dust and the soot of our great smoky cities." Similarly, the beard served as a "respirator" and a "comforter," protecting the neck against heat and cold.[29]

Mrs. White's general silence on male beards was more than offset by her outspoken criticism of the wigs and hair-pieces commonly worn by women. The artificial chignons and braids then so popular were particularly distasteful to her. The chignon or "waterfall" could be formed naturally by attaching a horsehair frame to the back of the head with an elastic band, brushing the hair down over it, and tucking the ends up underneath. But much time could be saved by simply purchasing one ready-made and securing it in place with hairpins. Braids, pinned up over the back of the head, were another favorite of the 1860s and could also be bought as hairpieces.[30]

---

28. EGW, "Simplicity in Dress," p. 635; EGW, unpublished MS (MS 106-1901, White Estate); EGW, "Words to Christian Mothers on the Subject of Life, Health, and Happiness — No. 1" *HR,* VI (September, 1871), 90; EGW, "Words to Christian Mothers on the Subject of Life, Health, and Happiness — No. 2," ibid., VI (October, 1871), 122; J. N. Andrews, "Business Proceedings of the Sixth Annual Session of the General Conference of Seventh-day Adventists," *R&H,* XXXI (May 26, 1868), 356.

29. "Fourth Annual Session of General Conference," *R&H,* XXVIII (May 22, 1866), 196; "Why We Should Wear Beards," *HR,* I (January, 1867), 93. At its 1866 session the General Conference approved an amended version of an eleven-point resolution on dress recently adopted by the Battle Creek Church. See "Resolutions on Dress," *R&H,* XXVII (May 8, 1866), 180.

30. EGW, "Words to Christian Mothers on the Subject of Life, Health, and Happiness — No. 2," p. 121; McClellan, *History of American Costume,* pp. 486, 495.

These "monstrosities" were known to be an excellent breeding ground for "pestiferous vermin," but Ellen White saw even more terrible consequences — "horrible disease and premature death" — resulting from wearing these contrivances. Addressing "Christian Mothers" in the *Health Reformer,* she described the dire physiological effects:

> The artificial hair and pads covering the base of the brain, heat and excite the spinal nerves centering in the brain. The head should ever be kept cool. The heat caused by these artificials induces the blood to the brain. The action of the blood upon the lower or animal organs of the brain, causes unnatural activity, tends to recklessness in morals, and the mind and heart is in danger of being corrupted. As the animal organs are excited and strengthened, the morals are enfeebled. The moral and intellectual powers of the mind become servants to the animal.
>
> In consequence of the brain being congested its nerves lose their healthy action, and take on morbid conditions, making it almost impossible to arouse the moral sensibilities. Such lose their power to discern sacred things. The unnatural heat caused by these artificial deformities about the head, induces the blood to the brain, producing congestion, and causing the natural hair to fall off, producing baldness. Thus the natural is sacrificed to the artificial.
>
> Many have lost their reason, and become hopelessly insane, by following this deforming fashion.[31]

Mrs. White's fears in this instance were based upon her understanding of the so-called science of phrenology, widely current among health reformers. According to phrenological theory (discussed in Chapter 3), the animal organs of the brain were located in the back and lower part of the head, while the organs of intellect and sentiment occupied the frontal region. Heating the back of the head thus stimulated the sexual passions — "amativeness," the phrenologist would say — and depressed the spiritual sentiments.

---

31. James Caleb Jackson, "The Hair," *HR,* V (May, 1871), 266; EGW, "Words to Christian Mothers on the Subject of Life, Health, and Happiness — No. 2," p. 121. Dr. Jackson's comments apparently inspired Mrs. White's writing on the subject five months later.

Her flirtation with phrenology seems to have begun during that first, critical visit to Dansville in 1864 when she took her two sons to Dr. Jackson for head readings and physical examinations. Only two years earlier she had denounced phrenology, along with psychology and mesmerism, as a tool of Satan. Although "good in their place," these sciences became in Satan's hands "his most powerful agents to deceive and destroy souls." In the years following her contacts with Dansville, however, phrenological allusions began appearing frequently in her writings. During her husband's extended illness, for instance, she complained that his "large and active" bumps of "cautiousness, conscientiousness, and benevolence," all assets in time of health, were in sickness "painfully excitable, and a hindrance to his recovery." And in an 1869 testimony regarding a brother's inordinate love of money, she attributed his problem to satanic excitation of "his organ of acquisitiveness."[32]

Ellen White's proclivity for phrenology was, of course, not atypical, especially for a health reformer. As one author has recently noted, the science had, "by the mid-1860's, filtered deeply into the common life of the country." Even among Adventists, it commanded widespread respect. Such prominent figures as William Miller and George I. Butler, twice president of the General Conference, unashamedly submitted to head readings, and the editors of the *Health Reformer* openly admired the work of the *American Phrenological Journal*. Mrs. White herself was reported to be "a woman of singularly well-balanced mental organization," notable for her traits of benevolence, spirituality, conscientiousness, and ideality.[33]

---

32. EGW to Bro. and Sister Lockwood, September [14], 1864; EGW, "Philosophy and Vain Deceit," *Testimonies*, I, 290, 296; EGW, "Our Late Experience," *R&H*, XXVII (February 27, 1866), 98; EGW, "Warnings to the Church," *Testimonies*, II, 238. It was not uncommon in the nineteenth century to distinguish between the philosophy of phrenology (thought to be materialistic and infidel) and its scientific content; see John D. Davies, *Phrenology, Fad and Science: A 19th-Century American Crusade* (New Haven: Yale University Press, 1955), p. 74.

33. Madeleine B. Stern, *Heads & Headlines: The Phrenological Fowlers* (Norman: University of Oklahoma Press, 1971), p. 214; "Phrenological Developments of Mr. Miller," *Advent Herald*, n.s., I (May 20, 1848), 127; Sylvester Bliss, *Memoirs of William Miller* (Boston: Joshua V. Himes, 1853), pp. 160-61; G. I. Butler to J. H. Kellogg, January 31, 1904 (Kellogg Collection, MSU); "Items for the Month," *HR*, I (March, 1867), 128; *American Biographical History of Eminent and Self-Made Men . . . Michigan Volume*

Phrenological theory also helps in understanding her sweeping statements on prenatal influences. It was her firm conviction — based on two divinely sent messages — that parents transmitted to their children not only physical characteristics but intellectual and spiritual ones as well. If they were selfish and intemperate, their children would likely tend toward selfishness and intemperance; while if they were loving and kind, these traits would be reflected in their offspring. Such notions, commonly found in the writings of health reformers, had long been a part of folklore, but nineteenth-century phrenology gave them a respectable scientific basis. The argument went this way: mental traits correspond with the physical organs of the brain; physical characteristics are known to be inheritable; therefore, mental traits can be passed from one generation to the next. Thus, in terms of both science and revelation, Mrs. White's statements made considerable sense to her contemporaries.[34]

Ellen White followed another well-marked trail when she ventured into the potentially hazardous field of sex. From the appearance of Sylvester Graham's *Lecture to Young Men on Chastity* in 1834 this subject had played an integral and highly visible role in health-reform literature. Alcott, Coles, Trall, and Jackson, among others, had all spoken out on the dangers of what they regarded as excessive or abnormal sexual activities, particularly masturbation, which was thought to cause a frightening array of pathological conditions ranging from dyspepsia and consumption to insanity and loss of spirituality. By carefully couching their appeal in humanitarian terms, they had largely avoided offending the sensibilities of a prud-

---

(Cincinnati: Western Biographical Publishing Co., 1878), Dist. 3, p. 108. Internal evidence suggests that this biographical sketch of Mrs. White was written by her niece, Mary Clough.

34. EGW, *The Ministry of Healing* (Mountain View, Calif.: Pacific Press, 1942; first published in 1905), pp. 371-73; O. S. Fowler, *Hereditary Descent: Its Laws and Facts Illustrated and Applied to the Improvement of Mankind* (New York: O. S. & L. N. Fowler, 1843), p. 127 et passim. On prenatal influences, see also Sylvester Graham, *Lectures on the Science of Human Life* (People's ed.; London: Horsell, Aldine, Chambers, 1849), pp. 211-14; and L. B. Coles, *Philosophy of Health* (rev. ed.; Boston: Ticknor, Reed, & Fields, 1853), p. 161.

ish public. Theirs was a genuinely moral crusade against what Jackson called *"the great, crying sin of our time."*[35]

Given this background, and the knowledge that she possessed both Trall's and Jackson's books on sex by late 1863, it is not surprising that Ellen White's very first book on health was a little volume entitled *An Appeal to Mothers: The Great Cause of the Physical, Mental, and Moral Ruin of Many of the Children of Our Time* (1864). As customary in such works, she began by emphasizing her strictly humanitarian and spiritual concern "for those children and youth who by solitary vice [masturbation] are ruining themselves for this world, and for that which is to come." Her explanation for writing on this delicate subject was a recent vision, apparently the one on June 5, 1863, in which her angel guide had directed her attention to the present corrupt state of the world. "Everywhere I looked," she recalled with obvious horror, "I saw imbecility, dwarfed forms, crippled limbs, misshapen heads, and deformity of every description." Sickened by the sight before her, she learned that it had resulted from the practice of solitary vice, so widespread that "a large share of the youth now living are worthless." And many adults, she might have added, for she was also shown a pitiful Adventist brother of her acquaintance who had been brought near death by this mind- and body-destroying habit.[36]

---

35. Sylvester Graham, *A Lecture to Young Men on Chastity* (10th ed.; Boston: Charles H. Peirce, 1848); William A. Alcott, *The Physiology of Marriage* (Boston: Dinsmoor and Company, 1855); Coles, *Philosophy of Health*, p. 126 et passim; Russell T. Trall, *Pathology of the Reproductive Organs, Embracing All Forms of Sexual Disorders* (Boston: B. Leverett Emerson, 1862); James C. Jackson, *The Sexual Organism, and Its Healthful Management* (Boston: B. Leverett Emerson, 1862), p. 11. On the humanitarian approach to sex, I am following Sidney Ditzion, *Marriage, Morals, and Sex in America: A History of Ideas* (New York: Bookman Associates, 1953), p. 317. On the development of attitudes toward masturbation, see Stephen W. Nissenbaum, "Careful Love: Sylvester Graham and the Emergence of Victorian Sexual Theory in America, 1830-1840" (Ph.D. diss., University of Wisconsin, 1968); and H. Tristram Engelhardt, Jr., "The Disease of Masturbation: Values and the Concept of Disease," *Bulletin of the History of Medicine*, XLVIII (Summer, 1974), pp. 234-48. As Vern L. Bullough and Martha Voght have recently pointed out, the term masturbation in the nineteenth century often denoted homosexuality as well; "Homosexuality and Its Confusion with the 'Secret Sin' in Pre-Freudian America," *Journal of the History of Medicine and Allied Sciences*, XXVIII (April, 1973), 143-55.

36. EGW, *An Appeal to Mothers* (Battle Creek: SDA Publishing Assn., 1864), pp. 17, 24-25.

AN

Appeal to Mothers.

THE

GREAT CAUSE

OF THE

PHYSICAL, MENTAL, AND MORAL RUIN OF MANY
OF THE CHILDREN OF OUR TIME.

BY ELLEN G. WHITE.

STEAM PRESS
OF THE SEVENTH-DAY ADVENTIST PUBLISHING ASSOCIATION.
BATTLE CREEK, MICH.:
1864.

Title page of Mrs. White's first book on health reform,
based on her vision of June 5, 1863
Courtesy Ellen G. White Estate, Inc.

To assist parents in detecting the presence of this vile practice, she offered a list of potentially incriminating symptoms: absent-mindedness . . . irritable disposition . . . forgetfulness . . . disobedience . . . ingratitude . . . impatience . . . disrespect for parental authority . . . lack of frankness . . . a strong desire to be with the opposite sex . . . a diminished interest in spiritual things. She also warned of dire physical consequences, calculated to strike fear in the most hardened of hearts. Continued masturbation, she warned, produced not only hereditary insanity and deformities, but a host of diseases, including "affection of the liver and lungs, neuralgia, rheumatism, affection of the spine, diseased kidneys, and cancerous humors." Not infrequently, it led its victims "into an early grave."[37]

She went on to offer a number of tips on combatting this terrible curse. Speaking as a parent, she wrote that it was vitally important to "teach our children self-control from their very infancy, and learn them the lesson of submitting their wills to us." Special care should be taken to protect the young from the contaminating influence of other children. In recent years she had come to view her crippling childhood accident as a blessing in disguise that had preserved her in pristine innocence. According to her account, she had grown up in "blissful ignorance of the secret vices of the young" and had learned about them only after marriage from "the private death-bed confessions of some females." To maintain the purity of her own offspring, she had never permitted them to associate with "rough, rude boys" or to sleep in the same bed or room with others their age. Her letters confirm that she did in fact keep a tight rein on their activities. In one note to sixteen-year-old Edson she forbade him from associating with a young Adventist friend suspected of keeping "dissolute company" and reprimanded him for going out riding with a girlfriend. "[Y]ou are well aware that we would not approve of your showing partiality or attention to any young miss at your age," she advised. "When you are old enough to begin to manifest a preference for any particular one we are the ones to be consulted and to choose for you."[38]

---

37. Ibid., pp. 6-9, 18.
38. Ibid., pp. 10-12; EGW to Edson White, October 19, 1865 (W-7-1865, White Estate). Dr. Jackson also warned of the dangers in letting children sleep together. Jackson, *The Sexual Organism*, p. 42.

Short Skirts and Sex

Like Graham before her, Ellen White regarded a bland diet as one of the best means of curbing the urge to masturbate. All stimulating substances like "Mince pies, cakes, preserves, and highly-seasoned meats, with gravies" were proscribed since they created "a feverish condition in the system, and inflame[d] the animal passions." In addition to watching their children's diets, parents were to be constantly on the lookout for overt signs of self-abuse. If apprehended in the act, the children were to be told "that indulgence in this sin will destroy self-respect, and nobleness of character; will ruin health and morals, and its foul stain will blot from the soul true love for God, and the beauty of holiness."[39]

Appended to Mrs. White's appeal was an anonymous twenty-nine page essay on "Chastity" citing persons "of high standing and authority in the medical world" who agreed with the prophetess. Among those quoted were many stalwarts of the reform movement: Sylvester Graham, L. B. Coles, James C. Jackson, Mary Gove Nichols, the phrenologist O. S. Fowler, and — for good measure — Dr. Samuel B. Woodward, superintendent of the Massachusetts Lunatic Hospital. So closely did the views of these individuals parallel those of Ellen White, the publishers felt it necessary to add a note denying prior knowledge on her part. Taking her word at face value, they asserted that "she had read nothing from the authors here quoted, and had read no other works on this subject, previous to putting into our hands what she has written. She is not, therefore, a copyist, although she has stated important truths to which men who are entitled to our highest confidence, have borne testimony."[40]

Ellen White's sexual attitudes, as even her publishers recognized, were far from unique. In fact, they rested squarely on the popular vitalistic physiology of Broussais that Sylvester Graham had been preaching since the early 1830s. Puzzled by the organic processes that sustained life, the vitalists had invented a mysterious "vital force" (or energy) that supposedly interacted with inanimate matter to produce the vital functions of the body. According

---

39. EGW, *An Appeal to Mothers*, pp. 13-14, 19-20. See also Graham, *A Lecture to Young Men on Chastity*, p. 147.

40. EGW, *An Appeal to Mothers*, p. 34. I have been unable to identify the author of the essay on chastity, but it might have been Horace Mann.

to Elder John Loughborough's necessarily vague definition, vital force was simply "that power placed in the human body, at its birth, which will enable the body, under favorable circumstances, to live to a certain age." Since the initial endowment was limited, and since each sexual act used up an irreplenishable amount, it behooved those who coveted a long life to keep their sexual activities to a minimum.[41]

To illustrate the concept of vital force, nineteenth-century authors frequently compared it to capital in a bank account, gradually depleted over the years by repeated withdrawals. Again Mrs. White was no exception. As she saw it, God had made the original deposit by granting each individual, according to sex, "a certain amount of vital force." (For some inscrutable reason he had been more generous with men than women.) Those who carefully budgeted their resources lived a normal lifetime, but those who by their intemperate acts used "borrowed capital," prematurely exhausted their account and met an early death. In her *Appeal to Mothers* she explained how continued self-abuse wasted "vital capital" and shortened life:

> The practice of secret habits surely destroys the vital forces of the system. All unnecessary vital action will be followed by corresponding depression. Among the young, the vital capital, the brain, is so severely taxed at an early age, that there is a deficiency, and great exhaustion, which leaves the system exposed to diseases of various kinds. But the most common of these is consumption. None can live when their vital energies are used up. They must die.[42]

---

41. Nissenbaum, "Careful Love," pp. 69-70; Sylvester Graham, *Lectures on the Science of Human Life*, pp. 155-56; J. H. Loughborough, *Hand Book of Health; or, A Brief Treatise on Physiology and Hygiene* (Battle Creek: SDA Publishing Assn., 1868), pp. 14-15. On Ellen White's use of vitalism, see Yvonne Tuchalski, "Vital Force as a Significant Factor in Ellen G. White's Health Reform Message" (unpublished paper submitted to the Department of History, Andrews University, August 14, 1970). Ellen White may not actually have read the works of other authors on sex, but she owned their manuals and assimilated their vocabularies; compare, for example, Mrs. White (*An Appeal to Mothers*, p. 6) with Jackson (*The Sexual Organism*, p. 69) on the "sievelike" memories of masturbators.

42. EGW, *An Appeal to Mothers*, pp. 27-28; EGW, *Christian Temperance and Bible Hygiene* (Battle Creek: Good Health Publishing Co., 1890), pp. 64-65; EGW, *Ministry*

Short Skirts and Sex

Although Ellen White could have acquired her knowledge of vitalism from any number of sources, a close examination of her writings reveals that she was particularly indebted to Horace Mann and L. B. Coles, whose works she had read no later than 1865.[43] Often she appropriated passages from them with only cosmetic changes, as the following parallel readings show:

Ellen G. White: Man came from the hand of God perfect in every faculty of mind and body; in perfect soundness, therefore in perfect health. It took more than two thousand years of indulgence of appetite and lustful passions to create such a state of things in the human organism as would lessen vital force.[44]

Horace Mann: Man came from the hand of God so perfect in his bodily organs . . . so surcharged with vital force, that it took more than two thousand years of the combined abominations of appetite and ignorance . . . to drain off his electric energies and make him even accessible to disease.[45]

Ellen G. White: If Adam, at his creation, had not been endowed with twenty times as much vital force as men now have, the race, with their present habits of living in violation of natural law, would have become extinct.[46]

Horace Mann: . . . if the race had not been created with ten times more vital force than it now possesses, its known violations of all the laws of health and life would, long ere this, have extinguished it altogether.[47]

---

of Healing, pp. 234-35. On the concept of vital force in nineteenth-century American thought, see Nathan C. Hale, Jr., *Freud and the Americans: The Beginnings of Psychoanalysis in the United States, 1876-1917* (New York: Oxford University Press, 1971), pp. 34-35.

43. *How to Live,* published in 1865, contains selections taken from both Mann and Coles.

44. EGW, "Indulgence of Appetite," *Testimonies,* IV, 29; first published in 1876.

45. Horace Mann, "Dedicatory and Inaugural Address," in *Life and Works* (Boston: Lee and Shepard Publishers, 1891), V, 335-36. The address was given in 1853.

46. EGW, "Proper Education," *Testimonies,* III, 138-39; first published in 1873.

47. Mann, "Dedicatory and Inaugural Address," p. 340. The two parallel readings given are excerpts from much longer passages taken from Mann. Ellen White's reliance on Mann can also be seen in her "Degeneracy-Education," *HR,* VII (November, 1872), 348; and *Christian Temperance,* pp. 7-8.

Her curious doubling of Adam's vital force no doubt stemmed from her reading of biblical history, which has early man living approximately twenty times longer than modern man.

Her reliance on Coles is evident in her discussion of a corollary to the doctrine of vitalism: the electrical transmission of vital force through the nervous system. In his *Philosophy of Health* Coles had shown how the nerves, branching out from the brain, acted "like so many telegraphic wires" carrying the electrical current to the various parts of the body. Ellen White not only employed the same simile, but followed the Millerite physician in positing an intimate electrical relationship between mind and body.[48]

Ellen G. White: The sympathy which exists between the mind and the body is very great. When one is affected, the other responds.[49]	*L. B. Coles:* The sympathy existing between the mind and the body is so great, that when one is affected, both are affected.[50]

On the basis of the reciprocal arrangement, she concluded that nine-tenths of all diseases originated in the mind.[51]

She also adopted Coles's electrical explanation of why masturbation deadened a person's spiritual sensibilities. In the *Philosophy of Health* he had argued that since God's only means of communicating with man was through the nervous system, any unnatural burden upon that system impeded the flow of divinely sent messages. Ellen White liked the idea so much that she worked it into an 1869 testimony on "Moral Pollution," but neglected, as she so often did, to cite her earthly source.

Ellen G. White: The brain nerves which communicate with the entire system are the only medium through which Heaven can communicate to man, and affect his inmost life. Whatever disturbs the	*L. B. Coles:* Whatever mars the healthy circulation of the electric currents in the nervous system, lessens the strength of the vital forces; and, through them, deadens the native susceptibilities of

---

48. Coles, *Philosophy of Health,* pp. 11-13; EGW, "Experience Not Reliable," *Testimonies,* III, 69.
49. EGW, "True Benevolence," ibid., IV, 60; first published in 1876.
50. Coles, *Philosophy of Health,* p. 127.
51. EGW, "Responsibilities of the Physician," *Testimonies,* V, 444.

circulation of the electric currents in the nervous system, lessens the strength of the vital powers, and the result is a deadening of the sensibilities of the mind.[52]

the soul. The nervous system is the only medium through which truth can reach Interior man. Divinity himself uses no other medium through which to reach the human heart.[53]

On October 2, 1868, five years after her first view of the world's corrupt state, Ellen White had a second major vision on sex, which left her confidence in humanity "terribly shaken." As the sordid lives of "God's professed people" passed before her, she became "sick and disgusted with the rotten-heartedness" of the church. Reputable brethren were shown leaving the "most solemn, impressive discourses upon the judgment" and returning to their rooms to engage "in their favorite, bewitching, sin, polluting their own bodies." Adventist children were pictured "as corrupt as hell itself." Speaking to the Battle Creek church in March, 1869, she reported that "Right here in this church, corruption is teeming on every hand." Privately, she estimated "that there is not one girl out of one hundred who is pure minded, and there is not one boy out of one hundred whose morals are untainted." So nearly universal seemed the practice of masturbation, she grew suspicious of almost everyone and even began refusing requests for prayers of healing for fear she might be asking the Lord's blessing upon a self abuser.[54]

In addition to the many who were abusing themselves there were others she learned who were abusing their spouses. In her second *How to Live* pamphlet she had urged couples to consider carefully the result of every privilege the marriage relation grants but until 1868 the brunt of her sexual advice had been directed to masturbators. Now, however she warned that even married persons were accountable to God "for the expenditure of vital energy which

52. EGW, "Moral Pollution," *Testimonies*, II, 347.
53. Coles, *Philosophy of Health*, pp. 266-67.
54. EGW, "An Appeal to the Church," *Testimonies*, II, 439, 468-69; EGW, "Christian Temperance," ibid., II, 360; EGW, "Moral Pollution," pp. 349-50; EGW to Dr. and Mrs. Horatio Lay, February 13, 1870 (L-30-1870, White Estate). The letter to the Lays was later published as "Labor Conducive to Health," *Testimonies*, IV, 96. Although Ellen White did not specifically attribute all the statements quoted in the paragraph to the 1868 vision, it seems certain that was the source.

weakens their hold on life and enervates the entire system." In phrenological language she counseled Christian wives not to "gratify the animal propensities" of their husbands but to seek instead to divert their minds "from the gratification of lustful passions to high and spiritual themes by dwelling upon interesting spiritual subjects." Husbands who desired "excessive" sex she regarded as "worse than brutes" and "demons in human form." Although she never defined exactly what she meant by excessive it seems likely — since she generally agreed with earlier health reformers in such matters — that she would have frowned on having intercourse more frequently than once a month. That was the maximum Sylvester Graham had condoned, and his disciple O. S. Fowler, who personally favored sex for procreation only, had stated that "to indulge, even in wedlock, as often as the moon quarters, is gradual but effectual destruction of both soul and body."[55]

The Whites seem to have agreed in principle with the New York phrenologist, for they reprinted this bit of marital advice in an expanded version of *Appeal to Mothers,* published in 1870 under the revealing title of *Solemn Appeal Relative to Solitary Vice, and the Abuses and Excesses of the Marriage Relation.* In addition to Fowler's essay and the material from the original edition, *Solemn Appeal* contained an account of how sexual disorders were treated at the Western Health Reform Institute, an article by a Dr. E. P. Miller on "The Cause of Exhausted Vitality," the complete second chapter of Ellen's "Disease and Its Causes" from *How to Live,* and several selections from testimonies based on the 1868 vision — with all references to their supernatural origin carefully edited out for non-Adventist consumption.[56]

Although Mrs. White never wrote specifically on contraception and family planning, her restrictions on the frequency of sexual intercourse no doubt served as a brake on unwanted pregnancies

---

55. EGW, *How to Live,* No. 2, p. 48; EGW, "An Appeal to the Church," pp. 472-75; Graham, *Lecture to Young Men on Chastity,* p. 83; Fowler, *Hereditary Descent,* p. 206; O. S. Fowler, "Evils and Remedy," in James White (ed.), *Solemn Appeal Relative to Solitary Vice, and the Abuses and Excesses of the Marriage Relation* (Battle Creek: SDA Publishing Assn., 1870), p. 200. For another example of marital advice phrased in phrenological terms, see EGW, "Sensuality in the Young," *Testimonies,* II, 391.

56. James White (ed.), *Solemn Appeal.*

Short Skirts and Sex

among Adventists, who had few other options. According to one 1865 manual, there were four known ways "to prevent child-getting": (1) withdrawing "the male organ just before the discharge of Semen takes place," (2) using a douche of cold water or white vitriol (zinc sulfate) immediately after coition, (3) inserting a walnut-sized sponge soaked in a weak solution of sulphate of iron and attached to a fine silk string, or (4) covering the penis with a sheath of India-rubber. Given these choices, and their respective liabilities, many families may have considered monthly intercourse an expedient and satisfactory policy.[57]

Following the spate of sex-oriented testimonies in 1869 and 1870, some of which she published with the guilty identified by name, Ellen White wrote surprisingly little on the subject for the rest of her life. Her volume on *Christian Temperance,* compiled in 1890 largely from her previously published writings, did include a chapter on "Social Purity," but the familiar topics of masturbation and marital excess were notably absent from *The Ministry of Healing* (1905), her last major work on health. In the meantime, Dr. John Harvey Kellogg kept Adventists sexually informed with his bestselling editions of *Plain Facts about Sexual Life,* a somewhat sadistic manual originally written in fourteen days that recommended such measures as frequent nighttime raids and circumcision without anesthesia to put an end to masturbation.[58]

Throughout her long life Ellen White remained generally antipathetic toward sex, though unlike Ann Lee and Jemima Wilkinson she always stopped short of advocating celibacy. In her waning years

---

57. James Ashton, *The Book of Nature* (New York: Brother Jonathan Office, 1865), pp. 38-41. On contraception, see John S. Haller and Robin M. Haller, *The Physician and Sexuality in Victorian America* (Urbana: University of Illinois Press, 1974), pp. 113-24.

58. EGW, *Testimony Relative to Marriage Duties, and Extremes in the Health Reform* (Battle Creek: SDA Publishing Assn., 1869); EGW, *Christian Temperance,* pp. 127-40; J. H. Kellogg, *Plain Facts about Sexual Life* (2nd ed.; Battle Creek: Good Health Publishing Co., 1879), pp. 336-37, 375-76; Richard W. Schwarz, "John Harvey Kellogg: American Health Reformer" (Ph.D. diss., University of Michigan, 1964), p. 233. It should be pointed out that drastic solutions to the problem of masturbation were not unusual; see Engelhardt, "The Disease of Masturbation," pp. 243-45; and John Duffy, "Masturbation and Clitoridectomy: A Nineteenth-Century View," *Journal of the American Medical Association,* CLXXXVI (October 19, 1963), 246-48.

she looked forward expectantly to an idyllic existence in the new earth free from such unpleasant activities. When some members inquired in 1904 if there would be any children born in the next life, she replied sharply that Satan had inspired the question. It was he, she said, who was leading "the imagination of Jehovah's watchmen to dwell upon the possibilities of association, in the world to come, with women whom they love, and of their raising families." As for herself, she needed no such prospects.[59]

---

59. EGW, Letter B-59-1904, quoted in J. E. Fulton, "Shun Speculative Theories," *Pacific Union Recorder,* XXXI (July 7, 1932), 2; EGW, MS 126, 1903, quoted in *The Adventist Home* (Nashville: Southern Publishing Assn., 1952), p. 121; Raymond Lee Muncy, *Sex and Marriage in Utopian Communities: 19th-Century America* (Bloomington: Indiana University Press, 1973), pp. 17, 33. Sex in the new earth was a position advocated by Elder E. J. Waggoner, who later divorced his wife to marry an English nurse. His story was sensationalized on the front page of the *Chicago American,* January 8, 1906. Mrs. White's 1904 statement was probably elicited by the spread of Waggoner's heresy to the South; see G. I. Butler to EGW, January 28, 1904 (White Estate).

CHAPTER SEVEN

Whatsoever Ye Eat or Drink

"We bear positive testimony against tobacco, spiritous liquors, snuff, tea, coffee, flesh-meats, butter, spices, rich cakes, mince pies, a large amount of salt, and all exciting substances used as articles of food."

Ellen G. White[1]

To the typical Seventh-day Adventist in the 1860s, health reform meant essentially a twice-a-day diet of fruits, vegetables, grains, and nuts. Since Ellen White's vision on June 5, 1863, meat, eggs, butter, and cheese had joined alcohol, tobacco, tea, and coffee on her index of proscribed items. The discontinuance of these articles was as much a religious as a physiological duty, for, as Mrs. White repeatedly said, health reform was as "closely connected with present truth as the arm is connected with the body." Many responded to the call for radical reform, and by the summer of 1870 James White was able to boast that Adventists from Maine to Kansas, "with hardly an exception," had discarded flesh-meats and suppers.[2]

During the early days of Adventist health reform the two-meal-a-day system shared equal billing with the vegetarian diet. Two

---

1. EGW, "Appeal for Burden-Bearers," *Testimonies*, III, 21.
2. EGW to Brother Aldrich, August 20, 1867 (A-8-1867, White Estate); James White, "Health Reform — No. 3: Its Rise and Progress among Seventh-day Adventists," *HR*, V (January, 1871), 130. On health reform as a religious duty, see also EGW, "Healthful Cookery," *Testimonies*, I, 682-84.

meals had long been the rule at places like Dr. Jackson's water cure in Dansville, but the Whites seem to have adopted the practice several months before their first visit to Our Home. What inspired them to do so is not entirely clear. Ellen indirectly tied the change to her June 5 vision, while James, never wanting to appear overly dependent on his wife, appealed to the Bible, arguing tenuously that "the New Testament recognizes but two meals a day." At any rate, by mid-1864 the Whites were taking breakfast at 7:00 A.M., dinner at 1:00 P.M., and no supper. Fruits, grains, and vegetables filled their pantry:

> *Vegetables.* — Potatoes, turnips, parsnips, onions, cabbage, squashes, peas, beans, &c., &c.
> *Grains.* — Wheat, corn, rye, barley, and oatmeal bread and puddings, rice, farina, corn starch, and the like.
> *Fruits.* — Apples, raw and cooked, pears, and peaches, canned and dried, canned strawberries, raspberries, blackberries, huckleberries, grapes, cranberries, and tomatoes.

In addition to these items, the Whites kept a supply of raisins for cooking purposes, and their family cow provided them with about ten quarts of fresh milk per day.[3]

Once or twice, for the children's sake, James and Ellen experimented with a light evening meal, but found that it resulted only in bad breath and unpleasant dispositions. To provide ample time for digestion Ellen White recommended spacing meals at least five hours apart and eating not "a particle of food" in between. According to countless testimonials in the *Health Reformer* and the *Review and Herald* her sparse regimen brought renewed vigor and strength to those who adopted it. "Praise God for the Health Reform" was the universal sentiment.[4]

---

3. EGW, *Spiritual Gifts: Important Facts of Faith, Laws of Health, and Testimonies Nos. 1-10* (Battle Creek: SDA Publishing Assn., 1864), pp. 153-54; James White, "Two Meals a Day," *HR,* XIII (June, 1878), 1; James White, "Health Reform — No. 3," p. 132.

4. EGW, "The Primal Cause of Intemperance: Second Paper," *HR,* XII (May, 1877), 139; EGW, MS-1-1876, quoted in EGW, *Counsels on Diet and Foods* (Washington: Review and Herald Publishing Assn., 1946), p. 179; M. E. Cornell, "Health Reform," *R&H,* XXIX (January 15, 1867), 66.

The rationale behind Mrs. White's ban on flesh-foods was not kindness to animals, which she never mentioned at this time, but her belief, expressed in *Appeal to Mothers* and subsequent writings, that meat caused disease and stirred up the "animal passions." The supposed relationship between diet and sexuality had been noted earlier by Sylvester Graham and others, but Ellen White seems to have learned of it primarily from Dr. L. B. Coles's *Philosophy of Health,* with which she was well acquainted.[5] In a testimony sent to a "Bro. and Sister H.," whose children she had seen in vision as having strong "animal propensities," she made free (and unacknowledged) use of Coles's phrenologically loaded language on the animalizing tendency of meat.

Ellen G. White: . . . flesh-meat is not necessary for health or strength. If used it is because a depraved appetite craves it. Its use excites the animal propensities to increased activity, and strengthens the animal passions. When the animal propensities are increased, the intellectual and moral powers are decreased. The use of the flesh of animals tends to cause a grossness of body, and benumbs the fine sensibilities of the mind.[6]	*L. B. Coles:* Flesh-eating is certainly not necessary to health or strength. . . . If it be used, it must be used as a matter of fancy . . . it excites the animal propensities to increased activity and ferocity. . . . When we increase the proportion of our animal nature, we suppress the intellectual . . . the use of flesh tends to create a grossness of body and spirit.[7]

Continuing to follow Coles, she went on in the same testimony to discuss the connection between meat-eating and disease:

Ellen G. White: Those who subsist largely upon flesh, cannot avoid eating the meat of animals which	*L. B. Coles:* When we feed on flesh, we not only eat the muscular fibres, but the juices or fluids of

---

5. EGW, *An Appeal to Mothers* (Battle Creek: SDA Publishing Assn., 1864), pp. 19-20; Sylvester Graham, *A Lecture to Young Men on Chastity* (10th ed.; Boston: Charles H. Peirce, 1848), p. 147.

6. EGW, "Flesh-Meats and Stimulants," *Testimonies,* II, 63. First published in 1868.

7. L. B. Coles, *Philosophy of Health: Natural Principles of Health and Cure* (rev. ed.; Boston: Ticknor, Reed, & Fields, 1853), pp. 64-67.

are to a greater or less degree diseased. The process of fitting animals for market produces in them disease; and fitted in as healthful manner as they can be, they become heated and diseased by driving before they reach the market. The fluids and flesh of these diseased animals are received directly into the blood, and pass into the circulation of the human body, becoming fluids and flesh of the same. Thus humors are introduced into the system. And if the person already has impure blood, it is greatly aggravated by the eating of the flesh of these animals. The liability to take disease is increased tenfold by meat-eating. The intellectual, the moral, and the physical powers are depreciated by the habitual use of flesh-meats. Meat-eating deranges the system, beclouds the intellect, and blunts the moral sensibilities.[8]

the animal; and these fluids pass into our own circulation — become our blood — our fluids and our flesh. However pure may be the flesh of the animals we eat, their fluids tend to engender in us a humorous state of the blood. . . . The very process taken to fit the animals for market, tends to produce a diseased state of their fluids. . . . Some of our meat is fatted in country pastures; but, by the time it reaches us, the process of driving to market has produced a diseased action of the fluids. . . . Animal food exposes the system more effectually to the causes of acute disease. Where the fluids are in a diseased state, the ordinary causes of disease find a more easy prey. . . . The objections, then, against meat-eating, are three-fold — intellectual, moral, and physical. Its tendency is to check intellectual activity, to depreciate moral sentiment, and to derange the fluids of the body.[9]

In view of Ellen White's indignant assertions that her testimonies were not subject to human influences — "I am as dependent upon the Spirit of the Lord in writing my views as I am in receiving them" — her manifest reliance on Coles is, to say the least, puzzling.[10]

The prohibition against meat-eating proved to be a trifle embarrassing for a church that put so much stock in biblical prophecies. Enemies pointed accusingly to the passage in Saint Paul's first epistle to Timothy (1 Tim. 4:1-3), where the apostle predicted that "in the latter times some shall depart from the faith, . . . commanding to ab-

---

8. EGW, "Flesh-Meats and Stimulants," p. 64.
9. Coles, *Philosophy of Health*, pp. 67-71.
10. EGW, "Questions and Answers," *R&H*, XXX (October 8, 1867), 260.

stain from meats, which God hath created to be received with thanksgiving of them which believe and know the truth." Were Seventh-day Adventists fulfilling that prophecy? Not at all, replied James White, for they did not *command* their members to refrain from eating meat, but simply *recommended* the change from "a physiological point of view." Besides, he added, the word *meats* really meant food, not flesh-meats. "The articles of food which God has permitted us to use are good; and they should be received with thanksgiving."[11]

For at least a decade after her June 5 vision Ellen White made little or no distinction between the use of meat and such animal products as butter, eggs, and cheese. They all aroused man's animal nature and were thus to be condemned indiscriminately. Her unyielding attitude toward these items is revealed in representative statements made between 1868 and 1873:

Cheese should never be introduced into the stomach.[12]

You place upon your tables butter, eggs, and meat, and your children partake of them. They are fed with the very things that will excite their passions, and then you come to meeting and ask God to bless and save your children. How high do your prayers go?[13]

No butter or flesh-meats of any kind come on my table.[14]

Children are allowed to eat flesh-meats, spices, butter, cheese, pork, rich pastry, and condiments generally.... These things do their work of deranging the stomach, exciting the nerves to unnatural action, and enfeebling the intellect. Parents do not realize that they are sowing the seed which will bring forth disease and death.[15]

---

11. James White, "Sermon on Sanctification, Delivered before the Congregation at Battle Creek, Michigan, March 16, 1867," *R&H*, XXIX (April 9, 1867), 207.
12. EGW, "Neglect of Health Reform," *Testimonies,* II, 68.
13. EGW, "Christian Temperance," ibid., II, 362.
14. EGW, "An Appeal to the Church," ibid., II, 487.
15. EGW, "Close Confinement at School," ibid., III, 136.

Eggs should not be placed upon your table. They are an injury to your children.¹⁶

These were hardly the words of a moderate; yet Mrs. White did not regard herself as an extremist. That epithet she reserved for the fanatics who wished to add milk, sugar, and salt to the list of forbidden foods. Throughout the early 1870s Adventist reformers argued incessantly over these three products. The disciples of Dr. Trall demanded their immediate discontinuance, while others professed to see no harm in them. In the middle stood Ellen White. She admitted that their free use was "positively injurious to health," and that it would probably be better never to eat them, but she refused to press additional restrictions on an unwilling church. Her husband, though obviously sympathetic to the Trall faction, concurred in this pragmatic decision and supported her policy of simply recommending a sparing use of all three articles, especially combinations of milk and sugar, which she considered to be worse than meat.¹⁷

Despite reservations about milk and her belief that the time would soon come when it would have to be discarded, she continued in her own home to use moderate amounts of both milk and sweet cream. At the same time she forbade butter, cheese, and eggs from appearing on her table. This apparent inconsistency toward dairy products actually placed her in good health-reform company. Years earlier, in his *Lectures on the Science of Human Life,* Sylvester Graham had made a similar distinction, arguing that cream was preferable to butter because its solubility made it more easily digestible, and that eggs were more objectionable than milk because they were "more highly animalized."¹⁸

The one item on which Ellen White broke with established

16. EGW, "Sensuality in the Young," ibid., II, 400.
17. EGW, "Appeal for Burden-Bearers," p. 21; EGW, "Christian Temperance," pp. 368-70; James White, "Western Tour: Kansas Camp-Meeting," *R&H,* XXXVI (November 8, 1870), 165; James White, "Health Reform — No. 4: Its Rise and Progress among Seventh-day Adventists," *HR,* V (February, 1871), 153-54; [James White], "Appetite Again," ibid., VII (July, 1872), 212.
18. EGW, Letter 1, 1873, quoted in EGW, *Counsels on Diet and Foods,* p. 330; EGW, Letter 5, 1870, quoted ibid., p. 357; EGW, *Spiritual Gifts* (1864), p. 154; Sylvester Graham, *Lectures on the Science of Human Life* (People's ed.; London: Horsell, Aldine, Chambers, 1849), pp. 226, 243.

health-reform opinion was salt. Her reason for this minor departure, she once wrote, was that God had given her special "light" showing its importance for the blood. Consequently she had disregarded Dr. Jackson's advice against its use. A private letter written in 1891, however, tells a somewhat different story:

> Many years ago, while at Dr. Jackson's, I undertook to leave it [salt] off entirely, because he advocated this in his lectures. But he came to me and said, "I request you not to come into the dining hall to eat. A moderate use of salt is necessary to you; without it you will become a dyspeptic. I will send your meals to your room." After a while, however, I again tried the saltless food, but was again reduced in strength and fainted from weakness. Although every effort was made to counteract the effect of the six-weeks' trial, I was all summer in so feeble a condition that my life was despaired of. I was healed in answer to prayer, else I should not have been alive today.

In this account the oft-maligned Dansville physician emerges as the source of inspiration for Mrs. White's tolerance of salt.[19]

Far worse than meat, eggs, butter, and cheese were what Ellen White called the "poisonous narcotics": tea, coffee, tobacco, and alcohol. With these items, she wrote, the "only safe course is to touch not, taste not, handle not."[20] Apparently she got the idea of classifying tea and coffee with alcoholic beverages from reading Coles's *Philosophy of Health,* in which all three are said to produce similar effects. Throughout her writings on the subject Coles's influence is unmistakable.

Ellen G. White: Tea is a stimulant, and to a certain extent produces intoxication.... Its first effect is exhilarating, because it quickens the motions of the living machinery; and the tea-drinker thinks that	*L. B. Coles:* Tea ... is a direct, diffusible, and active stimulant. Its effects are very similar to those of alcoholic drinks, except that of drunkenness. Like alcohol, it gives, for a time, increased vivacity of

---

19. EGW, Letter 37, 1901, quoted in EGW, *Counsels on Diet and Foods,* p. 344; EGW to H. C. Miller, April 2, 1891 (M-19a-1891, White Estate).

20. EGW, Unpublished MS (MS-5-1881, White Estate); EGW, "Power of Appetite," *Testimonies,* III, 488.

it is doing him a great service. But this is a mistake. When its influence is gone, the unnatural force abates, and the result is languor and debility corresponding to the artificial vivacity imparted.[21]

spirits. Like alcohol, it increases, beyond its healthy and natural action, the whole animal and mental machinery; after which there comes a reaction — a corresponding languor and debility.[22]

Still following Coles, she described the woeful effects of coffee on mind and body:

Ellen G. White: Through the use of stimulants, the whole system suffers. The nerves are unbalanced, the liver is morbid in its action, the quality and circulation of the blood are affected, and the skin becomes inactive and sallow. The mind, too, is injured. The immediate influence of these stimulants is to excite the brain to undue activity, only to leave it weaker and less capable of exertion. The after-effect is prostration, not only mental and physical, but moral.[23]

L. B. Coles: [Coffee] affects the whole system, and especially the nervous system, by its effects on the stomach. But, besides this, it creates a morbid action of the liver. . . . It affects the circulation of the blood, and the quality of the blood itself, so that a great coffee-drinker can generally be known by his complexion; it gives to the skin a dead, dull, sallow appearance. Coffee affects not only the body to its injury, but also the mind. It . . . excites the mind temporarily to unwonted activity. . . . [But afterward] come prostration, sadness, and exhaustion of the moral and physical forces.[24]

Certainly the most intriguing insight she borrowed from Coles was that tea and coffee were responsible for the rampant gossip at women's social gatherings:

21. EGW, *Christian Temperance and Bible Hygiene* (Battle Creek: Good Health Publishing Co., 1890), p. 34. A slightly different rendering of the same passage is found in EGW, "Flesh-Meats and Stimulants," p. 64.

22. Coles, *Philosophy of Health*, p. 80.

23. EGW, *Christian Temperance*, p. 35. See also EGW, "Flesh-Meats and Stimulants," p. 65.

24. Coles, *Philosophy of Health*, p. 79.

Ellen G. White: When these tea and coffee users meet together for social entertainment, the effects of their pernicious habit are manifest. All partake freely of the favorite beverages, and as the stimulating influence is felt, their tongues are loosened, and they begin the wicked work of talking against others. Their words are not few or well chosen. The tidbits of gossip are passed around, too often the poison of scandal as well.[25]

L. B. Coles: See a party of ladies met to spend an afternoon. . . . Toward the close of the afternoon . . . come the tea and eatables . . . the drooping mind becomes greatly animated, the tongue is let loose, and the words come flowing forth like the falling drops of a great shower. . . . Then is the time for small thoughts and many words; or, it may be, the sending forth of fire-brands of gossip and slander.[26]

Of all the "poisonous narcotics," tobacco struck Ellen White as being the most sinister. Even after most Adventists had given up smoking and chewing, she continued to remind them of the weed's pernicious effects. Writing in 1864 about her vision the previous year, she described tobacco as a "malignant" poison of the worst kind, responsible for the death of multitudes. She did not say specifically that it caused cancer, but she may well have had that thought in mind since Coles and others had already noted the relationship between prolonged tobacco use and carcinomas. Of equal, if not greater, concern to her was the fact (as she saw it) that tobacco created a thirst for strong drink and often laid "the foundation for the liquor habit."[27]

No health topic aroused Mrs. White to more fervent activity than abstinence from alcoholic drinks, or "temperance" as it was euphemistically called. Basically her position was that of a teetotaler, opposed even to a moderate consumption of fermented and distilled beverages. But on occasion both she and her husband grudgingly allowed a limited use of "domestic wine." In an 1869 testimony re-

---

25. EGW, *Christian Temperance,* p. 36.
26. Coles, *Philosophy of Health,* p. 82.
27. EGW, *Spiritual Gifts* (1864), p. 128; EGW, *The Ministry of Healing* (Mountain View, Calif.: Pacific Press, 1942), pp. 327-28; James White, "Health Reform — No. 2: Its Rise and Progress among Seventh-day Adventists," *HR,* V (December, 1870), 110; L. B. Coles, *The Beauties and Deformities of Tobacco-Using* (Boston: Ticknor, Reed, & Fields, 1853), p. 142.

proving a brother in Wisconsin for his extremist approach to health reform that had deprived his family of the necessities of life, she suggested that "a little domestic wine," or even a little meat, would have done his pregnant wife no injury. Presumably James went along with this advice, for only a few years earlier he had protested strenuously against the "disgusting" practice of substituting molasses and water for wine at communion. "This objecting to a few drops of domestic wine with which to only wet the lips at the Lord's supper, is carrying total-abstinence principles to great length," he commented in the *Review and Herald.* While not recommending that wine be purchased from local liquor-vendors, he saw nothing wrong with having the church deacons make it themselves. That way the purity and alcoholic content could be controlled.[28]

There were no signs of compromise, however, when Ellen White mounted the lecture platform, as she frequently did. In a clear, strong voice she vividly portrayed the horrors of alcoholism and carefully explained the cause-and-effect relationship between diet and drink. Temperance was her favorite theme, and she happily accepted the many speaking invitations that came her way. In the summer of 1874, for example, she joined the temperance forces in Oakland, California, and in several public appearances helped to defeat the liquor interests by the narrow margin of two hundred sixty votes. Three years later "fully five thousand persons" turned out in her hometown to hear her speak at a mass temperance rally co-sponsored by the Women's Christian Temperance Union and the Battle Creek Reform Club. But her greatest triumph as a temperance lecturer came in September, 1876, when she drew an estimated twenty thousand to a camp meeting in Groveland, Massachusetts. So impressed were the officers of the nearby Haverhill Reform Club, they invited her to talk again the next day in their city hall. Before a packed house of eleven

---

28. EGW, "Extremes in Health Reform," *Testimonies,* II, 384, originally published as *Testimony Relative to Marriage Duties, and Extremes in the Health Reform* (Battle Creek: SDA Publishing Assn., 1869); James White, "The Lord's Supper," *R&H,* XXIX (April 16, 1867), 222. According to Richard W. Schwarz, James White himself used domestic wine for medicinal purposes; "John Harvey Kellogg: American Health Reformer" (Ph.D. diss., University of Michigan, 1964), p. 144. For evidence of Ellen White's essentially uncompromising attitude toward alcoholic drinks, see EGW, "The Manufacture of Wine and Cider," *Testimonies,* V, 354-61.

hundred, including "the very *elite* of Haverhill's society," she "struck intemperance at the very root, showing that on the home table largely exists the fountain from which flow the first tiny rivulets of perverted appetite, which soon deepen into an uncontrollable current of indulgence, and sweep the victim to a drunkard's grave." Enthusiastic applause punctuated her talk.[29]

In addition to her lecturing, Ellen White was continually turning out temperance articles for various Adventist publications. Even the children were not forgotten. In her four-volume collection of *Sabbath Readings for the Home Circle* she included a selection of sentimental temperance stories with such titles as "Father, Don't Go," "Affecting Scene in a Saloon," and "The Major's Cigar." Typical was one tale entitled "Made a Drunkard by His Cigar," which told of a promising young clergyman whose intemperate habits killed his wife, made a beggar of his child, and eventually sent him to a mad-house.[30]

Adventist efforts on behalf of temperance culminated in 1879 in the formation of the American Health and Temperance Association, a denominational organization presided over by Dr. John H. Kellogg. The principal goal of the sponsors of the association was to acquire as many signatures as possible on their two pledges: a "teetotal pledge" for those swearing to abstain from "alcohol, tobacco, tea, coffee, opium, and all other narcotics and stimulants forever," and a less comprehensive "anti-liquor and tobacco pledge" for the faint-hearted. Ellen White was among the first to affix her name to the teetotal pledge and one of the most active in signing up others as she traveled from place to place.[31]

---

29. EGW, Diary entry for October 8, 1885, quoted in William Homer Teesdale, "Ellen G. White: Pioneer, Prophet" (Ph.D. diss., University of California, n.d.), p. 232; EGW, *Life Sketches* (Mountain View, Calif.: Pacific Press, 1915), pp. 220-21; J[ames] W[hite], "The Camp-Meetings," *R&H,* XLVIII (September 7, 1876), 84; U[riah] S[mith], "Grand Rally in New England," ibid.

30. EGW, (ed.), *Sabbath Readings for the Home Circle* (Oakland: Pacific Press, 1877-1881). "Made a Drunkard by His Cigar" appears in Vol. II, pp. 371-73. For a representative collection of Ellen's writings on temperance, see EGW, *Temperance* (Mountain View, Calif.: Pacific Press, 1949).

31. "American Temperance Society," *Seventh-day Adventist Encyclopedia,* ed. Don F. Neufeld (Washington: Review and Herald Publishing Assn., 1966), pp. 29-30; George I. Butler, "Camp-Meeting at Nevada City, Mo.," *R&H,* LIII (June 12, 1879), 188-89; EGW, "The Camp-Meeting at Nevada, Mo.," ibid., p. 188.

Kellogg's presidency of the American Health and Temperance Association symbolized his ascendancy to the leadership of the Adventist health-reform movement. From the time of his appointment in 1876 as superintendent of the Western Health Reform Institute, he had begun slowly to eclipse the prophetess as the church's health authority. By 1886 he could without embarrassment describe himself in a letter to Mrs. White as "a sort of umpire as to what was true or correct and what was error in matters relating to hygienic reform, a responsibility which has often made me tremble, and which I have felt very keenly." For her part, she seems to have willingly abdicated her previous role, having had her fill of trying to change the habits of a recalcitrant church. The noncontroversial temperance lectures continued, but there were few words about the short skirt, sex, or radical changes in diet. The less she said, the more her followers reverted to their former ways, and before long there were unmistakable signs of "a universal backsliding on health reform." As early as 1875 she noticed the drift and commented ruefully that "Our people are constantly retrograding upon health reform." Young Kellogg tried valiantly to stem the onrushing tide, but without Mrs. White's support, his efforts were doomed to failure.[32]

Evidence of dietary backsliding was particularly noticeable at the summer camp meetings, where provision stands prominently displayed "whole codfish, large slabs of halibut, smoked herring, dried beef and Bologna sausage." For years Kellogg waged a one-man crusade to cleanse the camps of these odious items, on occasion even buying up the entire stock and destroying it. But flesh-loving campers and ministers constantly hampered his efforts. At one statewide meeting in Indiana he paid fifteen dollars to have "the whole stock of meat, strong cheese and some detestable bakery stuff" thrown in the river, only to discover later that the conference ministers had surreptitiously salvaged the goods and divided the spoil among themselves.[33]

32. J. H. Kellogg to EGW, December 6, 1886 (White Estate); J. H. Kellogg to E. S. Ballenger, January 9, 1936 (Ballenger-Mote Papers); EGW, "Parents as Reformers," *Testimonies*, III, 569. On Kellogg's role in the Adventist reform movement, see also James and Ellen White, *Life Sketches* (Battle Creek: SDA Publishing Assn., 1880), p. 378.

33. Kellogg to Ballenger, January 9, 1936. Although there is no reason to doubt

Whatsoever Ye Eat or Drink

As this incident illustrates, the Adventist clergy were often the greatest enemies of reform. Many refused to preach against the evils of meat-eating and by their own example discouraged others who looked to them for guidance. At one point Kellogg estimated that all but "two or three" Adventist ministers ate meat. It was routinely served at their annual General Conference banquets, where even the leading brethren partook. Uriah Smith, the respected editor of the *Review and Herald,* was known to love a good steak and an occasional bowl of oyster soup, and others in the hierarchy apparently shared his tastes. By the turn of the century the reform movement had plunged to such depths, vegetarianism was more the exception than the rule in Adventist households.[34]

Although Ellen White liked to blame this great "backsliding" on extremists in the church who had given health reform a bad name, she herself was not guiltless. For when it came to meat-eating, she was for a time the most prominent backslider of all. (Charges that she also imbibed a little tea were resolutely denied.) We do not know precisely when she first resumed eating meat, but certainly it was not before March, 1869, when she assured the Battle Creek church that she had not changed her course "a particle" since first adopting the twice-a-day vegetarian diet: "I have not taken one step back since the light from Heaven upon this subject first shone upon my pathway." Only four-and-one-half years later, however, she was eating duck while vacationing in the Rockies. And by 1881 she was no longer willing to make an issue of eating meat and dairy products, against which she had once borne such "positive testimony." Meat, eggs, butter, and cheese, she now said, were not to be classed with

---

Kellogg's basic recollection, it should be remembered that the flamboyant doctor was writing about fifty years after the events described and may have had a tendency to embroider. See also EGW, Letter 40, 1893, quoted in EGW, *Counsels on Diet and Foods,* p. 369; and EGW, "Object-Lessons in Health Reform," *Testimonies,* VI, 112.

34. J. H. Kellogg to Willie White, April 12, 1875 (White Estate); Kellogg to Ballenger, January 9, 1936; Richard Julian Hammond, "The Life and Work of Uriah Smith" (MA. thesis, SDA Theological Seminary, 1944), pp. 147-48; "Interview between Geo. W. Amadon, Eld. A. C. Bourdeau, and Dr. J. H. Kellogg, October 7, 1907" (Ballenger-Mote Papers). According to family tradition, Uriah Smith liked to say that "God did not make oysters so good if he did not mean for them to be eaten"; personal interview with Mrs. Jane Smith Bonynge, March 31, 1974.

the poisonous narcotics — tea, coffee, tobacco, and alcohol — which were to be discarded entirely.[35]

According to Dr. John Kellogg, Mrs. White celebrated her return from Europe in 1887 with a "large baked fish." When she visited the doctor at the Battle Creek Sanitarium during the next several years, she "always called for meat and usually fried chicken," much to the consternation of Kellogg and the cook, both thoroughgoing vegetarians. At the various camp meetings she attended, her lax dietary habits became common knowledge, thanks in no small part to her own children, who were prone to indulge their "animal passions." Kellogg recalled once hearing Edson (J. E.) White,

> standing in front of his mother's tent, call out to a meat wagon that visited the grounds regularly and was just leaving, "Say, hello there! Have you any fresh fish?"
> "No," was his reply.
> "Have you got any fresh chicken?"
> Again the answer was "no," and J. E. bawled out in a very loud voice, "Mother wants some chicken. You had better get some quick."

It was obvious to Kellogg that Edson, never much of a health reformer, wanted the chicken every bit as much as his mother did.[36]

When the inevitable rumors began circulating that the prophetess had not always lived up to her own standards, Ellen White protested that she had indeed been "a faithful health reformer," as the members of her family could testify. But even her favorite son Willie related a different story. Years after his mother's death he told of the many setbacks in her struggle to overcome meat, of the difficulties

---

35. EGW, Letter 57, 1886, quoted in EGW, *Counsels on Diet and Foods,* p. 212; EGW, "A Consecrated Ministry" (MS-1a-1890, White Estate); EGW, "Christian Temperance," p. 371; EGW, Diary for October 5, 1873 (MS-12-1873, White Estate); EGW, MS-5-1881 (White Estate).

36. Kellogg to Ballenger, January 9, 1936. On Edson's attitude toward health reform, as seen by his mother, see EGW to Edson White, February 27, 1868 (W-5-1868, White Estate). Shortly after James White's death Dr. Kellogg advised Mrs. White to eat "a little fresh meat" for her health; J. H. Kellogg to EGW, September 17, 1881, quoted in Richard W. Schwarz, "The Kellogg Schism: The Hidden Issues," *Spectrum,* IV (Autumn, 1972), 36.

in finding competent vegetarian cooks, and of lunch baskets filled with turkey, chicken, and tinned tongue. Yet despite these lapses, both he and his mother seem to have regarded themselves as true vegetarians — in principle if not in practice.[37]

The rumors of Mrs. White's fondness for flesh were not based on hearsay alone; in 1890 she confessed in print to occasionally using meat. "When I could not obtain the food I needed, I have sometimes eaten a little meat," she admitted in the book *Christian Temperance*. She went on to add that she was "becoming more and more afraid of it" and was looking forward hopefully to the time when meat-eating would eventually disappear among those expecting the Second Coming of Christ. The very next year she advised a Brother H. C. Miller that "a little meat two or three times a week" would be preferable to "eating so largely of [Graham] gems and potatoes, and gravies, and strong sauce."[38]

It was not until January, 1894, that Ellen White finally gained the victory over her appetite for meat. She had just completed a temperance lecture in Brighton, Australia, when a Catholic admirer in the audience came forward and inquired if the speaker ate any meat. Upon hearing that she did, the woman fell on her knees at Mrs. White's feet and tearfully pleaded with her to have compassion on the unfortunate animals. The incident proved to be a turning point in the life of the prophetess, who described it in a letter to friends in the United States: "when the selfishness of taking the lives of animals to gratify a perverted taste was presented to me by a Catholic woman, kneeling at my feet, I felt ashamed and distressed. I saw it in a new light, and I said, I will no longer patronize the butchers. I will not have the flesh of corpses on my table." From that time until her death in 1915 she apparently never touched another piece of meat.[39]

---

37. EGW, "The Health Reform," *Testimonies*, IX, 159. Willie White's recollections are quoted verbatim in a letter from his son Arthur L. White to Anna Frazier, December 18, 1935 (Ballenger-Mote Papers). In 1884 Ellen White confessed that she "often" ate meat in California because the cook at St. Helena did not know how to prepare wholesome vegetarian dishes; EGW to Bro. and Sister Maxon, February 6, 1884 (Letter 4, 1884, White Estate).

38. EGW, *Christian Temperance*, pp. 118-19; EGW to H. C. Miller, April 2, 1891.

39. EGW, Letter 73a, 1896, quoted in Francis D. Nichol, *Ellen G. White and Her*

Now that she was once again in the vegetarian fold, Ellen White joined Dr. Kellogg in fighting the apathy and hostility that many members felt toward dietary reform. It seemed to her that the very success of the church depended upon an immediate "revival in health reform." In a 1900 testimony on the need for such a reawakening, she attributed the low state of the church to the fact that her earlier testimonies had "not been heartily received" and that many of the brethren were "in heart and practice opposed to health reform." "The Lord does not now work to bring many souls into the truth," she wrote, "because of the church-members who have never been converted [to health reform], and those who were once converted but who have backslidden." Ministers and conference presidents in particular were admonished to place themselves "on the right side of the question."[40]

By far the most controversial of her plans for reviving health reform was the so-called antimeat pledge, modeled after those used in the temperance work. In a March 29, 1908, letter to Elder A. G. Daniells, then president of the General Conference, she urged that a pledge be circulated requiring total abstinence from "flesh meats, tea, and coffee, and all injurious foods." Daniells, no vegetarian himself, balked at this unwelcome assignment, fearing that its implementation would unnecessarily divide the church and even split families. But not being anxious to offend the prophetess by an outright refusal, he countered with a less drastic proposal of his own calling for "an extensive well-balanced educational work . . . carried on by physicians and ministers instead of entering precipitately upon an Anti-Meat Pledge Campaign."[41]

Deferring to the president, Ellen White quietly withdrew her

Critics (Washington: Review and Herald Publishing Assn., 1951), pp. 388-89; Kellogg to Ballenger, January 9, 1936.

40. EGW, "A Revival in Health Reform," *Testimonies,* VI, 371-73.

41. EGW to A. G. Daniells, March 29, 1908; A. G. Daniells to W. C. White, July 17, 1908; and A. C. Daniells to [?], April 11, 1928; all quoted in "The Question of an Anti-Meat Pledge," prepared by the Ellen G. White Publications in September, 1951 (White Estate). On A. G. Daniells's dietary habits, see "Interview between Geo. W. Amadon, Eld. A. C. Bourdeau, and Dr. J. H. Kellogg, October 7, 1907." See also J. S. Washburn, *An Open Letter to Elder A. G. Daniells and an Appeal to the General Conference* (Toledo: Published by the author, 1922), pp. 27-28.

suggestion and took steps to prevent its publication. At the quadrennial session of the General Conference in 1909 she came out in support of Daniells's educational plan and pointedly discouraged any attempt to make the use of flesh food a "test of fellowship." Although her address closely paralleled her original communication to Daniells, there was no mention of a pledge this time. But the pledge episode did not end there. In 1911 some medical workers in California somehow obtained a copy of the March 29 letter and disclosed its contents at an Adventist camp meeting in Tulare. In harmony with its advice they circulated the following pledge: "In compliance with the revealed will of the Lord, and trusting in His help, we pledge ourselves to abstain from the use of tea, coffee, and flesh foods, including fish and fowl." Needless to say, this unauthorized version did not please either Mrs. White or her son Willie, who quickly saw to it that the pledge-signing movement died an early death.[42]

Ellen White's twentieth-century health-reform revival differed in many respects from the crusade she had originally launched in the 1860s. In the case of meat, the focus shifted from its animalizing tendencies to the diseased condition of animals and the "moral evils of a flesh diet," an argument made by her Catholic admirer in Australia. Nowhere is this change in emphasis more apparent than in *The Ministry of Healing* (1905), her last major work on health. Among the "reasons for discarding flesh foods" one searches in vain for any of the old references to animal passions or sexuality. In their place are two other arguments: that meat transmits cancer, tuberculosis, and "other fatal diseases" to man and is thus unfit for human consumption; and that meat-eating is cruel to the animals and destroys man's tenderness. In Australia Mrs. White had adopted a mongrel dog named Tiglath Pileser, and in her old age she grew increasingly fond of the intelligent and affectionate members of the animal kingdom. The thought of eating any of them now repulsed her. "What man with a human heart, who has ever cared for domes-

---

42. "The Question of an Anti-Meat Pledge." The 1909 general conference address was published as "Faithfulness in Health Reform," *Testimonies*, IX, 153-66. The White Estate still has not released portions of Ellen White's March 29, 1908, letter to Daniells.

tic animals, could look into their eyes, so full of confidence and affection, and willingly give them over to the butcher's knife?" she asked with obvious emotion. "How could he devour their flesh as a sweet morsel?"[43]

A similar evolution can be seen in her attitude toward eggs, butter, and other dairy products. In the early days she roundly condemned these items and indiscriminately lumped them together with meat and the poisonous narcotics. In 1872 she wrote:

> We bear positive testimony against tobacco, spirituous liquors, snuff, tea, coffee, flesh-meats, butter, spices, rich cakes, mince pies, a large amount of salt, and all exciting substances used as articles of food.

But just nine years later she refused to classify meat, eggs, butter, and cheese with the poisonous narcotics:

> Tea, coffee, tobacco, and alcohol we must present as sinful indulgences. We cannot place on the same ground, meat, eggs, butter, cheese and such articles placed upon the table.

By the turn of the century (1902) she was drawing a line between meat, on one hand, and milk, eggs, and butter on the other, even allowing that the latter three might have a salutary effect:

> Milk, eggs, and butter should not be classed with flesh-meat. In some cases the use of eggs is beneficial.

Again, in 1909, she cautiously recommended using eggs, butter, and milk to prevent malnutrition. By this time her greatest fear was the likelihood that these foods were diseased, not that they acted as aphrodisiacs.[44]

---

43. EGW, *Ministry of Healing*, pp. 313-17; Autograph album given to Ellen White in 1900 (White Estate). Mrs. White did occasionally mention the animalizing tendencies of meat after 1900 (see, e.g., "Health Reform," p. 159), but her emphasis was no longer on this aspect of meat eating. Over fifty years earlier L. B. Coles had also linked cancer with the eating of flesh; *Philosophy of Health*, p. 67.

44. EGW, "Appeal to Burden-Bearers," p. 21; EGW, MS-5-1881; EGW, "Educate the People," *Testimonies*, VII, 135; EGW, "Faithfulness in Health Reform," pp. 162-63. On

Mrs. White's intellectual development created "a good deal of controversy" among those who found the notion of progressive revelation difficult to understand. The gradual acceptance of butter was particularly troublesome in view of her once uncompromising stand against its use. At a meeting in 1904 Willie White helpfully explained to his aging mother why she had formerly condemned but now condoned the consumption of this product:

> Now, when that view was given you about butter [in 1863], there was presented to you the condition of things — people using butter full of germs. They were frying and cooking in it, and its use was deleterious. But later on, when our people studied into the principle of things, they found that while butter is not best, it may not be so bad as some other evils; and so in some cases they are using it.

Actually Mrs. White had not seen "germs" in 1863, only disease-producing humors. But in anachronistically substituting the more modern term, Willie was merely reflecting his mother's changing vocabulary. In her early writings she had described how flesh-meats filled the blood "with cancerous and scrofulous humors." Within a few decades, however, scientists like Louis Pasteur and Robert Koch had convinced the world of the existence of germs, and Mrs. White's language changed accordingly. The familiar humors disappeared from her works, and she began writing instead of meat filling the body with "tuberculous and cancerous germs."[45]

Many factors had a moderating effect on Mrs. White's dietary views. Her own struggle with meat had demonstrated that thoroughgoing reform was not easy, and her family's experience had taught her the impossibility of making "one rule for all to follow." Fanatics in the church, who carried reform to extremes, had shown her the

---

the benefits of eggs, see EGW to Dr. and Mrs. D. H. Kress, May 29, 1901, (K-37-1901, White Estate). In this letter Mrs. White recommends drinking a raw egg mixed in grape juice.

45. "Report of a meeting of the church school board, Sanitarium, California, January 14, 1904" (MS-7-1904, White Estate); EGW, *Spiritual Gifts* (1864), p. 146; EGW, "Parents as Reformers," p. 563; Howard D. Kramer, "The Germ Theory and the Early Public Health Program in the United States," *Bulletin of the History of Medicine*, XXII (May-June, 1948), 240-41.

potential for harm. Travels in Europe and the South Pacific had impressed on her the importance of international differences in a church rapidly expanding beyond the bounds of North America. But most significant of all were her frequent contacts with the growing number of Adventist physicians, especially her friend John Kellogg. Until his expulsion from the church in 1907 (discussed in the following chapter), Dr. Kellogg made a point of supplying the prophetess with the latest data from his laboratories and apprising her of developments in medicine and nutrition. Whenever visiting Battle Creek, she stopped by the doctor's office to learn of any new scientific discoveries relating to health. At other times, she relied on his multitudinous publications or corresponded with him by mail. Whatever his influence on her, it certainly was not negligible.[46]

Ellen White lived out her last years as a true health reformer, happily subsisting on a simple twice-a-day diet of vermicelli-tomato soup or thistle greens "seasoned with sterilized cream and lemon juice" — "horse feed" a companion good-naturedly called it. Meat, butter, and cheese never appeared on her table. She no longer objected to a moderate use of butter, but feared that if she ate a little, others would use it as an excuse to eat a lot. With the eating habits of a hundred thousand persons virtually hanging on her every bite, her fears were not unfounded. Once during an illness in Minneapolis she tried a small piece of cheese, only to have it "reported in large assemblies that Sister White eats cheese." It was taken for granted that whatever she ate, others were free to eat also. And at her age she had no desire to be a "stumbling block" to anyone.[47]

---

46. EGW, Letter 127, 1904, quoted in *Counsels on Diet and Foods*, p. 491; Alonzo L. Baker, "My Years with John Harvey Kellogg," *Spectrum*, IV (Autumn, 1972), 44; J. H. Kellogg to EGW, October 30, 1904 (White Estate); EGW, *Ministry of Healing*, p. 302.

47. Arthur L. White, "Ellen G. White the Person," *Spectrum*, IV (Spring, 1972), 11; EGW, Letter 10, 1902, quoted in EGW, *Counsels on Diet and Foods*, p. 324; EGW, Letter 45, 1903, ibid., p. 490; EGW, Talk in College Library, April 1, 1901 (MS-43-1901, White Estate); EGW to Brother and Sister Belden, November 26, 1905 (B-322-1905, White Estate).

CHAPTER EIGHT

Fighting the Good Fight

"In these letters which I write, in the testimonies I bear, I am presenting to you that which the Lord has presented to me. I do not write one article in the paper expressing merely my own ideas. They are what God has opened before me in vision — the precious rays of light shining from the throne."

Ellen G. White[1]

"We discard nothing that the visions have ever taught from beginning to end, from first to last. Whenever we give up any, we shall give up all; so let this point be once for all distinctly understood."

Uriah Smith[2]

The 1870s were among the best years of Ellen White's life. The previous decade, marred by perpetual sickness and strife, had not been a particularly happy one for the Whites. It had left their reputations so tarnished that the leaders of the church felt obliged in 1870 to publish a "vindication of their moral and Christian character," explaining James's new-found success and refuting libelous stories about

---

1. EGW, "The Testimonies Slighted," *Testimonies*, V, 67.
2. [Uriah Smith], *The Visions of Mrs. E. G. White: A Manifestation of Spiritual Gifts According to the Scriptures* (Battle Creek: SDA Publishing Assn., 1868), p. 40.

Ellen's having given birth to an illegitimate child named Jesus and having once proposed swapping husbands with Sister S. H. King. But by the mid-1870s the worst of their troubles had passed, and the Whites were again basking in the love and affection of the Advent believers. "We are appreciated here," the thankful prophetess wrote her son from Battle Creek. "We can do more good when we are appreciated than when we are not. We never had greater influence among our people than at the present time. They all look up to us as father and mother."[3]

While winning appreciation at home, Ellen White was also acquiring limited national recognition through her coast-to-coast lecturing on temperance — thanks in large part to her own niece, Mary L. Clough, who joined the White entourage in 1876 as press agent. It was Miss Clough's job to see that her aunt received favorable newspaper coverage wherever she went, instead of the silence or sneers that had formerly greeted her. Apparently she carried out her assignment well, for the *Health Reformer* reported at the close of the year that Mrs. White had receive "the highest encomiums from the press in nearly all parts of the United States," publicity her thrifty husband valued at over ten thousand dollars. Whatever fame Ellen White enjoyed outside the Adventist community seems to have come primarily from her temperance work rather than from her activities as a health reformer. Despite her personal acquaintances with Drs. Jackson, Trall, and Dio Lewis, whom she visited in 1871, she always remained an obscure and isolated figure in non-Adventist reform circles.[4]

The Whites spent much of the 1870s away from Battle Creek in the more relaxed surroundings of the Far West. In the summer of 1872 they took a much-needed vacation in the Colorado Rockies vis-

---

3. *Defense of Eld. James White and Wife: Vindication of Their Moral and Christian Character* (Battle Creek: SDA Publishing Assn., 1870), pp. 9-11, 104-6; EGW to W. C. White, October 26, 1876 (W-46-1876, White Estate).

4. J[ames] W[hite], "Our Camp-Meetings," *R&H*, XLVIII (October 19, 1876), 124; "Items for the Month," *HR*, XI (December, 1876), 381; EGW to Edson and Emma White, November 15, 1871 (W-15-1871, White Estate). Mary Clough, who never joined her aunt's church, was probably the author of a flattering biographical sketch of Mrs. White that appeared in *American Biographical History of Eminent and Self-Made Men . . . Michigan Volume* (Cincinnati: Western Biographical Publishing Co., 1878), Dist. 3, p. 108.

iting the family of Mary Clough's sister, Lou Walling. The climate was so invigorating that the Whites decided to purchase some property near Boulder and put up a small mountain cabin, to which they retreated in succeeding years. However, Mrs. White's first visit to Colorado almost proved to be her last. While riding horseback with relatives and friends through the Snowy Range, she was thrown from her frightened pony. When the others reached her, she could scarcely speak or breathe. Their first thought was to find water and towels and try "the virtues of hydropathy." The emergency treatments and prayer allowed the injured prophetess to continue her journey and taught her husband a valuable lesson: "Faith and hydropathy harmonize; faith and drugs, never."[5]

Shortly after this incident the Whites boarded a westbound train for northern California to meet with the growing number of believers in that state. On this first foray the Whites remained five months, then returned in late 1873 to take up residence, first in Santa Rosa and later near Oakland. Ellen White loved northern California and found sailing on San Francisco Bay the greatest pleasure of her life. With her encouragement, James established a western publishing house and launched a new weekly journal, *The Signs of the Times,* to aid in proselytizing the Pacific Coast. For the next several years the Whites divided their time between East and West and occasionally found themselves separated. Ellen never liked staying home by herself, and James's poor letter-writing did not make it any easier. "Dear Husband," she wrote in the spring of 1876:

> We received your few words last night on a postal card: "Battle Creek, April 11. No letter from you for two days. James White."
>
> This lengthy letter was written by yourself. Thank you for we know you are living.
>
> No letter from James White previous to this since April 6. . . . I have been anxiously waiting for something to answer.[6]

---

5. [James White], "The Summer in the Rocky Mountains," *HR,* VIII (January, 1873), 20-21.

6. Harold O. McCumber, *The Advent Message in the Golden West* (Mountain View, Calif.: Pacific Press, 1968), pp. 79-110; EGW, Letter 5, 1875, quoted in Arthur L. White, *Ellen G. White: Messenger to the Remnant* (Washington: Review and Herald Publishing Assn., 1969), pp. 100, 111.

The 1870s also marked the end of Ellen White's dramatic daytime visions, the last one coming about 1879 at age fifty-two. Years earlier Dr. Trall had privately predicted that the visions would end after menopause, and — whatever the cause — they did. In the summer of 1869 Mrs. White wrote Edson that she was going through the change of life and fully expected to die, as her sister Sarah had done.

> I am not in good health. . . . I have more indications of going down into the grave than of rallying. My vitality is at a low ebb. Your Aunt Sarah died passing through this critical time. My lungs are affected. Dr. Trall said I would probably go with consumption in this time. Dr. Jackson said I should probably fail in this time. Nature would be severly taxed, and the only question would be, were there vital forces remaining to sustain the change of nature. My lungs have remained unaffected until last winter. The fainting fit I had on the cars nearly closed my life. My lungs are painful. How I shall come out I cannot tell. I suffer much pain.

Somehow she survived the ordeal, which may have lasted until the mid-1870s; but thereafter her public visions apparently grew less and less frequent. For the remainder of her life she received her heavenly communications by means of dreams — "visions of the night" — unaccompanied by any outward physical manifestations. When her son Willie once asked how she knew that her dreams were not of the ordinary variety, she explained that the angel guide in her visions of the night was the same heavenly being who previously instructed her during her daytime trances. Thus she had no reason to doubt their divine origin.[7]

7. Merritt Kellogg to J. H. Kellogg, June 3, 1906 (Kellogg Collection, MSU); EGW to Edson White, June 10, 1869 (W-6-1869, White Estate); White, *Ellen G. White*, p. 7; D. M. Canright, *Life of Mrs. E. G. White, Seventh-day Adventist Prophet: Her False Claims Refuted* (Nashville: B. C. Goodpasture, 1953), p. 172. In "The Study of the Testimonies — No. 2," *Daily Bulletin of the General Conference*, V (January 29-30, 1893), 19, J. N. Loughborough places Mrs. White's last vision in 1884, but Merritt Kellogg in the letter cited above argues convincingly that 1879 is a more likely date. In *Ellen G. White and Her Critics* (Washington: Review and Herald Publishing Assn., 1951), pp. 43, 71, Francis D. Nichol suggests that the last public vision occurred in October, 1878, and that Ellen White went through menopause about 1875. We do not know

Fighting the Good Fight

On August 6, 1881, Ellen White suffered one of the severest blows of her life: the tragic loss of her husband, James. Only two weeks earlier he had seemed in perfect health. But a trip to Charlotte, Michigan, had chilled him, and the best efforts of Dr. Kellogg and the sanitarium staff proved in vain. Ellen's thirty-five-year marriage to James had been a good one, but not without its trials. On the one hand, James was not the easiest man to get along with. "He was of an eager, impetuous nature, and not seldom gave offense," wrote one pioneer Adventist historian. He was also excessively jealous of his wife's friendship with real or imagined rivals in the church hierarchy and refused on occasion to sleep in the same house with her. On the other hand, he was a person quick to forgive and to make amends, and he had his own cross to bear — living with a woman whose criticisms and reproofs came backed with divine authority.[8]

Whatever his failings, Ellen White loved and respected him and leaned on him in her hours of need. Without him, her career as a prophetess would probably never have gotten off the ground. Since the 1840s, publishing had been his passion — and the key to her success. In those early days it was he who insisted on printing her visions, after patiently correcting her grammar and polishing her style. It was through his journals and publishing houses that thousands received her testimonies and joined the church. And it was his efforts that culminated in a strong central organization, over which he served as president for ten critical years, founding both the Western Health Reform Institute and Battle Creek College. Seventh-day Adventism would not have been the same without Ellen White; it would not have existed without James.[9]

---

when menstruation actually ceased, but it is possible that Mrs. White experienced menopausal symptoms for years. It is also possible that the suggestions of physicians, which led her to expect significant changes in her life, contributed to the cessation of her daytime visions.

8. EGW, *Life Sketches* (Mountain View, Calif.: Pacific Press, 1915), pp. 247-52; M. Ellsworth Olsen, *A History of the Origin and Progress of Seventh-day Adventists* (Washington: Review and Herald Publishing Assn., 1925), p. 422; James White to D. M. Canright, May 24, 1881 (Ballenger-Mote Papers); "Interview between Geo. W. Amadon, Eld. A. C. Bourdeau, and Dr. J. H. Kellogg, October 7, 1907," p. 80 (Ballenger-Mote Papers).

9. EGW, "The Work at Battle Creek," *Testimonies*, III, 89; EGW, *Life Sketches*, pp. 248-49; EGW to Brother [?], July 8, 1906, quoted in Nichol, *Ellen G. White and Her*

Following her husband's death, the grief-stricken widow sank into a year-long depression. She struggled to remain active, but at nights "deep sorrow" came over her as she expectantly awaited her own demise. Then one night the Lord appeared to her in a dream and said: "LIVE. I have put My Spirit upon your son, W. C. White, that he may be your counselor. I have given him the spirit of wisdom, and a discerning, perceptive mind." Comforted by these words and the knowledge that her favorite son Willie would remain by her side, she resumed her ministry with renewed zeal.[10]

In her widowhood Ellen White literally followed the spread of Adventism around the world, from Europe to the South Pacific. From 1885 to 1887 she made her home in Switzerland, where John N. Andrews had gone in 1874 as the first Seventh-day Adventist missionary. Within two years he had founded a magazine, *Les Signes des Temps,* and set up headquarters in Basel, centrally located near France and Germany. By 1884 Switzerland alone had over two hundred Adventist believers, a publishing house was under construction, and the leaders in Europe were anxious for a visit from Mrs. White and her son Willie, who had been associated with the publishing work in Battle Creek and Oakland. Thus on August 8, 1885, Ellen White and family sailed from Boston on the steamer *Cephalonia,* and a month later were setting up housekeeping in an apartment above the new Basel press. For the next two years the thrill of sightseeing and speaking in new places tended to divert Mrs. White's attention from health reform, although she did squeeze in an occasional temperance lecture, drawing an estimated thirteen hundred in Christiania (Oslo), Norway.[11]

The years 1887 to 1891 found her back in the United States fighting a doctrinal battle to shift the focus of Adventist theology from the Ten Commandments to the love and righteousness of Christ.

Critics, p. 645; "James Springer White," *Seventh-day Adventist Encyclopedia,* ed. Don F. Neufeld (Washington: Review and Herald Publishing Assn., 1966), pp. 1419-25.

10. EGW, *Life Sketches,* pp. 252-54; EGW, *The Writing and Sending Out of the Testimonies to the Church* (Battle Creek: SDA Publishing Assn., 1913), pp. 19-20.

11. EGW, *Life Sketches,* pp. 281-308; Olsen, *History of the Origin and Progress of Seventh-day Adventists,* pp. 303-14; "Switzerland," *Seventh-day Adventist Encyclopedia,* p. 1282.

Fighting the Good Fight

But late in 1891, in response to an earnest appeal for her presence, she departed with a clutch of assistants for Australia and New Zealand, where she remained until 1900. Adventist missionaries had arrived in Melbourne only six years earlier and had, as usual, immediately set about to start a periodical and publishing house. By the time of Mrs. White's arrival the greatest need was for a school to train workers, and it was this task to which the sixty-four-year-old prophetess put her hand. One night in a dream the Lord showed her the ideal spot for a Bible training school, and a short time later it was discovered in the country about seventy-five miles north of Sydney. There in rural Cooranbong Mrs. White served as a true "medical missionary," opening her home as "an asylum for the sick and afflicted." (Her favorite remedy for everything from fevers to bruises was the charcoal poultice.) Her frequent acts of kindness won the love and affection of all around her and prompted one grateful recipient of a sack of flour to follow her back to America to take care of her farm.[12]

A painful bout of rheumatism during her first year in Australia caused her to wonder at times why she had ever left the comforts of home. But she refused to let her suffering curtail her writing, and produced twenty-five hundred pages of manuscript under the most awkward conditions: "First my hair-cloth chair is bolstered up with pillows, then they have a frame, a box batted with pillows which I rest my limbs upon and a rubber pillow under them. My table is drawn up close to me, and I thus write with my paper on a cardboard in my lap."[13]

With the exception of this rheumatic attack, which lasted about eleven months, Ellen White enjoyed remarkably good health for a woman her age and with her history. When illness did come, she no

---

12. A. V. Olson, *Through Crisis to Victory: 1888-1901* (Washington: Review and Herald Publishing Assn., 1966); EGW, *Life Sketches*, pp. 331-40; Olsen, *History of the Origin and Progress of Seventh-day Adventists,* pp. 379-87; EGW to O. A. Olsen, January 30, 1905 (O-55-1905, White Estate); EGW to J. A. Burden and Others, March 24, 1908 (B-90-1908, White Estate); Autograph album given to Ellen White when she left Australia in 1900 (White Estate).

13. EGW, Letters 16c and 18a, 1892, quoted in White, *Ellen G. White,* pp. 102, 110; EGW, MS 8, 1904, quoted in EGW, *Selected Messages* (Washington: Review and Herald Publishing Assn., 1958), I, 104.

longer followed her former practice of calling in the brethren to pray for her recovery. Since she was never healed outright as a result of such prayers, she feared that allowing others to pray for her would only produce disappointment and skepticism, as she explained to the General Conference committee in 1890: "I never yet have been healed out and out; and that is why I do not call on any one to pray for me, because they will expect that I will be healed, and I know from the past I will not be healed; that is, that I shall not have the work done right then and there...." Through the years she had also grown reluctant to pray for the sick herself because those healed often turned out to be unworthy: "One, after having grown to years, became a notorious thief; another became licentious, and another, though grown to manhood, has no love for God or his truth."[14]

While living in Australia, Mrs. White noted that the medical work was an excellent means of breaking down prejudice toward Adventism. From time to time prominent citizens, who had little or no interest in doctrine, would come to the Seventh-day Adventists with a request to establish a sanitarium or treatment room in their town. Once in operation these institutions created a positive image for Adventists and made it easier for their evangelists to come in and preach what was commonly called "the third angel's message." So successful was this approach, Ellen White declared in 1899 that nothing converted "the people like the medical missionary work." The following year she published a volume of testimonies urging that the health work be used as "an entering wedge, making a way for other truths to reach the heart." Henceforth, gospel and medical workers were to join hands in converting the world.[15]

Upon returning to America in 1900, Mrs. White purchased a comfortable farm near St. Helena, California, and returned to the

14. EGW, "Talk before the General Conference Committee," Lake Goguac, July 14, 1890 (C. Burton Clark Collection); EGW to J. H. Kellogg, March 11, 1892 (C. Burton Clark Collection).

15. EGW, Letter 76, 1899 (White Estate); EGW, "Object-Lessons in Health Reform," *Testimonies*, VI, 112-13; EGW, "The Medical Missionary Work and the Third Angel's Message," ibid., p. 289; EGW, "United Effort in Canvassing," p. 327. It should be pointed out that even before going to Australia, Ellen White recognized the potential uses of the health work; see, e.g., EGW, *Christian Temperance and Bible Hygiene* (Battle Creek: Good Health Publishing Co., 1890), p. 121.

mountains north of San Francisco to live on her royalties and her ministerial salary. Now well past seventy, she appeared to be nearing the end of a long and colorful career. But instead of quietly fading away, she entered one of her most productive periods, writing voluminously and directing a major campaign to establish Adventist sanitariums "near every large city." In addition to the main sanitarium in Battle Creek, the church was already operating several other hydropathic institutions. In 1878 Dr. Merritt Kellogg, hoping to attract invalids and pleasure seekers from the San Francisco Bay area, had opened a Rural Health Retreat in St. Helena. The success of his venture and especially that of his brother in Battle Creek encouraged others, and by 1900 Adventists were running medical centers of one kind or another in more than a half-dozen locations, including Portland, Oregon; Boulder, Colorado; Copenhagen, Denmark; and Sydney, Australia. Behind all these early efforts Ellen White's influence could be seen, but it was not until the first decade of this century that she began sanitarium-building in earnest.[16]

The event that triggered her twentieth-century campaign was the burning of the Battle Creek Sanitarium early in the morning of February 18, 1902. To Dr. Kellogg and his colleagues, the fire was a personal and denominational tragedy, but Ellen White saw it as a sign of divine displeasure with overcentralization in Battle Creek. Instead of supporting Kellogg's plan to rebuild in the same location, she seized this God-given opportunity to push for the opening of many smaller sanitariums in rural settings outside large cities. "My warning is: keep out of the cities," she declared in 1903. This insistence on country settings stemmed partially from a desire to return to nature — "God's physician" — and partially from a deep-seated fear of the labor unions that were beginning to infest urban areas. The Lord had shown her that these organizations would be used by Satan to bring about the "time of trouble" predicted for God's people in the last days, and she wanted "nothing to do with them." Union membership is a violation of the commandments of God, she

---

16. EGW to Brother and Sister Kress, August 9, 1905 (C. Burton Clark Collection); McCumber, *The Advent Message in the Golden West,* pp. 124-25; White, *Ellen G. White,* p. 122. On the early history of Adventist sanitariums, consult the *Seventh-day Adventist Encyclopedia.*

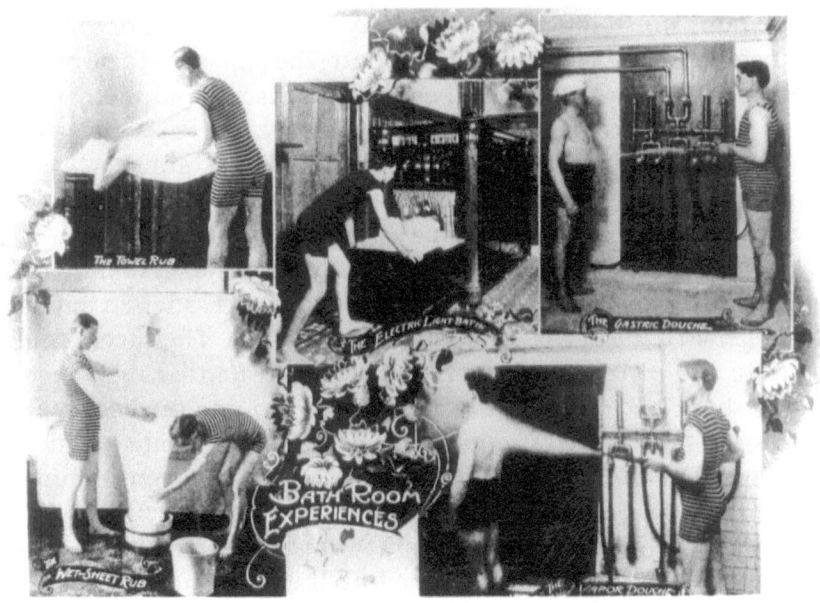

Water treatments at the Battle Creek Sanitarium near the turn of the century

told the church, "for to belong to these unions means to disregard the entire Decalogue."[17]

The scene of Mrs. White's most intensive sanitarium-building was Southern California, where the financial disaster of 1887 had sent real-estate prices plummeting. By the turn of the century defunct tourist and health resorts littered the landscape, priced at a fraction of their original cost. Guided by revelations from the Lord "in the night season," Ellen White helped to select three choice sanitarium sites in the years 1904 and 1905: in Paradise Valley outside San Diego, in Glendale on the outskirts of Los Angeles, and in Loma Linda near Redlands and Riverside. During the same decade she also assisted, directly or indirectly, in establishing sanitariums near

17. EGW to the General Conference Committee and the Medical Missionary Board, July 6, 1902 (B-128-1902, White Estate); EGW, "The Value of Outdoor Life," *Testimonies,* VII, 76-78; EGW, *Medical Practice and the Educational Program at Loma Linda* (Washington: Ellen G. White Publications, 1972), p. 57; EGW, "Avoiding Labor Conflicts," *Selected Messages,* II, 141-44.

the cities of Washington (Takoma Park), Chicago (Hinsdale), Boston (Melrose), and Nashville (Madison), as well as in several other places both in America and abroad.[18]

Her involvement with these new institutions went far beyond mere verbal encouragement. She personally inspected many of the locations and sometimes helped raise the necessary funds. When the Southern California conference officers hesitated to purchase property in drought-stricken Paradise Valley, Ellen White herself borrowed two thousand dollars to help close the deal and later took a keen interest in the sanitarium's day-to-day operations. She was also intimately connected with the financing and staffing of the Loma Linda Sanitarium, where she was a frequent and popular visitor.[19]

Even this late in her life she advised sanitarium personnel to use only natural, drugless remedies, and to avoid such newfangled (and expensive) electrical devices as the X-ray machine, which God had shown her was "not the great blessing that some suppose it to be."[20] Her sanitariums were not intended to compete with "worldly" hospitals and health resorts, but were to serve as unique medical missionary centers ministering as much to spiritual as physical needs. "Our sanitariums," she stressed over and over again, "are to be established for one object, — the advancement of present truth." If they failed in that mission, she could see no reason for their existence. On this point she parted company with Dr. John Kellogg, who had been fighting this "narrow sectarian spirit" for years. As early as 1893 he had spoken out against the feeling in some Adventist quarters "that work for the needy and suffering unless done with a direct

---

18. McCumber, *Advent Message in the Golden West*, pp. 156-71; EGW to the Workers in the Glendale Sanitarium, March 14, 1904 (C. Burton Clark Collection); *Seventh-day Adventist Encyclopedia*, passim.

19. D. E. Robinson, *The Story of Our Health Message* (3rd ed.; Nashville: Southern Publishing Association, 1965), pp. 335-402.

20. EGW to Brother Burden, June 17, 1906 (C. Burton Clark Collection). Physicians recognized the possible dangers of x-rays almost immediately after their therapeutic introduction; see, for example, David L. Edsall, "The Attitude of the Clinician in Regard to Exposing Patients to the X-Ray," *Journal of the American Medical Association*, XLVII (November 3, 1906), 1425-29. About 1911 x-ray therapy successfully removed a black spot on Mrs. White's forehead; EGW to J. E. White, Letter 30, 1911, quoted in EGW, *Selected Messages*, II, 303.

proselytizing motive was of no account and that it was not in the interests of the cause."[21]

To "serve as feeders to the sanitariums located in the country," Ellen White advocated setting up an urban network of hygienic restaurants and treatment rooms. These establishments would not only recruit patients but, more important, would acquaint city dwellers with the principles of Adventism. According to her divine instructions, "one of the principal reasons why hygienic restaurants and treatment-rooms should be established in the centers of large cities is that by this means the attention of leading men will be called to the third angel's message." However, the restaurant business never lived up to her early expectations, largely because proprietors tended to place economic above spiritual interests. As the prophetess put it, they "lost the science of soul saving." When vegetarian restaurants in Los Angeles and San Francisco failed to win many converts during their first years of operation, her enthusiasm for this phase of the health work began to flag noticeably.[22]

Because of her undying belief in the imminent return of Christ, Ellen White found it difficult to support projects not directly related to hastening that longed-for event. And in that category fell Dr. John Kellogg's numerous "health food" inventions. Dissatisfied with the sanitarium's "meager and monotonous" vegetarian diet, in the 1880s he launched a lifetime search for palatable supplements, ultimately inventing peanut butter, dry cereals, and "meat substitutes" made from nuts and wheat gluten. One of his first creations, a multigrained cereal named Granola, turned out to be nutritious and pleasant tasting — but also tough enough to crack dentures. After one irate patient

---

21. EGW to the General Conference Committee and the Medical Missionary Board, July 6, 1902; EGW, "Not for Pleasure Seekers," *Testimonies,* VII, 95-97; EGW, Letter 11, 1900, quoted in EGW, *Medical Practice and the Educational Program at Loma Linda,* p. 15; J. H. Kellogg to EGW, March 21, 1893 (White Estate). For a few years Ellen White even had hopes of infiltrating the Women's Christian Temperance Union and converting those temperance workers to "the Sabbath truth." See EGW to Dr. Lillis Wood Starr, September 5, 1907, and September 19, 1907 (S-278-1907 and S-302-1907, White Estate).

22. EGW, "Extent of the Work," *Testimonies,* VII, 60; EGW, "The Restaurant Work," ibid., VII, 115-22; EGW, "Object-Lessons in Health Reform," p. 113; EGW to Brother and Sister Burden, September 27, 1905 (C. Burton Clark Collection).

demanded ten dollars for her broken false teeth, he returned to his laboratory to develop a product more easily masticated. Assisted by his younger brother Will Keith, he finally came up with a flaked wheat cereal, Granose Flakes, for which he obtained a patent in 1894.[23]

When the commercial value of his Granose Flakes became apparent, as it soon did, Kellogg unselfishly offered to turn over production rights to the Adventist church, accurately predicting that it could "make enough money out of it to support the entire denominational work." But Mrs. White ignored his offer, and a decade later vetoed a chance to obtain the rights to the even more successful corn flakes. She feared tying up so much time and talent in manufacturing mere temporal foods when they might better be spent supplying "the multitudes with the bread of life." Besides, she was not especially fond of Dr. Kellogg's cereals. "When a thing is exhalted, as the corn flakes has been, it would be unwise for our people to have anything to do with it," she warned. "It is not necessary that we make the corn flakes an article of food." Her decision cost the church a fortune, which ultimately went into the pockets of Kellogg's enterprising brother, W. K.[24]

To staff their ever-growing collection of health-related institutions, Seventh-day Adventists found it necessary to set up their own educational programs. The leader in this work was also Dr. Kellogg. Beginning in 1877, he organized a school of hygiene at the Battle Creek Sanitarium, where in a twenty-week course students could either prepare for medical school or learn how to become health lecturers. In 1883 he added a second school to train young women in "nursing, massage, the use of electricity, and other branches of the practical medical department." And just six years later he opened still a third school which offered nontechnical training for hygienic cooks and health missionaries.[25]

---

23. Richard W. Schwarz, "John Harvey Kellogg: American Health Reformer" (Ph.D. diss., University of Michigan, 1964), pp. 277-86. See also Gerald Carson, *Cornflake Crusade* (New York: Rinehart, 1957).

24. J. H. Kellogg to EGW, June 10, 1896 (White Estate); EGW to J. A. Burden, November [?], 1906 (C. Burton Clark Collection); EGW, MS-10-1906, quoted in EGW, *Counsels on Diet and Foods* (Washington: Review and Herald Publishing Assn., 1946), p. 277.

25. S. N. Haskell, "The Hygienic School," *R&H*, L (December 20, 1877), 197; "The

But always the most pressing need was for qualified Adventist physicians. For almost twenty years, from about 1875 to the early 1890s, Kellogg simply tutored promising pupils at Battle Creek for a year and then sent them on to some "outside" medical school like the University of Michigan at Ann Arbor to complete their education. Each summer they were expected to return to Battle Creek and keep the sanitarium supplied with cheap help. Eventually the Adventists had so many of their young people going through Ann Arbor, the church purchased a home near the university where their students could live with fellow believers and get proper vegetarian meals. To prevent opportunists from taking advantage of this work-study plan and then turning their backs on the church, it finally became necessary to have prospective students sign a pledge swearing to work for the denomination at least five years after graduation and to "uphold by precept and example, the principles of hygienic and temperance reform presented in the Testimonies of Sister White, and promulgated by the Sanitarium and its managers."[26]

Try as they might, Adventist leaders were incapable of shielding their medical students from all heterodox influences. Time and again young doctors returned from their stay at Ann Arbor tainted by heretical medical or theological views. The risk was so great that Mrs. White finally advised not sending any more Adventists to the University of Michigan "unless it is a positive necessity." Even Kellogg began to have doubts about his arrangement with Ann Arbor. After laboring repeatedly to correct "errors" — like the use of "strychnia and other poisonous drugs" — imbibed at the university, he concluded it would be less trouble to train the physicians himself. Earlier, when James White had made a similar suggestion, Kellogg had wanted

---

Sanitarium Medical Mission and Training School," *Medical Missionary,* II (November-December, 1892), 217-19; E. H. W., "A Review of Our Work," ibid., IV (January, 1895), 9-13; "Health and Temperance Missionary School," *Seventh-day Adventist Encyclopedia,* pp. 506-8.

26. Ellet J. Waggoner to Willie White, July 8, 1875 (White Estate); "A Medical Course," *Good Health,* XVI (September, 1881), 288; J. H. Kellogg, "Wanted at Once," *R&H,* LXVI (November 12, 1889), 720; "The Missionary Medical Course," *Medical Missionary,* II (November-December, 1892), 225-26; J. H. Kellogg, "The Sanitarium Home for Medical Missionary Students, Ann Arbor, Michigan," ibid., I (November, 1891), 92-93; "An Important Meeting," ibid., I (August, 1891), 154-56.

nothing to do with what would obviously be a second-rate institution, but now he was convinced he could offer a respectable four-year curriculum "equal to that of the best medical schools in the country." Instruction in the basic sciences would be given at Battle Creek, while much of the clinical work would be taken in Chicago, where there were several large hospitals and an Adventist dispensary. By the fall of 1895 he had obtained a charter from the State of Illinois and was welcoming first-year students to the American Medical Missionary College. During its fifteen-year existence, before being absorbed by the University of Illinois, Kellogg's medical school awarded a total of 194 doctorates in medicine and furnished the Adventist church with a generation of much-needed physicians.[27]

For over a quarter century Ellen White and her protégé John Kellogg had worked harmoniously to turn an obscure Midwestern water cure into the center of a rapidly expanding international medical organization, which by the turn of the century controlled more employees than the General Conference. True, they had had their occasional differences, but a bond of mutual affection had always drawn them together. "I have loved and respected you as my own mother," the doctor wrote in 1899. "I have the tenderest feeling toward you," the prophetess replied a short time later. Though he found the scientific accuracy of her testimonies more persuasive than their visionary origin, he had since youth accepted her claims to divine inspiration. He had appreciated her counsel and tolerated her rebukes. But in the late 1890s, when she started accusing him of pride, selfishness, and other sins, the relationship began to sour noticeably. On November 10, 1907, Dr. Kellogg was disfellowshipped from the Seventh-day Adventist Church. The charges: being antagonistic "to the gifts now manifest in the church" and allying himself "with those who are attempting to overthrow the work for which this church existed."[28]

27. EGW to Brother and Sister Prescott, November 14, 1893 (P-50-1893, White Estate); J. H. Kellogg to EGW, May 26, 1895, and June 6, 1895 (White Estate); J. H. Kellogg, "A Medical Missionary College," *R&H,* LXXII (June 11, 1895), 381-82; J. H. Kellogg, "The American Medical Missionary College," *Medical Missionary,* V (October, 1895), 289-92; "American Medical Missionary College," *Seventh-day Adventist Encyclopedia,* pp. 28-29.

28. J. H. Kellogg to EGW, March 8, 1899 (Kellogg Collection, MSU); EGW to J. H. Kellogg, November 11, 1902 (K-174-1902, White Estate); Richard W. Schwarz, "The

The story behind Kellogg's sensational excommunication is a complex affair, replete with unsubstantiated charges of doctrinal heresy and sexual misconduct. In retrospect it appears to have been basically an unfortunate personal and political struggle between the sometimes haughty czar of the Adventist medical institutions and a group of ministers that included A. G. Daniells, General Conference president and former associate of Mrs. White's in Australia; W. W. Prescott, editor of the *Review and Herald;* and Willie White. Caught in the middle was an aging and sometimes bewildered prophetess, whose authority became the focal point of the conflict.[29]

No later than the first months of 1906 Mrs. White became aware that certain doctors and ministers in Battle Creek were raising embarrassing questions about the validity of her testimonies. In a nighttime "vision" she saw the faces of many of her critics, including Dr. Kellogg, Elder A. T. Jones, and William S. Sadler, an ordained preacher recently graduated from the American Medical Missionary College. "I was directed by the Lord to request them and any others who have perplexities and grievous things in their minds regarding the testimonies that I have borne, to specify what their objections and criticisms are," she related, adding that the Lord had also promised to help her answer their queries. Accordingly, she sent a letter to several of those she had seen, as well as to Kellogg's associate Dr.

Kellogg Schism: The Hidden Issues," *Spectrum,* IV (Autumn, 1972), 23-39; Schwarz, "John Harvey Kellogg," pp. 360-76. For Kellogg's views on the scientific accuracy of Mrs. White's testimonies on health, see his introduction to EGW, *Christian Temperance and Bible Hygiene,* pp. iii-iv.

29. Irving Keck to A. G. Daniells, December 3, 1906 (Ballenger-Mote Papers); J. S. Washburn, *An Open Letter to Elder A. G. Daniells and an Appeal to the General Conference* (Toledo: Published by the author, 1922), pp. 11-12; "Interview between Geo. W. Amadon, Eld. A. C. Bourdeau, and Dr. J. H. Kellogg, October 7, 1907," p. 97 (Ballenger-Mote Papers). This interview to determine the grounds for Kellogg's dismissal from the church is discussed in G. W. Amadon to A. G. Daniells, October 16, 1907 (Archives of the General Conference of Seventh-day Adventists). Among Daniells's concerns was the decline of membership and spirituality among Adventists shortly after the turn of the century, a loss he attributed partially to the commercializing and secularizing influence of the medical work; see, for example, A. G. Daniells to W. C. White, May 17, 1903, and August 9, 1903 (White Estate). Contrary to Keck's testimony, Daniells denied ever believing that Dr. Kellogg "was immoral in his relations to women"; Daniells to G. I. Butler, June 21, 1907 (White Estate).

Charles E. Stewart, asking them to "place upon paper a statement of the difficulties that perplex their minds." Kellogg refused to reply, but both Sadler and Stewart obliged Mrs. White by sending in long lists of "perplexities," which — regardless of their accuracy — shed considerable light on the puzzling estrangement between Ellen White and her former friends in Battle Creek.[30]

Uppermost in the minds of both Sadler and Stewart were the apparent inconsistencies and manipulations of her purportedly divine messages, called testimonies. For example, in 1899 or 1900 Mrs. White, disgruntled with Dr. Kellogg for not sending her sufficient money to support the work in Australia, wrote a testimony reproving him for squandering sanitarium funds on an elaborately furnished building in Chicago. In one of her special dreams she had seen "a large building in Chicago, which in its erection and equipment, cost a large sum of money." Kellogg protested his innocence, but to no avail. The prophetess insisted her information was correct and cited an article in the *New York Observer* as proof. Upon returning to America, she reportedly even asked to visit the Chicago building the Lord had shown her. Only when it could not be found did she concede that perhaps a slight mistake had been made. After learning from Judge Jesse Arthur, legal counsel for the sanitarium, that plans for the erection of a large building in Chicago had indeed been discussed (while Kellogg was away in Europe), she suggested that the real purpose of her vision had not been to condemn an accomplished fact, as she had previously thought, but to serve as "an object-lesson for our people, warning them not to invest largely of their means in property in Chicago, or any other city." But the damage had been done. A man had been falsely accused on the basis of a vision, and Stewart, for one, was not willing to blame God for the mistake.[31]

---

30. Charles E. Stewart to EGW, May 8, 1907, published as *A Response to an Urgent Testimony from Mrs. Ellen G. White* (Riverside, Calif.: E. S. Ballenger, n.d.); W. A. Sadler to EGW, April 26, 1906 (Kellogg Collection, MSU). Ellen White's letter "To Those Who Are Perplexed Regarding the Testimonies Relating to the Medical Missionary Work," March 30, 1906, appears in full in the Stewart letter. A third reply to Mrs. White's request is David Paulson to EGW, April 19, 1906 (Kellogg Collection, MSU).

31. Stewart to EGW, May 8, 1907; "Interview between Geo. W. Amadon, Eld. A. C. Bourdeau, and Dr. J. H. Kellogg, October 7, 1907," pp. 44-45; M. C. Kellogg, "Statement," [1908] (Kellogg Collection, MSU); EGW to Brother and Sister Haskell, March

Another point of contention related to the handling of testimonies regarding the building of the Battle Creek Sanitarium following the disastrous fire of February 18, 1902. After four new stories had gone up, a testimony appeared in 1905 publicly censuring Kellogg and his colleagues for going against "the expressed will of God" in rebuilding another large sanitarium instead of several smaller ones. At the same time Mrs. White released an earlier testimony, dated just two days after the fire, indicating divine opposition to raising another "mammoth institution." Kellogg was mystified. He knew he had received no such testimony; yet the impression was deliberately being given that he had. On being asked to explain what was going on, Mrs. White's secretary confirmed that the earlier testimony, though written in manuscript form on February 20, 1902, had never been sent to him and in fact had never left the office until December, 1905, when it had been taken to the printers. "It is difficult to comprehend," said Stewart in his letter to Mrs. White, "why such a vital message as this should have been withheld, and since it was withheld, it is still quite difficult to imagine what good purpose was served by publishing it three years later . . . especially when a false impression has been created by its appearance in this connection."[32]

In view of Ellen White's continuing insistence that "There is, throughout my printed works, a harmony with present teaching," it was practically inevitable that questions would also be asked about her inconsistency as a health reformer. Predictably, Dr. Stewart inquired not only about her apparently contradictory statements on the use of milk, butter, and eggs, but also about her personal eating habits. How, he asked, did she harmonize her own years of meat-eating with her assertion that "God gave the light on health reform

---

8, 1903 (H-135-1903, White Estate); "Dr. Kellogg's Work in Chicago," *New York Observer,* LXXIV (August 6, 1896), 212. W. C. White offered one explanation of the Chicago building testimony in a letter to Dr. Charles E. Stewart, April 10, 1906 (White Estate). The earliest extant testimony relating to the mysterious Chicago building is dated February 27, 1900, but Richard W. Schwarz has suggested that Mrs. White may have first written to Kellogg about this matter in 1899; Schwarz, "John Harvey Kellogg," p. 370.

32. Stewart to EGW, May 8, 1907; "Interview between Geo. W. Amadon, Eld. A. C. Bourdeau, and Dr. J. H. Kellogg, October 7, 1907," pp. 14-15. Mrs. White's testimonies are quoted in the Stewart letter.

and those who rejected it, rejected God"? Was he to conclude that testimonies written during "the period between 1868 and 1894 in which you ate meat and oysters and served meat on your table . . . contrary to the light God had given you" were not truly of the Lord?[33]

The Battle Creek dissidents were also perplexed by Mrs. White's practice of appropriating the writings of others and passing them off as her own. In one of her own books alone, *Sketches from the Life of Paul* (1883), Stewart had discovered "over two hundred places" that corresponded remarkably with passages from Conybeare and Howson's *Life and Epistles of the Apostle Paul* (3rd ed., 1855). Similar parallels existed between her volume on *The Great Controversy* and certain histories of the Protestant Reformation. He had even found a few sentences from testimonies on health reform that seemed to be lifted right out of L. B. Coles's *Philosophy of Health*. "Is that special light you claim to have from God revealed to you, at least to some extent through reading the various commentaries and other books treating of religious subjects?" he queried.[34]

The parallels between Mrs. White's writings and the works of others, so disturbing to Stewart, scarcely bothered most Adventists, including some of the doctor's colleagues at Battle Creek. When Dr. Daniel Kress stumbled onto a copy of Coles's *Philosophy of Health* in the 1890s, he readily explained the puzzling similarities to Ellen White's *How to Live* in terms of multiple inspiration. Isn't it wonderful, he remarked to Dr. Kellogg, "that the Lord should put this into two minds at different times." Kress's reaction is reminiscent of the response of Jemima Wilkinson's disciples to the discovery that she had copied one of her books almost word for word from a Quaker

---

33. EGW, "Journey to Southern California," *R&H,* LXXXIII (June 14, 1906), 8; Stewart to EGW, May 8, 1907.

34. Ibid. For contemporary reactions to Ellen's alleged plagiarizing, see F. E. Belden to E. S. Ballenger, January 28, 1938 (Ballenger-Mote Papers); and "Interview between Geo. W. Amadon, Eld. A. C. Bourdeau, and Dr. J. H. Kellogg, October 7, 1907," pp. 32-33. Adventists were outraged in 1864 when a Luthera B. Weaver "borrowed" a favorite hymn by Annie Smith; "Plagiarism," *R&H,* XXIV (September 6, 1864), 120. On the writing of *The Great Controversy,* see William S. Peterson, "A Textual and Historical Study of Ellen White's Account of the French Revolution," *Spectrum,* II (Autumn, 1970), 57-69; and Ronald Graybill, "How Did Ellen White Choose and Use Historical Sources?" ibid., IV (Summer, 1972), 49-53.

preacher named Isaac Penington. "Could not the Spirit dictate to her the Same Word as it did to Isaac?" asked one of her followers hopefully.[35]

According to one of Mrs. White's former literary assistants, Frances (Fanny) Bolton, many of her employer's publications were not only paraphrased from other sources but written in their final form by privately hired editors. The material coming from Ellen White's own hand she described as being "illogically written, full of illiteracies, awkward writing, and often wrong chronology."[36] Upon divulging these secrets, she promptly lost her job. As Dr. Merritt Kellogg, who was in Australia with Mrs. White at the time, described the incident, Fanny came to him one day and said:

> "Dr. Kellogg I am in great distress of mind. I come to you for advice for I do not know what to do. I have told Elder [George B.] Starr what I am going to tell you, but he gives me no satisfactory advice. You know," said Fanny, "that I am writing all the time for Sister White. Most of what I write is published in the *Review and Herald* as having come from the pen of Sister White, and is sent out as having been written by Sister White under inspiration of God. I want to tell you that I am greatly distressed over this matter for I feel that I am acting a deceptive part. The people are being deceived about the inspiration of what I write. I feel that it is a great wrong that anything which I write should go out as under Sister White's name, as an article specially inspired of God. What

---

35. "Interview between Geo. W. Amadon, Eld. A. C. Bourdeau, and Dr. J. H. Kellogg, October 7, 1907," p. 33; Herbert A. Wisbey, Jr., *Pioneer Prophetess: Jemima Wilkinson, the Publick Universal Friend* (Ithaca, N.Y.: Cornell University Press, 1964), pp. 32-33. Mrs. White's unacknowledged use of the works of others is indeed puzzling. Since she borrowed from sources familiar to many of her readers, conscious deception seems unlikely. Yet one psychiatrist has noted that "imposters" often fail to protect adequately against detection because of unconscious guilt and other psychological factors; Phyllis Greenacre, "The Impostor," *Psychoanalytic Quarterly*, XXVII (1958), 363-64. Fawn M. Brodie has used Dr. Greenacre's theory in explaining the behavior of Joseph Smith; see her *No Man Knows My History: The Life of Joseph Smith, the Mormon Prophet* (2nd ed.; New York: Alfred A. Knopf, 1971), pp. 418-19.

36. Frances E. Bolton to George Mattison, February 24, 1926 (Ballenger-Mote Papers).

I write should go out over my own signature, then credit would be given where credit belongs." I gave Miss Boulton [sic] the best advice I could, and then soon after asked Sister White to explain the situation to me. I told her just what Fanny had told me. Mrs. White asked me if Fanny told me what I had repeated to her, and my affirming that she did she said, "Elder Starr says she came to him with the same thing." Now said Sister White, with some warmth, "Fanny Boulton shall never write another line for me. She can hurt me as no other person can." A few days later Miss Boulton was sent back to America.[37]

In reply to such accusations, Mrs. White admitted that her husband had routinely edited her writings and that after his death "faithful helpers joined me, who labored untiringly in the work of copying the testimonies, and preparing articles for publication." But it was absolutely untrue, she insisted, "that any of my helpers are permitted to add matter or change the meaning of the messages I write out."[38]

For Dr. Sadler, the "most serious of all the difficulties" concerning the testimonies was Willie White's alleged influence over them. "I have been hearing it constantly," he wrote Mrs. White, "from leaders, ministers, from those sometimes high in Conference authority, that Willie influenced you in the production of your Testimonies." For a long time he had simply passed it off as loose gossip, but recently someone had shown him a letter written by Mrs. White herself telling of how Willie had talked her out of sending a particular message to Elder A. G. Daniells. His suspicions were aroused further by a conversation with Edson White in which "he spoke very positively against his brother Willie and his relation to you, and [told] how Willie was seeking to manage things in his way, and make them come his way, by his influence over you." Family relationships had deteriorated to such an extent that Willie was refusing to let his older brother even talk to his mother in private. If the Lord did not

---

37. M. B. Kellogg, "Statement," [1908]. Mrs. White's side of the Fanny Bolton story is given in W. C. White and D. E. Robinson, *The Work of Mrs. E. G. White's Editors* (St. Helena, Calif.: Elmshaven Office, 1933). Miss Bolton was a talented but troubled young woman, who later spent some time in a state mental hospital.

38. EGW, *The Writing and Sending Out of the Testimonies to the Church*, p. 4.

do something to prevent Willie and others from perverting his mother's gift, Edson told Dr. Sadler, he thought "it would be necessary for him to expose his brother, and others who were doing those things."[39]

Ellen White freely granted that someone had been manipulating her writings — but it was not Willie. "It is One who is mighty in counsel, One who presents before me the condition of things." Her position had not changed since 1867 when she had said: "I am as dependent upon the Spirit of the Lord in writing my views as I am in receiving them, yet the words I employ in describing what I have seen are my own, unless they be those spoken to me by an angel, which I always enclose in marks of quotation." For his part, Willie steadfastly denied ever trying to affect his mother's testimonies. If her views were similar to his, he explained, it was because he had been influenced by her. But in spite of these denials, some of the most respected Adventist brethren remained unconvinced. Dr. John Kellogg, a confessed manipulator himself, even saw a kind of poetic justice in now being the target of her testimonies: "I have doubtless been myself guilty with others in this matter, and it is right that I should be punished as I am being punished."[40]

The pointed criticisms of Stewart and Sadler were apparently more than Mrs. White had bargained for when she solicited them. Instead of answering their perplexities, as she had promised the

---

39. Sadler to EGW, April 26, 1906. Sadler, an embarrassed Edson told Willie, "very much misrepresents me and he has gone far beyond any thought I ever had in regard to this matter; but I desire to let this do also. I do not feel inclined to go into explanations which can only result in statements which will again be misconstrued, and will bring me into greater trial." J. E. White to W. C. White, May 21, 1906 (White Estate).

40. EGW, Letter 52, 1906, quoted in White, *Ellen G. White*, p. 17; EGW, "Questions and Answers," *R&H*, XXX (October 8, 1867), 260; W. C. White in a note appended to *The Writing and Sending Out of the Testimonies to the Church*, pp. 29-30; J. H. Kellogg to G. I. Butler, April 1, 1906 (Kellogg Collection, MSU). See also R. S. Owen to J. H. Kellogg, June 16, 1907, and June 21, 1907 (Kellogg Collection, MSU); G. I. Butler to J. H. Kellogg, June 11, 1905 (Kellogg Collection, MSU); James White to D. M. Canright, May 24, 1881 (Ballenger-Mote Papers); Uriah Smith to D. M. Canright, April 6, 1883, July 31, 1883, and August 7, 1883 (Ballenger-Mote Papers); A. T. Jones, *The Final Word and a Confession* (n.p., n.d.), p. 27.

Lord would help her to do, she remained silent, saying only that "a messenger from heaven" had directed her "not to take the burden of picking up and answering all the sayings and doubts that are being put into many minds."[41]

The very frankness of the Battle Creek letters played directly into the hands of Kellogg's enemies. Willie White saw to it that a copy of Stewart's confidential communication reached his friend A. G. Daniells, who in turn used it to incite the church against the so-called apostates in Battle Creek. When the contents of his letter began leaking out and he had still received no reply, Stewart arranged for its anonymous publication. This called for a strategy session among Mrs. White's associates, who judiciously decided not to issue a formal reply. However, in regard to the specific charge of plagiarism, it was agreed "that W. C. White shall prepare quite a full and frank statement of the plans followed in preparing manuscripts for publication in book form, including (if Sister White gives her consent) a statement of the instruction which Sister White received in early days as to her use of the productions of other writers." Unfortunately, the precise nature of Ellen White's divine literary license was never revealed.[42]

The Battle Creek schism profoundly altered the Seventh-day Adventist church, doctrinally as well as institutionally. As a result of the clash between the forces of Daniells and Kellogg, acceptance of Mrs. White's testimonies for the first time became an accepted "test of fellowship," a development unthinkable in the early days of the church. But this innovation had its price. Besides creating widespread internal dissension, the new test directly or indirectly resulted in the loss of the Battle Creek Sanitarium, the American Medical Missionary College, and a number of leading ministers and

---

41. A. T. Jones to EGW, n.d., published in pamphlet form by The Gathering Call, Riverside, California (Ballenger-Mote Papers).

42. Ibid.; Preface to Stewart, *A Response to an Urgent Testimony from Mrs. White;* "Memorandum of Plans Agreed upon in Dealing with 'The Blue Book'" (DF 213, White Estate). Willie White once asked J. H. Kellogg: "Don't you think that when Mother sees things, runs across things that agree with what she has seen in vision, that it is all right for her to adopt it?" "Interview between Geo. W. Amadon, Eld. A. C. Bourdeau, and Dr. J. H. Kellogg, October 7, 1907," p. 32. For A. G. Daniells's reaction to Stewart's charges, see Daniells to W. C. White, June 24, 1907 (White Estate).

physicians, including Drs. Stewart, Sadler, and Kellogg, the most prominent Seventh-day Adventist in the world.[43]

Kellogg's fall from grace was not, however, without its humor. During the heat of the controversy Merritt Kellogg learned that Mrs. White had predicted that his brother, "like Nebuchadnezzar . . . would be humbled, and driven out to eat grass like an ox." "I think it is a good thing for you that you have been a vegetarian so many years," Merritt told John. "You will not miss the savory roasts and juicy joints at that time, as will many of the S.D.A. preachers when they have to eat grass like an ox, as many of them will, or starve, when the fallacies of their teaching is revealed, as it will be in God's own good time."[44]

Without the Battle Creek Sanitarium and the American Medical Missionary College, "orthodox" Adventists had no place to send their young people who aspired to medical careers. Thus Mrs. White determined in 1906 to turn the Loma Linda Sanitarium into an educational center, beginning with a College of Evangelists to train "gospel medical missionaries." At first there was no course for physicians because she felt it was folly "to spend years in preparation" when time on this earth was so short. But the need for a continuing supply of doctors became so acute that she finally decided it would be wiser to set up an Adventist medical school than to send students to some worldly institution or, God forbid, to the American Medical Missionary College. On September 29, 1910, the College of Medical

---

43. Ibid., p. 69; F. E. Belden to W. A. Colcord, October 17, 1929 (Ballenger-Mote Papers). In 1883 the influential Uriah Smith wrote: "I still hold that Sr. W. has been shown things in vision, and that this is a manifestation of Spiritual gifts; but they do not stand on a level with the Scriptures, and should not be made a test of fellowship"; Smith to D. M. Canright, August 7, 1883 (Ballenger-Mote Papers). James White, though always reluctant to make his wife's visions a test, did concede that under certain circumstances rejection of her gift was grounds for separation. Seventh-day Adventists do not, he wrote, "make a belief in this work a test of Christian fellowship. But, after men and women have had evidence that the work is of God, and then join hands with those who fight against it, our people claim the right to separate from such, that they may enjoy their sentiments in peace and quiet." [James White], "Western Tour," *R&H,* XXXVII (June 13, 1871), 205.

44. M. C. Kellogg to J. H. Kellogg, May 3, 1906 (Kellogg Collection, MSU). Daniells's alleged meat-eating was a source of great irritation to John Kellogg; see Schwarz, "The Kellogg Schism," p. 30.

Evangelists, as the Loma Linda school was now called, opened its classrooms to a student body of ninety-two: ten second-year medical, twenty-four first-year medical, six cooks and bakers, and fifty-two nurses. The American Medical Association deemed it worthy of only a "C" rating, but at least it was legally chartered and doctrinally orthodox. Under the guidance of Dean (later President) Percy Magan it evolved into a respectable and thoroughly regular institution, which today, as part of Loma Linda University, has the distinction of being the only medical school in America to have come out of the hydropathic tradition.[45]

During the last few years of her life Ellen White labored incessantly to ensure that the College of Medical Evangelists fulfilled its divinely appointed mission. Repeatedly she urged its graduates to pattern themselves after Christ, the Great Physician, and to stick by three of the reforms Adventist medicine had come to represent. First, it meant "treating the sick without the use of poisonous drugs." Since her vision of June, 1863, she had discovered no better remedies than those freely provided by nature: pure air, sunlight, rest, exercise, proper diet, water, and perhaps some "simple herbs and roots." Second and "just as important as the discarding of drugs," it meant that Adventist doctors were not to "follow the world's methods of medical practice, exacting large fees that worldly physicians demand for their services." The Christian physician, she wrote, "has no more right to minister to others requir-

---

45. EGW, "A Plea for Medical Missionary Evangelists," *Testimonies,* IX, 172; EGW, "The Loma Linda College of Evangelists," ibid., IX, 173; EGW and Others, "The Relation of Loma Linda to Medical Institutions," September 20, 1909 (C. Burton Clark Collection); "A Medical School at Loma Linda," *R&H,* LXXXVII (May 19, 1910), 17-18; S. P. S. Edwards, "College of Medical Evangelists," ibid., LXXXVII (October 27, 1910), 17-18; Merlin L. Neff, *For God and C.M.E.: A Biography of Percy Tilson Magan* (Mountain View, Calif.: Pacific Press, 1964), pp. 158-70. Although CME's first curricula included the traditional medical school subjects, hydrotherapy was "the center of the vast system of physiologic therapeutics" taught in the school; *Second Annual Announcement of the College of Medical Evangelists, Loma Linda, California, 1910-1911,* p. 19. Early graduates often struggled to overcome the school's sectarian image, and twelve students in the class of '17 finally petitioned that their diplomas specifically identify them as "Regular Physicians and Surgeons"; Petition to the Faculty of the College of Medical Evangelists, April 22, 1917 (Loma Linda University Archives).

ing a large remuneration than has the minister of the gospel a right to set his labors at a high money value." Third, it meant following "the Lord's plan" of having men treat men and women treat women. The custom of ignoring sexual distinctions in the practice of medicine was the source of "much evil" and an offense to God. Times were rapidly changing, however, and it was not long before scarcely a trace of these three reforms could be found among Seventh-day Adventist physicians, many of whom continued to revere the prophetess.[46]

On July 16, 1915, five months after a broken thigh bone confined her to a wheelchair, Ellen White, age 87, passed away. After a lifetime of illness and frequent brushes with death she finally succumbed to chronic myocarditis, complicated by arteriosclerosis and asthenia resulting from her hip injury. In a fundamental way her life had been a paradox. Although consumed with making preparations for the next world, she nevertheless devoted much of her energy toward improving life and health in this one. Despite the Battle Creek tragedy, she left behind at the time of her death thirty-three sanitariums and countless treatment rooms on six continents. Over 136,000 devoted followers mourned her passing. In a fitting tribute to the fallen health reformer, the women of the Seventh-day Adventist church pledged themselves in 1915 to raise funds for an Ellen G. White Memorial Hospital in Los Angeles, which served for years as the principal clinical facility of the College of Medical Evangelists.[47]

At the time of Ellen White's death only one other woman — Mary Baker Eddy — had contributed more to the religious life of

---

46. EGW, "The Loma Linda College of Evangelists," pp. 175-76; EGW, *The Ministry of Healing* (Mountain View, Calif.: Pacific Press, 1942), pp. 126-27; EGW to Edgar Caro, October 2, 1893 (C-17a-1893, White Estate); EGW, "Two Important Interviews Regarding Physicians' Wages," December 4, 1913 (C. Burton Clark Collection); EGW to J. H. Kellogg, December 24, 1890 (C. Burton Clark Collection); EGW, *Medical Practice and the Educational Program at Loma Linda*, p. 52-e; EGW to J. A. Burden, June 7, 1911 (C. Burton Clark Collection); EGW to J. A. Burden and Others, March 24, 1908 (B-90-1908, White Estate).

47. Death certificate of Ellen G. White, July 16, 1915 (Office of the County Recorder, Napa County, California); H. E. Rogers (ed.), *1915 Year Book of the Seventh-day Adventist Church* (Washington: Review and Herald Publishing Assn., 1915), pp. 202-11; McCumber, *Advent Message in the Golden West*, pp. 176-82.

America. Yet the Adventist leader died relatively unknown outside her church, having never sought or received the worldly recognition accorded Mrs. Eddy. Although she never thought highly of the founder of Christian Science, whom she regarded as little better than a spiritualist, she had much in common with her. Both women were born in New England in the 1820s. As children they both experienced debilitating illnesses, which curtailed their formal schooling; and as young women they suffered from uncontrollable spells that left them unconscious for frighteningly long periods of time. They both sought cures in Grahamism and hydropathy. Early in 1863 Mrs. White found hers through Dr. Jackson's essay on diphtheria, but just six months earlier Mrs. Eddy had left a New Hampshire water cure in disappointment. Abandoning hydropathy for the mind cure of Phineas P. Quimby, she did for Quimbyism what Ellen White did for health reform: she made a religion out of it. Both she and Mrs. White claimed divine inspiration, and both succeeded in establishing distinctive churches. But despite their many similarities, the two women had basically different goals: Ellen White longed for a mansion in heaven, Mary Baker Eddy wanted hers here on earth. Thus while Mrs. Eddy died one of the richest and most powerful women in America, Mrs. White lived her last days in comfortable, but unpretentious surroundings, still waiting for the Lord to come.[48]

Today the memory of Ellen White lives on in the lives of nearly two and one-half million Seventh-day Adventists, many of whom continue to believe "that she wrote under the inspiration of the Holy Spirit, that her pen was literally guided by God." In the years since her death sales of her two most popular health books, *The Ministry of Healing* and *Counsels on Diet and Foods,* have topped a quarter-million. Most of her disciples abstain entirely from alcohol and tobacco, and many will not touch meat, tea, or coffee; and, if we are to

---

48. Robert Peel, *Mary Baker Eddy: The Years of Discovery* (New York: Holt, Rinehart, and Winston, 1966), pp. 13, 44-46, 172; Edwin Franden Dakin, *Mrs. Eddy: The Biography of a Virginal Mind* (New York: Charles Schribner's Sons, 1929), pp. 51-52, 337; EGW, *The Story of Prophets and Kings* (Mountain View, Calif.: Pacific Press, 1917), p. 210. On the creative function of illness in the life of Mary Baker Eddy, see George Pickering, *Creative Malady* (New York: Oxford University Press, 1974), pp. 183-205.

believe recent scientific reports, they enjoy better health for it. As of 1970, Seventh-day Adventists were operating a worldwide chain of 329 medical institutions stretching from Kingston to Karachi, from Bangkok to Belém — each a memorial to the life and work of Ellen G. White, prophetess of health.[49]

---

49. Jerome L. Clark, *1844* (Nashville: Southern Publishing Assn., 1968), II, 255; Hugh J. Forquer to R.L.N., January 16, 1973; M. E. Maud Seeley to R.L.N., February 20, 1973; *Seventh-day Adventist Health Care Facilities around the World* (Washington: Department of Health, General Conference of Seventh-day Adventists, 1972). On the health of Seventh-day Adventists, see, for example, R. T. Walden and Others, "Effect of Environment on the Serum Cholesterol-Triglyceride Distribution among Seventh-day Adventists," *American Journal of Medicine,* XXXVI (February, 1964), 269-76; E. L. Wynder and F. R. Lemon, "Cancer, Coronary Artery Disease, and Smoking," *California Medicine,* LXXXIX (October, 1958), 267-72; F. R. Lemon and Others, "Cancer of the Lung and Mouth in Seventh-day Adventists," *Cancer,* XVII (April, 1964), 486-97; F. R. Lemon and R. T. Walden, "Death from Respiratory System Disease among Seventh-day Adventist Men," *Journal of the American Medical Association,* CXCVIII (October, 1966), 137-46.

AFTERWORD

Ellen White on the Mind and the Mind of Ellen White

RONALD L. NUMBERS AND JANET S. NUMBERS

When Ellen Harmon was about fourteen years old, she suffered an excruciating bout of depression, brought on by anxiety about the fate of her soul. "Almost total darkness settled upon me, and there seemed no way out of the shadows," she later recalled. "My sufferings of mind were intense." At times she feared she was losing her mind. Eventually she survived the ordeal with her sanity intact, but as an adult she came to suspect that "many inmates of insane asylums were brought there by experiences similar to my own."[1] This adolescent episode and her interpretation of it poignantly illustrate the two

---

1. EGW, *Life Sketches of Ellen G. White* (Mountain View, Calif.: Pacific Press, 1915), pp. 29-31; EGW, "Biographical Sketch," *Testimonies,* I, 25.

Earlier versions of this paper were presented in 1982 at a conference on Adventist psychiatry organized by Ronald Geraty and held in conjunction with the annual meeting of the American Psychiatric Association in Toronto; in 1985 at an education meeting of the Adult Outpatient Department, The Menninger Foundation, Topeka, Kansas, and at a meeting of the Mid-America Psychosocial Study Group hosted by The Menninger Foundation; and in 1987 at a psychiatry and religion seminar sponsored by the Department of Psychiatry, Medical College of Georgia. On each occasion we benefited immensely from the criticisms and suggestions offered. The late Paul W. Pruyser, of The Menninger Foundation, was particularly helpful. In addition, a number of friends — historians, psychologists, and psychiatrists — kindly critiqued our manuscript: Barbara J. Brigham, Jonathan M. Butler, Peter J. Clagnaz, Lawrence J. Friedman, Catherine A. Mayer, Mary Jo Peebles, Richard J. Roberts, Rennie B. Schoepflin, and Samuel B. Thielman. We thank them for their advice and absolve them of any blame for our remaining mistakes.

AFTERWORD

interrelated themes of this afterword: Ellen White's views of human psychology and her own sometimes precarious mental health.

The original edition of this book said virtually nothing about either topic, but subsequent publications have focused considerable attention on both. A year after *Prophetess of Health* appeared, the Ellen G. White Estate issued a two-volume compilation of her writings on mental health, not to memorialize her Victorian views but to serve as a practical guide for the late twentieth century. The compilers, believing that "Ellen G. White wrote under the influence of the Spirit of God," expressed confidence that "as research in psychology and mental health progresses, her reputation for setting forth sound psychological principles will be still more firmly established." They made virtually no effort to place White's statements in their historical context. In contrast, in exploring in the first part of this essay what she thought and taught about the causes and cures of mental illness, we emphasize the ways in which the Bible, contemporary medical ideas, and her own experiences may have influenced her opinions.[2]

In the second part we examine perhaps the most sensitive issue of all in Ellen G. White scholarship: her own mental health. During the first half of the 1980s two Adventist physicians, Delbert Hodder, a pediatrician with subspecialty interest in neurology, and Molleurus Couperus, a dermatologist, scandalized Seventh-day Adventists by suggesting that Ellen White suffered from complex partial seizures, formerly known as temporal-lobe or psychomotor epilepsy. They argued that this condition, a result of her childhood head injury, explained not only her visions but a host of other abnormalities. The Ellen G. White Estate immediately rushed to her defense, convening a committee of Adventist mental-health experts to rebut these charges. After reviewing the available evidence, the doctors gave White a clean bill of health, concluding "that (1) there is no convincing evidence that Ellen G. White suffered from any type of epilepsy, and (2) there is no possibility that complex partial seizures could account for Mrs. White's visions or for her role in the develop-

---

2. Unpaginated Foreword to EGW, *Mind, Character, and Personality: Guidelines to Mental and Spiritual Health*, 2 vols. (Nashville, Tenn.: Southern Publishing Association, 1977). The discussion in the first section closely follows our article on "The Psychological World of Ellen White," *Spectrum*, XIV (August, 1983), 21-31.

ment of the Seventh-day Adventist Church."³ We tend to agree with this verdict — but not because Ellen White enjoyed optimal mental health. We believe that the extant evidence, including her own voluminous testimony (presented in Appendix 1), indicates that from youth onward she suffered from recurrent episodes of depression and anxiety to which she responded with somatizing defenses and a histrionic personality style. These allowed her to transform debilitating and destructive forces into creative and productive ones.

Ellen White on the Mind

In harmony with the prevailing psychiatric opinion of her time Ellen White generally regarded mental illness as a somatic condition: a diseased brain. According to her understanding of human physiology, two channels connected the brain with the rest of the body. The nervous system, like a telegraph network, transmitted "vital force" or "electrical energy" from the brain to other organs, while the vascular system carried blood to the brain. A healthy brain needed a constant supply of pure blood. "If by correct habits of eating and drinking the blood is kept pure," she wrote, "the brain will be properly nourished." A "mysterious and wonderful relation" thus united mind and body, with the vast majority of diseases originating in the brain, the "seat" of all mental activity.[4]

---

3. Delbert H. Hodder, "Visions or Partial-Complex Seizures?" *Evangelica* (November, 1981), 30-37; Molleurus Couperus, "The Significance of Ellen White's Head Injury," *Adventist Currents*, I (June, 1985), 17-23; "Ellen G. White and Epilepsy," *Ministry*, LVII (August, 1984), 24-25. See also Donald I. Peterson, *Visions or Seizures: Was Ellen White the Victim of Epilepsy?* (Boise, Idaho: Pacific Press, 1988). Bernadine L. Irwin, who served on the White Estate committee, has written "A Psychohistory of the Young Ellen White: A Founder of the Seventh-day Adventist Church" (Ph.D. diss., United States International University, 1984), a quasi-apologetical Eriksonian analysis that sheds no new light on White's psycho-logical development. The phrases complex partial seizures and partial complex seizures are sometimes used interchangeably.

4. EGW, "Responsibilities of the Physician," *Testimonies*, V, 444; "Power of Appetite," ibid., III, 485. On the relationship between mind and brain, see EGW, "Experience Not Reliable," ibid., III, 69; and Anita Clair Fellman and Michael Fellman, *Making Sense of Self: Medical Advice Literature in Late Nineteenth-Century America* (Philadelphia: University of Pennsylvania Press, 1981), pp. 57-71.

Afterword

By the early nineteenth century the notion that demonic possession caused insanity had largely disappeared from both medical and theological literature. Although some religious writers continued to invoke the power of Satan, more commonly, orthodox ministers admitted "the theoretical possibility of demonological possession but denied its actual presence in the mentally ill." According to the historian Norman Dain, "This position enabled clergymen to accept the concept of somatic pathology and to sanction medical treatment of insanity."[5] White assumed a similar stance. She knew from the Bible that demonic possession could cause insanity; but whenever she discussed mental illness in her own time, she tended to invoke natural rather than supernatural causes. Even in relating the story of how Jesus cured the "maniac of Capernaum" by rebuking the "demon" that possessed him, she suggested that the maniac had lost his mind because of intemperance and frivolity.[6]

Most mid-century American physicians who cared for the mentally ill separated the causes of insanity into two categories: predisposing and exciting. Predisposing causes included such factors as inherited tendencies and neglect of personal health, which, though not directly the cause of insanity, could make a person vulnerable to the disease. Exciting causes allegedly precipitated abnormal behavior. In their annual reports asylum superintendents listed among exciting causes everything from excessive study, disappointed ambition, and physical abuse to Mormonism, Millerism, mesmerism, and spiritualism. Some physicians distinguished between "physical" and "moral" causes of insanity, but it was never clear which label to apply to such conditions as masturbation. In determining etiology, admitting physicians customarily relied on accounts of relatives and friends, but they remained well aware of the hazards of such an approach, including the possibility that they might be confusing cause with effect.[7]

---

5. Norman Dain, *Concepts of Insanity in the United States, 1789-1865* (New Brunswick, N.J.: Rutgers University Press, 1964), p. 187.

6. EGW, *The Desire of Ages: The Conflict of the Ages Illustrated in the Life of Christ* (new ed.; Mountain View, Calif.: Pacific Press, 1940), pp. 255-56.

7. See, e.g., Amariah Brigham, *First Annual Report of the Superintendent of the New York State Lunatic Asylum at Utica* (1843), pp. 20-22. A common system of classification divided insanity into mania, melancholia, dementia, and idiocy; but, as Brigham noted (ibid., p. 25), no system of classification seemed to be "of much prac-

Ellen White on the Mind and the Mind of Ellen White

Ellen White never systematically discussed the etiology of mental illness, but her scattered comments on the subject eclectically reflected the prevailing opinions of her time. Like many physicians, especially those writing after the Civil War, she suspected that a large percentage of mental illness was attributable to inheritance. Typical of her many statements was one written shortly after her major health-reform vision in 1863. "As the result of wrong habits in parents," she asserted, "disease and imbecility have been transmitted to their offspring." In her opinion, no habits were more insidious than those that violated the laws of health:

> Our ancestors have bequeathed to us customs and appetites which are filling the world with disease. The sins of the parents, through perverted appetite, are with fearful power visited upon the children to the third and fourth generations. The bad eating of many generations, the gluttonous and self-indulgent habits of the people, are filling our poorhouses, our prisons, and our insane asylums. Intemperance, in drinking tea and coffee, wine, beer, rum, and brandy, and the use of tobacco, opium, and other narcotics, has resulted in great mental and physical degeneracy, and this degeneracy is constantly increasing.

Fortunately for the great majority of humans — and the doctrine of free will — right living could overcome a predisposition to insanity inherited from one's parents. Thus, as the mental hygienists of the late nineteenth century insisted, insanity was a preventable disease. But persons predisposed to mental illness by their inheritance had a "duty to ascertain wherein their parents violated the laws of their being" and to make sure that they did not continue in the same course.[8]

One's own intemperance could also induce madness. In fact,

---

tical utility." On the allegedly debilitating effects of excessive study on women, see Edward H. Clarke, *Sex in Education; or, A Fair Chance for Girls* (Boston: Houghton, Mifflin and Co., 1873), and the response by Julia Ward Howe, ed., *Sex and Education: A Reply to Dr. E. H. Clarke's "Sex in Education"* (Boston: Roberts Brothers, 1874).

8. EGW, *Selected Messages* (Washington: Review and Herald Publishing Assn., 1958), I, 465; EGW, *Mind, Character, and Personality,* I, 144; EGW, "Duty to Know Ourselves," *HR,* I (August, 1866), 2. On the prevention of insanity, see Barbara Sicherman, *The Quest for Mental Health in America, 1880-1917* (New York: Arno Press, 1980), pp. 79-152. See also Dain, *Concepts of Insanity,* p. 109.

AFTERWORD

White assigned the "main cause" of insanity to "improper diet, irregular meals, a lack of physical exercise, and careless inattention in other respects to the laws of health." Her enthusiasm for health reform following her 1863 vision no doubt encouraged her in this belief, but her own experience confirmed it. "When my brain is confused," she wrote in 1900, "I know that I have been making some mistake in my diet." As shown in Chapter 6, White especially stressed the link between masturbation and insanity. In *An Appeal to Mothers* she gruesomely described the physical effects of self-abuse on the brains of girls: "the head often decays inwardly. Cancerous humor, which would lay dormant in the system their life-time, is inflamed, and commences its eating, destructive work. The mind is often utterly ruined, and insanity takes place."[9]

In addition to the various physical causes of insanity, White at one time or another identified a host of "moral" causes: frustrated ambition, excessive grief, guilt, gossip, and novel reading, the excitement of which weakened the "delicate machinery of the brain." "Thousands are today in the insane asylum," she observed, "whose minds became unbalanced by novel reading." White was not alone in seeing this activity as a threat to the nation's mental health. The superintendent of the Mount Hope Institution in Baltimore warned parents in his annual report for 1846 to "guard their young daughters" against the pernicious practice of reading works of fiction. "We have had several cases of moral insanity, for which no other cause could be assigned than excessive novel reading."[10]

During times of religious enthusiasm and revivalism, asylum physicians often listed religious anxiety and excitement among the leading causes of insanity. Shortly after the Millerite disappoint-

---

9. EGW, *Mind, Character, and Personality*, II, 382; *Guidelines to Mental Health: Materials Assembled from the Writings of Ellen G. White* (Washington: Ellen G. White Estate, 1966), p. 217; EGW, *An Appeal to Mothers* (Battle Creek: SDA Publishing Assn., 1864), pp. 17, 27. According to White, even the wearing of wigs could cause insanity; see p. 205 of this book.

10. EGW, *Mind, Character, and Personality*, II, 399, 674; *Guidelines to Mental Health*, pp. 72, 159; EGW, *Selected Messages*, II, 64; EGW, "Responsibilities of the Physician," *Testimonies*, V, 444; EGW, *The Ministry of Healing* (Washington: Review and Herald Publishing Assn., 1905), p. 446; William H. Stokes, *Fourth Annual Report of the Mount Hope Institution for the Year 1846*, p. 34.

ment in 1844, for example, Amariah Brigham, superintendent of the New York State Lunatic Asylum in Utica, noted that thirty-two Millerites had been committed during the past year alone. "The nervous system of many of those who have been kept in a state of excitement and alarm for months," he explained, "has received a shock that will predispose them to all the various and distressing forms of nervous disease and to insanity, and will also render their offspring born hereafter, liable to the same."[11]

The nature of the relationship between religion and insanity generated considerable debate in the nineteenth century, and Ellen White resented the "infidels" who attributed insanity to religion. "The religion of Christ," she argued, "so far from being the cause of insanity, is one of its most effectual remedies; for it is a potent soother of the nerves." Nevertheless, she conceded that under certain conditions remorse for sin could unbalance the mind and that "erroneous doctrines," such as "an eternally burning hell," could have the same effect. Her own experiences in the 1840s made these connections seem plausible and later caused her to suspect, as we noted in the introduction to this essay, that "many inmates of insane asylums were brought there by experiences similar to my own."[12]

White claimed to possess first-hand knowledge of Millerites who had lost their minds during the turmoil following the Great Disappointment:

> ... after the passing of the time in 1844, fanaticism in various forms arose.... I went into their meetings. There was much excitement, with noise and confusion.... Some appeared to be in vision, and fell to the floor.... As the result of fanatical movements such as I have described, persons in no way responsible for them

---

11. [Amariah Brigham], "Millerism," *American Journal of Insanity*, I (1845), 250. See also Ronald L. Numbers and Janet S. Numbers, "Millerism and Madness: A Study of 'Religious Insanity' in Nineteenth-Century America," in *The Disappointed: Millerism and Millenarianism in the Nineteenth Century*, ed. Ronald L. Numbers and Jonathan M. Butler (Bloomington: Indiana University Press, 1987), pp. 92-117.

12. EGW, "Responsibilities of the Physician," *Testimonies*, V, 444; EGW, "Biographical Sketch," ibid., I, 25-26. Elizabeth Cady Stanton tells a similar story about the effects of Charles G. Finney's sermons on her physical and mental health in *Eighty Years and More: Reminiscences, 1815-1897* (reprinted ed.; New York: Schocken Books, 1971).

have in some cases lost their reason. They could not harmonize the scenes of excitement and tumult with their own past precious experience; they were pressed beyond measure to receive the message of error; it was represented to them that unless they did this they would be lost; and as the result their mind was unbalanced, and some became insane.

Exactly how much of this account paralleled her own experience we cannot determine. We do know, however, that during this same time *she* experienced visions and fell to the floor and became so mentally distraught that "for two weeks my mind wandered," an episode she later referred to as her "extreme sickness." We also know, from recently discovered trial records involving a Millerite charged with disturbing the peace, that in the months following the Disappointment she joined in some of the same "fanatical" activities she soon afterwards vociferously condemned in others.[13]

During White's formative years, American physicians who cared for the mentally ill expressed great optimism about curing insanity with what they called "moral therapy." This form of treatment involved removing patients from the environments that had caused their illnesses and placing them in an asylum, where their lives could be restructured. Asylum superintendents reported remarkable — and undoubtedly inflated — cure rates, ranging as high as 90 percent. In the latter decades of the century, as mental institutions filled up with chronically ill patients and increasingly assumed a custodial function, optimism gave way to realism. Although White took no note of these trends, she did express herself from time to time on the best — and worst — means of treating mental illness. Unlike her writings on etiology, which rarely went beyond natural causes, her discussions of therapy often referred to the supernatural. The physician who treats mental problems, she said in a representative statement, can be efficacious only if he is aware of "the power of divine grace. . . . [I]f he has a firm hold upon God, he will be

---

13. EGW, *Selected Messages*, II, 34-35; EGW, *Spiritual Gifts: My Christian Experience, Views and Labors in Connection with the Rise and Progress of the Third Angel's Message* (Battle Creek: James White, 1860), pp. 51, 69; Frederick Hoyt, ed., "Trial of Elder I. Dammon Reported for the *Piscataquis Farmer*," *Spectrum*, XVII (August, 1987), 29-36. See Appendix 3 of this book.

able to help the diseased, distracted mind." Early in her ministry White occasionally relied on prayer alone to cure mental illness. For example, upon encountering one Adventist sister suffering from "fit," she called upon "the name and strength of Jesus . . . put my arms around her, and lifted her up from the bed, and rebuked the power of Satan, and bid her, 'Go free.' She was instantly brought out of the fit, and praised the Lord with us." In her later years, however, White recommended that religious healing should supplement medical therapy, not supplant it.[14]

More for theological than therapeutic reasons White roundly condemned using the so-called mind cure — "the most awful science which has ever been advocated" — to treat physical or mental problems. The intensity of her feeling stemmed from her association of mind cures with the much-feared activities of spiritualists and mesmerists (mentioned in Chapter 1). "At the beginning of my work," she wrote in 1901,

> I had the mind-cure science to contend with. I was sent from place to place to declare the falseness of this science, into which many were entering. The mind cure was entered upon very innocently — to relieve the tension upon the minds of nervous invalids. But, oh, how sad were the results! God sent me from place to place to rebuke everything pertaining to this science.

She did not indicate whether the dire consequences of using the mind cure were physical or spiritual, but it seems likely that she cared less about the efficacy of the treatment than about the propriety of exposing oneself to Satan's "electric currents."[15]

Both to prevent and to cure mental disorders, especially depression, White prescribed physical and mental exercise. Like many Victorian mental-health writers who wished to avoid the pitfalls of physiological determinism, she stressed the importance of exercis-

---

14. Dain, *Concepts of Insanity*, p. 113; *Guidelines to Mental Health*, p. 485; EGW, *Spiritual Gifts* (1860), pp. 71-72. See also Gerald N. Grob, *Mental Institutions in America: Social Policy to 1875* (New York: Free Press, 1973).

15. EGW, *Medical Ministry: A Treatise on Medical Missionary Work in the Gospel* (Mountain View, Calif.: Pacific Press, 1932), pp. 113, 116; EGW, "Spiritualist Physicians," *Testimonies*, V, 193-98.

ing the will, the mental faculty that most markedly set humans apart from animals. "The power of the will is not valued as it should be," she wrote in one of her testimonies. "Exercised in the right direction, it would control the imagination and be a potent means of resisting and overcoming diseases of both mind and body." She did not elaborate on the physiological processes involved, but she once asserted that exercising the will would give "tone and strength" to the mind and nerves. Her apparently successful application of the exercise cure during her husband's mental breakdown in the mid-1860s (see Chapter 4) convinced her that she had indeed found the best method for treating the mentally disturbed, and she urged the physicians at the Western Health Reform Institute to follow her example. "Lead the patients along step by step, step by step," she counseled, "keeping their minds so busily occupied that they have no time to brood over their own condition."[16]

The Mind of Ellen White

In her correspondence and autobiographical writings Ellen White reported a dazzling array of physical and psychological problems (see Appendix 1); yet despite even repeated expectations of imminent death, she lived to the ripe age of eighty-seven. A self-described "great sufferer from disease" and "lifelong invalid," she from time to time complained of weakness and fainting, episodes of unconsciousness, breathing difficulties, "heart disease," pain in her lungs, "pressure of blood on the brain," intense headaches and "inflammation on the brain," dropsy, weak back, lameness, "tenderness of the stomach," nosebleeds, pleurisy, and rheumatism. On occasion she experienced dimmed eyesight, paralysis, lack of sensation, and muteness — to say nothing of repeated visions and hallucinations. She frequently suffered from depression and despondency.[17]

For understandable reasons, Ellen White attributed all of her vi-

---

16. EGW, *Ministry of Healing* (Washington: Review and Herald Publishing Assn., 1905), p. 246; EGW, "Parents and Children," *Testimonies*, I, 387; EGW, *Selected Messages*, II, 306-8. On nineteenth-century views of the will, see Fellman and Fellman, *Making Sense of Self*, pp. 115-33.

17. See Appendix 1 of this book.

sions and many of her ailments to supernatural causes, thus deviating from her customary reliance on etiological naturalism. But what should we make of them? If she were to seek medical assistance today, how would she be diagnosed and treated? What explanations would be offered? The diagnosis of mental problems can be difficult under the best of circumstances and becomes increasingly problematic with the passage of time. Nosologies have changed over the years in response to both scientific and social developments. For example, neurasthenia, "the national disease" of Victorian America, disappeared as a diagnosis when physicians, aided by new medical techniques, began interpreting exhaustion as a mere symptom of other diseases; and in 1973 the American Psychiatric Association, responding to social and political concerns, defined homosexuality out of existence as a mental illness.[18] But despite changing nomenclatures, many psychological disorders, such as depression and anxiety, seem to be relatively constant across time and space.

For the historian, retrospective diagnosis also raises the specter of imposing present-day categories on past behavior. And psychiatric labels are particularly subject to abuse. In a recent essay on "Psychohistory As History" Thomas A. Kohut censures those who write what he calls "pathographies," descriptive psychiatric histories of notable persons that often degenerate into character assassination by diagnosis. He offers the useful criterion that "information about the personal life of a historical figure should only be presented if that information either directly or indirectly has relevance for the understanding of his historical significance."[19] We agree. And precisely because so much of Ellen White's self-identity and ministry revolved around visions and ill health, we feel that we cannot adequately understand her without exploring the underlying causes. We have no desire to reduce her experience to a mere diagnostic label; in fact, we readily grant that cultural and religious explanations account for much of her behavior. Nevertheless, we hope to enhance our comprehension of a complex life by delineating per-

18. Judith Walzer Leavitt and Ronald L. Numbers, eds., *Sickness and Health in America: Readings in the History of Medicine and Public Health* (2nd ed.; Madison: University of Wisconsin Press, 1985), p. 11.

19. Thomas A. Kohut, "Psychohistory As History," *American Historical Review*, XCI (1986), 341.

sonality patterns that gave meaning to her experience, colored her thinking, informed her emotional responses, and guided her behavior. Ultimately, the better we get to know White and to comprehend the ways in which she coped with her cornucopia of mental and physical afflictions, the more empathic we become and the more we admire what she accomplished.

As mentioned above, two physicians have speculated recently that Ellen White suffered from complex partial seizures, the result of the childhood injury she received when struck in the face by a rock. Such seizures, often entailing altered consciousness, auditory or visual hallucinations, automatic movements, staring, and perseveration of speech, occur in roughly 10 percent of cases involving a serious head injury. To be sure, White in vision displayed many of these symptoms; however, her behavior also differed in significant ways from what might be expected of someone experiencing complex partial seizures. She apparently spoke clearly and lucidly during her visions, emerged from them with a clear mind, and did not suffer the amnesia, disorientation, or terror so often associated with complex partial seizures.[20]

Besides, it seems unlikely that the childhood injury to her nose damaged her brain sufficiently to cause complex partial seizures. Although the accident produced severe bleeding and left her in "a stupid state" for about three weeks, there is no conclusive evidence that it induced a prolonged coma suggestive of severe brain injury. The neurologist Donald I. Peterson thinks it more likely that she suffered from a prolonged case of pneumonia: "If, while she was unconscious, Ellen aspirated blood and secretions from her nose and

---

20. Hodder, "Visions or Partial-Complex Seizures?" 30-37; Couperus, "The Significance of Ellen White's Head Injury," 17-23. On complex partial seizures, see Bernard H. Smith, *Differential Diagnosis: Neurology* (New York: Arco, 1979), pp. 164-68; Charles E. Wells and Gary W. Duncan, *Neurology for Psychiatrists* (Philadelphia: F. A. Davis, 1980), pp. 120-24; Sir John Walton, *Brain's Diseases of the Nervous System* (9th ed.; New York: Oxford University Press, 1985), p. 615; and Raymond D. Adams and Maurice Victor, *Principles of Neurology* (4th ed.; New York: McGraw-Hill, 1989), 252-54. On personality changes often associated with brain damage, see Wells and Duncan, *Neurology for Psychiatrists,* pp. 195-97. On the relationship between hysteria and organic brain disease, see Alex Roy, "Hysterical Neurosis," in *Hysteria,* ed. Alex Roy (New York: John Wiley and Sons, 1982), pp. 93-96.

throat (not an unlikely possibility, given the lack of adequate first aid knowledge in those days), she probably contracted pneumonia. Thus blood loss and pneumonia, *not severe brain injury,* is the more reasonable explanation of what she referred to as 'my sickness.'"[21]

Complex partial seizures also shed little light on her manifold physical complaints, and they inadequately account for the degree to which her visions depended on the approval of others. But most telling of all, this diagnosis fails to recognize the large number of White's contemporaries who claimed to have had visionary episodes similar to hers — but reported no brain-damaging injuries. Thus we must look beyond complex partial seizures for an adequate explanation of her distinctive medical history.[22]

A more convincing diagnosis, which not only accounts for many of her physical and psychological symptoms but acknowledges the importance of social and cultural factors, is what mental-health experts today call somatization disorder with an accompanying histrionic personality style. These categories encompass the behaviors and symptoms formerly grouped together under the now-discarded label "hysteria." According to the current edition of the diagnostician's guidebook, the *Diagnostic and Statistical Manual of Mental Disorders* put out by the American Psychiatric Association, the essential features of somatization disorder "are recurrent and multiple somatic complaints, of several years' duration, for which medical attention has been sought, but that apparently are not due to any physical disorder." In other words, persons suffering from this disorder repeatedly complain of a wide range of physical problems and believe themselves to be sickly but are not physically ill. Symptoms,

---

21. Peterson, *Visions or Seizures,* pp. 12-13. For an equally skeptical opinion on the diagnosis of complex partial seizures, by a non-Adventist neurologist, see Thomas Babb, Letter to the Editor, *Adventist Currents,* I (June, 1985), 37.

22. On nineteenth-century visionaries, see pp. 58-60 of this book. Recent historical discussions include Jean M. Humez, "'My Spirit Eye': Some Functions of Spiritual and Visionary Experience in the Lives of Five Black Women Preachers, 1810-1880," in *Women and the Structure of Society,* ed. Barbara J. Harris and JoAnn K. McNamara (Durham, N.C.: Duke University Press, 1984), pp. 129-43; and J. P. Williams, "Psychical Research and Psychiatry in Late Victorian Britain: Trance as Ecstasy or Trance as Insanity," in *The Anatomy of Madness: Essays in the History of Psychiatry,* vol. 1: *People and Ideas,* ed. W. F. Bynum, Roy Porter, and Michael Shepherd (London: Tavistock Publications, 1985), pp. 233-54.

which range from gastrointestinal difficulties, chest pains, shortness of breath, palpitations, and dizziness to loss of voice, blurred or double vision, fainting, paralysis, difficulty walking, and amnesia, usually begin in the teens and occur most commonly in females. Although often described in a dramatic or exaggerated manner, the symptoms are neither intentional nor conscious; the typical sufferer has no sense of controlling them and sincerely believes them to be of organic origin. However, it is possible, as the historian Carroll Smith-Rosenberg has suggested, that some women diagnosed as hysterics unconsciously succumbed to this malady as a way of opting out of the traditional roles society assigned to them.[23]

The *Diagnostic and Statistical Manual of Mental Disorders* describes persons with a histrionic personality disorder as presenting "a pervasive pattern of excessive emotionality and attention-seeking, beginning by early adulthood and present in a variety of contexts. . . . People with this disorder constantly seek or demand reassurance, approval, or praise from others and are uncomfortable in situations in which they are not the center of attention." They may also dramatize personal experiences, interpret nonsexual situations sexually yet be fearful of sex, display dependent and demanding interpersonal behavior, indulge in role-playing, easily fall prey to the suggestions of others, and overly react to disappointments. They typically deny internal conflicts or externalize them by attributing unacceptable emotions to others, blaming someone or something else, or somatizing, which shifts the conscious focus of attention from inner psychological conflicts to outer physical discomfort. Histrionic personality disorder often coexists with somatization disorder.[24]

---

23. American Psychiatric Association, *Diagnostic and Statistical Manual of Mental Disorders* (3rd ed. rev.; Washington: American Psychiatric Association, 1987), pp. 261-64; Carroll Smith-Rosenberg, "The Hysterical Woman: Sex Roles and Role Conflict in 19th-Century America," *Social Research*, XXXIX (1972), 652-78. On the history of hysteria, see Ilza Veith, *Hysteria: The History of a Disease* (Chicago: University of Chicago Press, 1965).

24. American Psychiatric Association, *Diagnostic and Statistical Manual*, pp. 348-49. See also Alan Krohn, *Hysteria: The Elusive Neurosis,* vol. XII, nos. 1/2 of *Psychological Issues* (New York: International Universities Press, 1978), pp. 54, 64; and George W. Fenton, "Hysterical Alterations of Consciousness," in Roy, ed., *Hysteria,* pp. 233-38.

Ellen White on the Mind and the Mind of Ellen White

As described by the psychologist Alan Krohn, histrionic persons often appear to be relatively "normal" and rarely go "far enough to be considered substantially deviant." Their self-identity commonly incorporates desirable roles and pleasing behaviors, but this is done unconsciously, not deliberately or deceptively. "This identity, . . . though seldom overlooked and often flamboyant, remains within the bounds of convention," writes Krohn. "Indeed, this flamboyance, rarely iconoclastic, resides in novel, fashion-setting modifications of what is *in vogue*."[25]

In this diagnostic context, which, for our purposes, possesses greater heuristic than deterministic value, White's frequent dreams and visions shrink to mere epiphenomena. Histrionic persons today rarely report seeing visions, largely because such experiences have gone out of fashion. In the nineteenth century, however, trances and visions were the order of the day for a host of mesmerists, spiritualists, and religious enthusiasts. Self-proclaimed seers not only modeled themselves after the biblical writers, particularly Daniel and John the Revelator, but saw themselves as the fulfillment of the prophecy that "in the last days . . . your sons and your daughters shall prophesy, and your young men shall see visions, and your old men shall dream dreams" (Acts 2:17). In view of White's suggestibility and the attention and reinforcement her dissociative experiences elicited from others, her claim to visions is hardly surprising. The exact mechanism that triggered these apparently self-hypnotic episodes is of less historical interest than the fact that phenomenologically her visions in no way differed from the trances of the run-of-the-mill mesmerist or spiritualist. The proof of this claim is White's own inability to distinguish empirically between her visions and those of her contemporaries. She distanced herself from other trance mediums not on the basis of physical evidence, but spiritual content.[26]

From White's own testimony we are convinced that beginning in childhood she suffered from episodes of depression and anxiety that often left her debilitated and at times even crippled. Unfortunately, little is known about the biological or social matrix in which

---

25. Krohn, *Hysteria*, pp. 160-63.
26. See p. 67 of this book.

AFTERWORD

these disorders developed and in which her personality was rooted. It seems likely, however, that her unhappiness stemmed at least in part from insufficiently gratifying relationships with parents and siblings, perhaps aggravated by the experience of being a twin. Her inadequate sense of identity left her vulnerable to fluctuations in self-esteem and consequently dependent on others to enhance her sense of self. Within a few years, certainly by adolescence, she was responding to outer stress and inner distress by unconsciously constructing a defensive system that allowed her to ward off unpleasant conflict through poor health. This gained her the supportive attention of others, who tended to see external rather than internal problems. By her adult years she had developed a full-fledged somatization disorder and a histrionic personality style.[27]

Let us now examine some of the evidence that favors this assessment. In describing her childhood "misfortune" nearly a quarter-century after the event, White dramatically emphasized the severity of the injury, claiming that it threatened her life, turned her into an invalid, and destroyed her "natural looks." Seeing herself in a mirror left her dismayed: "Every feature of my face seemed changed. The sight was more than I could bear. . . . The idea of carrying my misfortune through life was insupportable."[28] In all likelihood the accident caused ugly bruising and swelling but produced greater psychological than physical trauma. Its occurrence at a time when children are commonly becoming self-conscious about their bodies undoubtedly heightened her distress and embarrassment, though later photographs give no indication of facial disfigurement or permanent damage. Her greatest trauma probably resulted from the narcissistic wound she received from being publicly assaulted by a schoolmate. Her own words (given in Appendix 1) reveal a socially insecure child in the grips of recurrent and at times severe anxiety, no doubt exacerbated by the memory of her humiliating injury and the anticipation of further ridicule. Her professed love of learning and eagerness to continue her education caught her on the horns of a classic wish-fear dilemma: wanting desperately to do something

---

27. On the relationship between depression and histrionic defenses, see Gerald L. Klerman, "Hysteria and Depression," in Roy, ed., *Hysteria,* pp. 211-28.

28. EGW, *Spiritual Gifts* (1860), pp. 7-9.

but too afraid to do it. Indeed, severe anxiety about school rather than physical disability seems to account for the hand trembling, blurred vision, sweating, faintness, and dizziness that plagued her when she attempted to resume her education. Interpreting these symptoms as medical problems allowed her to skip school and avoid an unpleasant situation — a dynamic critical to the development of her somatization disorder.[29]

By the age of fourteen or fifteen she seems also to have been in the throes of a major clinical depression. Her autobiography lists all the classic symptoms: feelings of hopelessness, worthlessness, guilt, despair, and melancholy; loss of appetite, weight, the ability to concentrate, and a sense of pleasure; sleeplessness and nightmares; a lack of energy; social withdrawal; and morbid preoccupations, with recurrent thoughts of death and hell. Five of these symptoms alone would today warrant a diagnosis of major depression.[30] To cope with this unspeakable anguish, she unconsciously hid behind histrionic defenses constructed out of the fragments of her own religious experience. By attributing her suffering to a passion for salvation — both her own and others' — she externalized the source of conflict and diffusely projected personal concerns onto religious ones. In the process she also denied other troubling sources of anxiety, such as sexuality and interpersonal relationships, common to adolescents.

Ellen's first public prayer, during which she apparently fainted, marks the beginning of another critical stage in the development of her histrionic style. At the time, her mother and "other experienced Christians" attributed her prostration to "the wondrous power of God."[31] The significance of such social reinforcement can hardly be exaggerated. Her accident and her anxieties had removed her from the society of her schoolmates and had truncated the normal

---

29. These symptoms are all indicative of a generalized anxiety disorder; see American Psychiatric Association, *Diagnostic and Statistical Manual*, pp. 251-53. The evidence presented in Appendix 1 of this book suggests that she continued to suffer from occasional anxiety episodes in her adult life.

30. EGW, *Life Sketches*, pp. 29-31. The diagnostic criteria for major depression are given in American Psychiatric Association, *Diagnostic and Statistical Manual*, pp. 222-24.

31. EGW, *Life Sketches*, p. 38.

developmental routes to social acceptance and approval. At home she had to compete with her twin sister and other siblings for the limited attention of her busy parents — and do so while feeling handicapped by her physical appearance. In the contest for parental nurturance an unconsciously assumed sick role could only be an advantage. Psychological studies of twins show them to be particularly sensitive to issues of identity and independence, especially as they journey through adolescence. As God's chosen messenger, Ellen definitively separated herself from her twin sister, Elizabeth, and acquired an enviable identity — though not one her sister acknowledged.[32]

Ellen's early fainting spells connected her emotionally with others, brought her attention and special notice, and thrust upon the socially awkward youth — "naturally so timid and retiring that it was painful for me to meet strangers" — a positive role by which she could relate to others.[33] The onset of visions a couple of years later seems to have brought temporary freedom from depression, thus further reinforcing the trances. Perhaps most important, her visionary visits with heavenly beings endowed her with a positive self-image that surely helped to dissipate the feelings of low self-esteem that had tormented her for so long. Years later she described her feelings of exhilaration and exaltation: "An unspeakable awe filled me, that I, so young and feeble, should be chosen as the instrument by which God would give light to His people."[34]

For a period of six months in 1843-44 Ellen repeatedly fell under the power of "the Spirit of the Lord" and consequently enjoyed improved mental and physical well-being. But following the Great Disappointment of October 22, 1844, her health declined rapidly. She complained primarily of cardiopulmonary symptoms, which reportedly caused even her physician to fear that she might die suddenly. In writing of this period, she admitted to harboring dark thoughts about the world, but in the exaggerated manner of the histrionic she chose to highlight her physical rather than depressive symptoms:

32. See Ricardo C. Ainslie, *The Psychology of Twinship* (Lincoln: University of Nebraska Press, 1985). We have been unable to determine whether the twins were identical. As far as we know, Elizabeth never accepted Ellen's religious claims.
33. EGW, *Life Sketches*, p. 69.
34. Ibid., p. 69.

intense suffering, imminent death, and gory detail. A short time later the criticism of others left her literally speechless. Clearly, by this time illness had become an important part of her defensive repertoire against depression. Given the attention and adoration of others, she felt healthy and whole; without them, she slipped into a psychosomatic slough.

Ellen White's close identification with the sufferings of Christ undoubtedly colored the way she viewed her episodes of poor health. In fact, she grandiosely predicted for herself the same fate that had befallen him:

> For forty years, Satan has made the most determined efforts to cut off this testimony from the church; but it has continued from year to year to warn the erring, to unmask the deceiver, to encourage the desponding. My trust is in God. I have learned not to be surprised at opposition in any form or from almost any source. I expect to be betrayed, as was my Master, by professed friends.[35]

In this context suffering became a virtue.

It seems likely that White's somatization helped her to avoid conscious feelings of anxiety, by repressing emotional needs and conflicts, and to externalize depression, by blaming others for her suffering. It may also have salved the narcissistic wounds inflicted by the verbal barbs of skeptics, which caused as much pain and humiliation in adulthood as the stone had caused her in childhood. Physical pain, which made her the object of sympathetic attention rather than derision, thus served to mask emotional anguish. Besides, in a culture that regarded assertive and ambitious women with considerable ambivalence, White's poor health allowed her to project a nonthreatening image of vulnerability while she relentlessly fought to stay on top of a male-dominated subculture. As a prophet, she could sublimate unacceptable and competitive urges in a socially acceptable and divinely sanctioned role. In denying any personal striving for success and in externalizing the source of her ambition — God made her do it — she displayed common histrionic characteristics.

---

35. Quoted in Arthur L. White, *Ellen G. White*, 6 vols. (Washington: Review and Herald Publishing Assn., 1981-1986), III, 229.

Afterword

In reading White's autobiographical accounts, one is immediately struck by the exaggerated, dramatic manner in which she portrays personal events. For example, she tells of how in 1858, following her vision of the "Great Controversy" between Christ and Satan, she suffered from temporary paralysis and loss of speech, followed by several weeks of unsteadiness and impaired sensation. Her explanation: "Satan designed to take my life to hinder the work I was about to write; but angels of God were sent to my rescue, to raise me above the effects of Satan's attack."[36]

White hungered for the attention that attached to her role as a latter-day prophet. As early as 1845, public questioning of the divine nature of her visions so filled her with anguish her family thought she would die — at least that's what she reported. Later, in the mid-1850s, when her self-conscious husband refused to publish her testimonies and fellow believers neglected them, her visions dwindled and she sank into despair.[37] As her fame spread, the utility of illness in gaining and holding an audience became increasingly apparent. At times she experienced miraculous cures while addressing a crowd. In 1877, for example, ill health almost forced her to cancel a dreaded appointment in Danvers, Massachusetts, where she would be preaching to a hostile audience. Though almost too weak to stand, she mounted the platform and attempted to speak:

> Like a shock of electricity I felt [the Spirit of the Lord] upon my heart, and all pain was instantly removed. I had suffered great pain in the nerves centering in the brain; this also was entirely removed. My irritated throat and sore lungs were relieved. My left arm and hand had become nearly useless in consequence of pain in my heart; but natural feeling was now restored. My mind was clear; my soul was full of the light and love of God. Angels of God seemed to be on every side, like a wall of fire.[38]

Several years later she attended a camp meeting so indisposed she asked for a sofa near the speaker's stand to lie on. At the close of the

---

36. EGW, *Spiritual Gifts* (1860), II, 271-72.
37. EGW, *Life Sketches*, p. 69; "Communication from Sister White," *R&H*, VII (1856), 118.
38. EGW, "Experience and Labors," *Testimonies*, IV, 280-81.

sermon she mustered the energy to rise to her feet. As she began to speak, the "power of God" swept over her, healing her instantly. "It cannot be attributed to imagination," she insisted. "The people saw me in my feebleness, and many remarked that to all appearance I was a candidate for the grave. Nearly all present marked the change which took place in me while I was addressing them."[39] Such public healings not only highlighted and validated her ministry but served as a substitute for more conventional healing services, in which ailing members of the audience were restored to health.

Ellen White often relied on her visions and ill health to control the distasteful behavior of family members and followers, at times even holding her own children responsible for her indispositions. Writing of her offspring in the mid-1850s, she said: "I was keenly sensitive to faults in my children, and every wrong they committed brought on me such heartache as to affect my health." Blaming her sons for her suffering may not have changed their behavior, but it undoubtedly induced considerable guilt. Even for relatively mundane matters she invoked the threat of becoming sick. When congregations failed to meet her demands for the ventilation of buildings, she on one occasion "fell very sick with nervous prostration ... suffering much with inflammation of head, stomach, and lungs," and on another she refused to speak altogether out of fear that the poisonous air "would cost me my life," in effect saying, "Open the windows, or I'll die."[40]

White's visions, like her ailments, served to keep family and followers in line. For how could they acknowledge her as God's inspired messenger and still dispute her messages, whether theological or personal? Those audacious enough to challenge her authority found themselves the objects of divinely sent reprimands. When Fannie Bolton, one of White's literary assistants, raised embarrassing questions about her boss's writings, White heard a voice saying, "Beware and not place your dependence upon Fannie to prepare articles or to make books. . . . She is your adversary. . . . She is not true

---

39. EGW, *Life Sketches*, p. 264.
40. EGW, *Spiritual Gifts* (1860), pp. 211-12; A. L. White, *Ellen G. White*, III, 353; V, 50-51.

to her duty, yet flatters herself she is doing a very important work." Similar warnings discredited the claims of rival prophets, present and future. "I have been shown," said White, that there will be "many who will claim to be especially taught of God, and will attempt to lead others, and they will undertake a work from mistaken ideas of duty that God has never laid upon them; and confusion will be the result."[41]

Indirect evidence suggests that Ellen White experienced deep-seated conflicts over sexuality and aggression. Her accident confined her to bed for "many months" and left her an invalid for years. At about age twelve — often the onset of puberty — she described herself as feeling terribly guilty, unworthy, and sinful. One might suspect that these guilt feelings arose as a result not only of the sexual fantasies common to children of this age, but also from the first sexual stirrings of pre-adolescence — and possibly from the sexual exploration of her own body as well, though White later insisted that she did not discover the fact of female masturbation until adulthood, when Adventist sisters began confessing their sins to her. During periods of her adult life she found sexuality a morbidly fascinating topic: both her 1863 health-reform vision and her first booklet on health focused on the horrors of masturbation. Her occasional testimonies about the secret sins of others, given under the cloak of divine immunity, smacked of voyeurism and possibly served to displace personal guilt about sexual fantasies and behavior.

Unacceptable aggressive and competitive impulses may also have induced guilt. Her conscious self-image is reflected in the following passage: "All through my life, it has been terribly hard for me to hurt the feelings of any, or disturb their self-deception. . . . It is contrary to my nature. It costs me great pain, and many sleepless nights."[42] Such protests notwithstanding, her visions often betrayed a distinctly aggressive quality — so much so that others sometimes criticized her for unnecessary harshness in reproving her followers. The visions allowed her to deny her aggression in two

---

41. EGW, Letter 59, 1894, quoted in A. L. White, *Ellen G. White,* IV, 241; EGW, Letter 54, 1893, quoted ibid., pp. 126-27.

42. EGW, "Camp-Meeting Address," *Testimonies,* V, 19-20.

ways: she could externalize the impulse by pointing outside herself to the sins of others, and she could silence her critics by asserting that she was not responsible for the content of her messages because she was only acting as God's instrument. "In no case have I given my own judgment or opinion," she wrote in 1882. "I have enough to write of what has been shown me without falling back on my own opinions."[43]

Finally, to what extent does Ellen White's histrionic personality help us understand her tendency to appropriate the writings of others as her own? Recent research has shown in embarrassing detail the extent to which she lifted substantial portions of her published works, especially on biblical history, from contemporary sources.[44] Was she a self-conscious plagiarist or a self-deceived copyist? We lean toward the latter view, though the two interpretations are not mutually exclusive. In analyzing White's behavior, we need to keep in mind psychologist David Shapiro's observation that the histrionic style of thinking is generally "global, relatively diffuse, and lacking in sharpness, particularly in sharp detail. In a word, it is *impressionistic*." Thus, when pressed for specific answers to questions, the histrionic person is more likely to give vague impressions than hard facts and to ignore such conventions as crediting one's sources and telling the exact truth. In assuming her prophetic role, White no doubt suppressed conscious knowledge of the extent to which she was borrowing the language of others and actually came to believe that the words were her own. When quizzed about the similarity of her writings to those of others, she defended herself in characteristic fashion. By both denying her indebtedness and blaming her ac-

---

43. EGW, *Testimony for the Battle Creek Church*, quoted in A. L. White, *Ellen G. White*, III, 199-20.

44. The most searching published expose of White's plagiarisms is Walter T. Rea, *The White Lie* (Turlock, Calif.: M & R Publications, 1982). But see also Eric Anderson, "Ellen White and Reformation Historians," *Spectrum*, IX (July, 1978), 23-26; Donald R. McAdams, "Shifting Views of Inspiration: Ellen G. White Studies in the 1970s," ibid., X (March, 1980), 27-41; Donald Casebolt, "Ellen White, the Waldenses, and Historical Interpretation," ibid., XI (February, 1981), 37-43; and Jonathan Butler, Review of *The White Lie*, by Walter T. Rea, ibid., XII (June, 1982), 44-48. The best recent study of plagiarism is Thomas Mallon, *Stolen Words: Forays into the Origins and Ravages of Plagiarism* (New York: Ticknor & Fields, 1989).

cusers for acting inappropriately, she deflected disapproval from her to her critics.[45]

In a compelling book called *Creative Malady* the distinguished British physician Sir George Pickering has explored the relationship between creativity and illness in the lives of such eminent Victorians as Charles Darwin, Florence Nightingale, and Mary Baker Eddy, the founder of Christian Science. Despite debilitating illnesses, which Pickering attributes in most cases to psychological causes, all made significant contributions to their chosen fields; and they did so, he argues, *because* of their ailments, which they used variously to protect themselves from unwanted intrusions, to manipulate those around them, or, as in the case of Eddy, to create a new system of healing.[46] Ellen White's life conforms to a strikingly similar pattern. Rather than falling victim to illness, she used it to escape anxiety-provoking or unwanted tasks, to elicit sympathy and support, to fashion a rewarding career, and to construct a religious system that prominently featured the ministry of healing. Hers was truly a creative malady.

---

45. David Shapiro, *Neurotic Styles* (New York: Basic Books, 1965), p. 111. See also George Pickering, *Creative Malady: Illness in the Lives and Minds of Charles Darwin, Florence Nightingale, Mary Baker Eddy, Sigmund Freud, Marcel Proust, Elizabeth Barrett Browning* (New York: Oxford University Press, 1974), pp. 297-309; and Phyllis Greenacre, "The Impostor," *Psychoanalytic Quarterly*, XXVII (1958), 359-82.

46. Pickering, *Creative Malady*. For a psychoanalytic interpretation of the Mormon prophet Joseph Smith, see Fawn M. Brodie, *No Man Knows My History: The Life of Joseph Smith* (2nd ed.; New York: Alfred A. Knopf, 1971), pp. 405-25. See also Fawn M. Brodie, "Ellen White's Emotional Life," *Spectrum*, VIII (January, 1977), 13-15.

APPENDIX 1

Physical and Psychological Experiences of Ellen G. White: Related in Her Own Words

1827	Born in Gorham, Maine, on November 26; a twin.
1836?	Response to an article predicting the imminent end of the world: "In contemplating the event predicted, I was seized with terror.... Such a deep impression was made upon my mind by the little paragraph on the scrap of paper, that I could scarcely sleep for several nights, and prayed continually to be ready when Jesus came." [*Life Sketches*, pp. 20-21]
1836-37	Hit on the nose with a stone: "I was stunned by the blow, and fell senseless to the ground.... When [after about three weeks] I again aroused to consciousness, it seemed to me that I had been asleep.... a great cradle had been made for me, and in it I lay for many weeks. I was reduced almost to a skeleton.... For two years I could not breathe through my nose, and was able to attend school but little. It seemed impossible for me to study and to retain what I learned.... My nervous system was prostrated, and my hand trembled so that I made but little progress in writing, and could get no farther than the simple copies in coarse hand. As I endeavored to bend my mind to my studies, the letters in the page would run together, great drops of perspiration would stand upon my brow, and a faintness and dizziness would seize me. I had a bad cough, and my whole system seemed debilitated." [*Life Sketches*, pp. 17-19]

APPENDIX 1

1840	Joined the Millerites, who believed that Christ would return to earth about 1843, later October 22, 1844.
1842	Concern about salvation: "The mental anguish I passed through at this time was very great. . . . I was in deep despair. I feared that I should be lost, and that I should live throughout eternity suffering a living death. . . . [While listening to sermons describing hell] my imagination would be so wrought upon that the perspiration would start, and it was difficult to suppress a cry of anguish, for I seemed already to feel the pains of perdition. . . . Almost total darkness settled upon me, and there seemed no way out of the shadows. . . . My sufferings of mind were intense. Sometimes for a whole night I would not dare to close my eyes, but would wait until my twin sister was fast asleep, then quietly leave my bed and kneel upon the floor, praying silently, with a dumb agony that cannot be described. The horrors of an eternally burning hell were ever before me. . . . I frequently remained bowed in prayer nearly all night, groaning and trembling with inexpressible anguish, and a hopelessness that passes all description." [*Life Sketches,* pp. 29-32] Regarding this episode she later wrote: "I have since thought that many inmates of insane asylums were brought there by experiences similar to my own." [*Testimonies,* vol. I, p. 25]
1842	Religious agitation: "I settled in a melancholy state which increased to deep despair. In this state of mind I remained three weeks, with not one ray of light to pierce the thick clouds of darkness around me. My sufferings were very great. . . . I remained bowed before the Lord nearly all night, groaning, and all I had any confidence to utter was, 'Lord, have mercy.' Such utter hopelessness would seize me that I would fall upon my face with such agony of feelings as cannot be described. . . . I became much reduced in flesh. My friends looked upon me as one sinking in a decline. At length a dream was given me which sunk me still lower in despair, if possible. . . . The horror of my mind could not be described. I awoke, and it was some time before I could convince myself it was not a reality.

	Surely, thought I, my doom is fixed. . . ." A second dream gave her hope. [*Spiritual Gifts,* vol. II, pp. 16-18]
1842	First public prayer: "As the others knelt for prayer, I bowed with them, trembling, and after a few had prayed, my voice arose in prayer before I was aware of it. . . . As I prayed, the burden and agony of soul that I had so long endured, left me, and the blessing of the Lord descended upon me like the gentle dew. . . . Everything seemed shut out from me but Jesus and His glory and I lost consciousness of what was passing around me. The Spirit of God rested upon me with such power that I was unable to go home that night. . . . When I was first struck down, some of those present were greatly alarmed, and were about to run for a physician, thinking that some sudden and dangerous indisposition had attacked me, but my mother bade them let me alone, for it was plain to her, and to the other experienced Christians, that it was the wonderous power of God that had prostrated me." [*Life Sketches,* p. 38]
1843-44	Spirit possessed: "For six months not a cloud intervened between me and my Saviour. . . . At times the Spirit of the Lord rested upon me with such power that my strength was taken from me. This was a trial to some who had come from the formal churches, and remarks were often made that grieved me much. Many could not believe that one could be so overpowered by the Spirit of God as to lose all strength. . . . My mind was in great perplexity in consequence of this opposition. . . . [After her opponents, under the influence of the Holy Spirit, began falling to the floor, they all] confessed that they had grieved the Holy Spirit by so doing, and they united in sympathy with me in love for the Saviour. . . . The Spirit of God often rested upon me with great power, and my frail body could scarcely endure the glory that flooded my soul." [*Testimonies,* vol. I, pp. 44-55]
Late 1844	Following the Great Disappointment of October 22: "My health failed rapidly. I could only talk in a whisper, or broken tone of voice. One physician said my disease was dropsical consumption; that my right lung was gone, and

my left affected. He thought I could not live long, might die very suddenly. It was very difficult for me to breathe lying down, and nights was bolstered almost in a sitting posture, and would often awake with my mouth full of blood." [*Spiritual Gifts,* vol. II, p. 30]

Late 1844 "Visions" began: "While we were praying, the power of God came upon me as I had never felt it before. I seemed to be surrounded with light, and to be rising higher and higher from the earth.... After I came out of vision, everything seemed changed; a gloom was spread over all that I beheld. Oh, how dark this world looked to me! I wept when I found myself here, and felt homesick. I had seen a better world, and it had spoiled this for me.... An unspeakable awe filled me, that I, so young and feeble, should be chosen as the instrument by which God would give light to His people." [*Life Sketches,* pp. 64-68] "... when the Lord sees fit to give a vision, I am taken into the presence of Jesus and angels, and am entirely lost to earthly things. I can see no farther than the angel directs me. My attention is often directed to scenes transpiring upon earth." [*Spiritual Gifts,* vol. II, p. 292]

Late 1844 "My health was so poor that I was in constant bodily suffering, and to all appearance had but a short time to live. I was only seventeen years of age, small and frail, unused to society and naturally so timid and retiring that it was painful for me to meet strangers." [*Life Sketches,* p. 69]

1844-45 An angel assures her that physical afflictions would preserve humility: "One great fear that had oppressed me was that if I obeyed the call of duty, and went out declaring myself to be one favored of the Most High with visions and revelations for the people, I might yield to sinful exaltation.... I now entreated that if I must go and relate what the Lord had shown me, I should be preserved from undue exaltation. Said the angel: 'Your prayers are heard, and shall be answered. If this evil that you dread threatens you, the hand of God will be stretched out to save you; by affliction He will draw you to Himself, and preserve your humility....'" [*Life Sketches,* pp. 71-72]

Physical and Psychological Experiences of Ellen G. White

1845	Charges of mesmerism: ". . . if it pleased the Lord to give me a vision in meeting, some would say that it was the effect of excitement and mesmerism. . . . All these things weighed heavily upon my spirits, and in the confusion I was sometimes tempted to doubt my own experience. While at family prayers one morning, the power of God began to rest upon me, and the thought rushed into my mind that it was mesmerism, and I resisted it. Immediately I was struck dumb, and for a few moments was lost to everything around me. I then saw my sin in doubting the power of God, and that for so doing I was struck dumb, but that my tongue should be loosed in less than twenty-four hours. . . . After I came out of vision, I beckoned for the slate, and wrote upon it that I was dumb. . . . I was unable to speak all day. Early the next morning my soul was filled with joy, and my tongue was loosed to shout the high praises of God. . . . Up to this time I could not write; my trembling hand was unable to hold a pen steadily. While in vision, I was commanded by an angel to write the vision. I obeyed, and wrote steadily. My nerves were strengthened, and from that day to this my hand has been steady." [*Life Sketches,* pp. 88-90]
1845	Response to negative rumors about her: "Discouragements pressed heavily; and the condition of God's people so filled me with anguish that for two weeks my mind wandered. My relatives thought I could not live. . . ." [*Spiritual Gifts,* vol. II, p. 51] Later she referred to "the two weeks of my extreme sickness, when my mind wandered." [ibid., p. 69]
1845	Concern about the reactions of persons she was correcting: "It was very crossing for me to relate to individuals what I had been shown concerning their wrongs. It caused me great distress to see others troubled or grieved. And when obliged to declare the messages, I often softened them down and related what I had seen as favorable for the individuals as I could, and then would go by myself and weep in agony of spirit. . . . such distress hung upon my soul, I often felt that death would be a welcome mes-

Appendix 1

senger, and the grave a sweet resting-place. I did not realize that I was so unfaithful, and did not see the danger and sin of such a course, until I was taken in vision into the presence of Jesus. He looked upon me with a frown, and turned his face from me. It is not possible to describe the terror and agony I then felt." [*Spiritual Gifts,* vol. II, pp. 60-61]

1846　Healing in Gorham, Maine: ". . . I was taken very sick, and suffered extremely. My parents, husband and sister, united in prayer for me; but still I suffered on for three weeks. Our neighbors thought I could not live. I often fainted like one dead; but in answer to prayer, revived again. . . . After others had prayed, Bro. Henry [Nichols] commenced praying, and seemed much burdened, and with the power of God resting upon him, rose from his knees, came across the room, and laid his hands upon my head, saying, 'Sister Ellen, Jesus Christ maketh thee whole,' and fell back prostrated by the power of God. I believed that the work was of God, and the pain left me. . . . The next day we rode thirty-eight miles to Topsham." [*Spiritual Gifts,* vol. II, pp. 83-85] A few months later James White reported that "Ellen has enjoyed the best state of health for six weeks past that she has for so long a time for six years." [James White to S. Howland, March 14, 1847, quoted in A. L. White, *Ellen G. White,* vol. I, p. 117]

1847　Continued sickness and fainting spells: In August James wrote that "She has been out of health for years, and suffers much at this time. . . . For years Ellen has been subject to fainting spells. She has had many the year (last Monday) that we have been married. It was the opinion of our unbelieving neighbors that she would die in one of her faint spells, but to the astonishment of all she has not had a faint spell for two weeks." [James White to Elvira Hastings, Aug. 25 and Sept. 1, 1847, quoted in A. L. White, *Ellen G. White,* vol. I, pp. 133-34]

Late 1840s　An angel's touch: "For two or three years my mind continued to be locked to an understanding of the Scriptures. . . . [Then, after she healed a man,] Light seemed to shine all through the house, and an angel's hand was laid upon my head. From that time to this I have been able to understand the Word of God." [*Selected Messages,* vol. I, p. 207]

1851 "You remember I was not very well when we parted. I continued to grow feeble and all day Sabbath was very weak, not able to sit up; in the eve I fainted quite away. The brethren prayed over me and I was healed and taken off in vision. I had a deep plunge in the glory. . . ." [Letter 8, 1851, White Estate]

1853-54 "In the winter and spring I suffered much with heart disease. It was difficult for me to breathe lying down, and I could not sleep unless raised in nearly a sitting posture. My breath often stopped, and fainting fits were frequent. But this was not all my trouble. I had upon my left eye-lid a swelling which appeared to be a cancer. . . . In about three weeks I fainted and fell to the floor, and remained unconscious about thirty-six hours. It was feared that I could not live; but in answer to prayer again I revived. . . . For months I had suffered such constant pain in my heart that I did not have one joyful feeling, but my spirits were constantly depressed." [*Spiritual Gifts,* vol. II, pp. 184-86]

1855 "In December, 1855, I fell and sprained my ankle, which confined me to crutches six weeks. The confinement was an injury to my lungs. . . . I have not been entirely free from pain in the left lung since that time [writing in 1860]. After this I suffered with a dull, heavy pain in my head for three weeks, when the pain became intense. . . . It was inflammation on the brain. . . . I did not expect to live. . . . My husband called for a few who had faith to pray for me. The Spirit of the Lord rested upon me, and my grateful thanks ascended to our great Physician who had mercifully relieved me." [*Spiritual Gifts,* vol. II, pp. 206-7]

Mid 1850s Concern for her children, whom she often left with others while she traveled: "I felt grieved. My greatest anxiety had been for my children, to bring them up free from evil habits. . . . Henry had been from us five years, and Edson had received but little of our care. . . . I was keenly sensitive to wrongs in my children, and every wrong they committed

Appendix 1

	brought on me such heartache as to affect my health." [*Spiritual Gifts,* vol. II, pp. 211-12]
Mid 1850s	Unappreciated, the visions temporarily cease: "For some months past my spirit has been much depressed. God has seen fit to use me, a feeble instrument, for a few years past by giving me visions. . . . when I have seen how little the visions have been heeded, I have been discouraged. The visions have been of late less and less frequent, and my testimony for God's children has been gone." ["Communication from Sister White," *Review and Herald,* VII (1856), 118]
1858	Events in Jackson, Michigan, following her vision of the "Great Controversy" between Christ and Satan: "We had been in the house but a short time, when, as I was conversing with Sr. P[almer], my tongue refused to utter what I wished to say, and seemed large and numb. A strange, cold sensation struck my heart, passed over my head, and down my right side. For a while I was insensible; but was aroused by the voice of earnest prayer. I tried to use my left arm and limb, but they were perfectly useless. For a short time I did not expect to live. It was the third shock I had received of paralysis. . . . For several weeks I could not feel the pressure of the hand, nor the coldest water poured upon my head. In rising to walk, I often staggered, and sometimes fell to the floor. In this condition I commenced to write the Great Controversy. . . . [In June she was shown in vision] that in the sudden attack at Jackson, Satan designed to take my life to hinder the work I was about to write; but angels of God were sent to my rescue, to raise me above the effects of Satan's attack. I saw, among other things, that I should be blest with better health than before the attack at Jackson." [*Spiritual Gifts,* vol. II, pp. 271-72]
Late 1850s	"Disease has pressed heavily upon me. For years I have been afflicted with dropsy and disease of the heart, which has had a tendency to depress my spirits and destroy my faith and courage. . . . my perplexity of mind has been great. Disease seemed to make continual progress upon

	me, and I thought that I must lie down in the grave. I had no desire to live.... Often when I retired to rest at night, I realized that I was in danger of losing my breath before morning.... [In a vision] I saw that Satan had been trying to drive me to discouragement and despair, to make me desire death rather than life." [*Testimonies,* vol. I, p. 185]
1860	Three weeks after the difficult birth of a son on September 20 her husband left on a trip. On October 29 she wrote: "I have felt so lonesome that I could not prevent two or three crying spells." On November 2 she wrote: "I have a long cry now and then, and it does me good, I feel better afterward.... My back is weak and I am so lame I cannot get around much, I want upstairs once on my knees to get these things together for the poor." [Paul Gordon and Ron Graybill, "Letters to Lucinda," *Review and Herald,* CL (Aug. 23, 1973), 4-7]
1860	Following the death of her baby: "When my child was dying, I would not weep. I fainted at the funeral.... despondency and gloom settled upon me." [*Spiritual Gifts,* vol. II, p. 296]
Early 1860s	"... for years I have suffered peculiar trials of mind.... In my last vision I inquired of my attending angel why I was left to suffer such perplexity of mind, and was so often thrown upon Satan's battleground.... Then our past life was presented before me, and I was shown that Satan had sought in various ways to destroy our usefulness.... I saw that in our journeying from place to place, he had frequently placed his evil angels in our path to cause accident which would destroy our lives; but holy angels were sent upon the ground to deliver. Several accidents have placed my husband and myself in great peril, and our preservation has been wonderful. I saw that we had been the special objects of Satan's attacks...." [*Testimonies,* vol. I, pp. 346-47]
1861	"The cause of God is a part of us. Our experience and lives are interwoven with this work. We have had no separate existence. It has been a part of our very being. The believers in present truth have seemed as near as our children.

APPENDIX 1

	When the cause of God prospers we are happy, but when wrongs exist among the people of God we are unhappy, and nothing can make us glad." [Letter 5a, 1861, in R. D. Graybill, "The Power of Prophecy," p. 17]
1863	"When the [health] message first came to me [in a vision on June 5, 1863], I was weak and feeble, fainting once or twice a day." [MS-50-1904, White Estate]
1863	To preserve her health, she must cut back on domestic chores: In a vision "I saw that now we should take special care of the health God has given us. . . . I saw that I had spent too much time and strength in sewing and waiting upon and entertaining company. I saw that home cares should be thrown off. The preparing of garments is a snare; others can do that. God had not given me strength for such labor. We should preserve our strength to labor in His cause, and bear our testimony when it is needed." [MS 1, 1863, quoted in A. L. White, *Ellen G. White,* vol. II, pp. 18-19]
1865	Continued to suffer from poor health, especially "tenderness of the stomach." [Ellen G. White, "Our Late Experience," *Review and Herald,* XXVII (1866), 98]
1866	Cares for her ailing husband as he has cared for her: "I did not consider this a task — it was to me a privilege. I have been nearly all my life an invalid, and tenderly and patiently has he sympathized with and watched over and taken care of me when I was suffering, and now my turn had come to repay in a small measure the attention and kind offices I had received." [Quoted in A. L. White, *Ellen G. White,* vol. II, p. 124]
1866-67	Response to criticism: ". . . I felt an inexpressible depression of spirits, amounting to agony of mind, which seemed for a short period to palsy my vital energies. For three nights I scarcely slept at all. . . . The blood rushed to my brain, frequently causing me to reel and nearly fall. I had the nosebleed often, especially after making an effort to write. . . . [Experienced difficulty in writing] because of pressure of blood to the brain. . . . I supposed that after resting a few days I could again resume my writing. But to

Physical and Psychological Experiences of Ellen G. White

my great grief I found that the condition of my brain made it impossible for me to write.... Grieved in spirit beyond measure, I remained at home, dreading to go anywhere among the church for fear of being wounded.... When friends and relatives had despaired of my life, because disease was preying upon me, I had been borne in my husband's arms to the boat or cars." [*Testimonies,* vol. I, pp. 576-81]

1867 "I had for four weeks suffered much with my lungs, and it was with difficulty that I spoke to the people. Sabbath evening a fomentation was applied over my throat and lungs, but the head-cap was forgotten, and the difficulty of the lungs was driven to the brain. As I arose in the morning, I felt a singular sensation upon the brain. Voices seemed to vibrate, and everything appeared to be swinging before me. As I walked, I reeled, and came near falling to the floor.... I grew very sick, and could not sit up.... I could not gather or retain a sentence in my mind.... I staggered to the tent with a strangely confused brain, but told the preaching brethren on the stand that if they would sustain me by their prayers, I would speak.... Since that meeting, my lungs have been greatly relieved, and I have been improving in health." [*Testimonies,* vol. I, pp. 604-5]

1867 Denies discouragement: "Do you ever see me gloomy, desponding, complaining? I have a faith that forbids this.... It is the want of genuine religion that produces gloom, despondency, and sadness.... Those who follow Christ the most closely have not been gloomy." [MS 1, 1867, quoted in A. L. White, *Ellen G. White,* vol. II, p. 122]

1867 Her role required freedom of expression: "The relation which I sustain to this work demands of me an unfettered expression of my views." [*Testimonies,* vol. I, p. 562]

1867 On her "remarkable dreams": "The multitude of dreams arise from the common things of life, with which the Spirit of God has nothing to do. There are also false dreams, as well as false visions, which are inspired by the spirit of Satan. But dreams from the Lord are classed in the word of God with visions, and are as truly the fruits of

Appendix 1

the spirit of prophecy as visions. Such dreams, taking into the account the persons who have them, and the circumstances under which they are given, contain their own proofs of their genuineness." [*Testimonies,* vol. I, pp. 569-70]

1868 "A feeling of discouragement came over me, and I sank into a feeble state, and remained so several days, frequently fainting.... On the evening of February 5 ... I was in a fainting, breathless condition, supported by my husband." Healed by prayer and a dream. [*Testimonies,* vol. II, p. 10]

1869 Criticism undermines Ellen White's health: "I have seen no less than four evil angels controlling members of the family [of critics]. . . . We have labored and toiled and tugged. We have prayed and wept at home. We could not rest or sleep. . . . I wrote testimony after testimony at the expense of health, and I feared of life, hoping to arouse the consciences of the people at Battle Creek." [Letter 3, 1869, quoted in A. L. White, *Ellen G. White,* vol. II, p. 268]

1869 Letter to her son, Edson, regarding menopause: "I am not in good health.... I have more indications of going down into the grave than of rallying. My vitality is at a low ebb. Your Aunt Sarah died passing through this critical time. My lungs are affected. Dr. Trall said I would probably go with consumption in this time. Dr. Jackson said I should probably fail in this time. Nature would be severely taxed, and the only question would be, were there vital forces remaining to sustain the change of nature. My lungs have remained unaffected until last winter. The fainting fit I had on the cars nearly closed my life. My lungs are painful. How I shall come out I cannot tell. I suffer much pain." [W-6-1869, White Estate]

1870 Letter to her son, Willie, describing the drama of traveling when ill: "Your father rushed out [onto a crowded railroad platform] with me on his arm. He put his shoulder against men and women, crying out, 'Make way for a sick woman. Clear the track for a sick woman.' He rushed through the crowd, took me to one side, and found me a

	seat." [Letter 13, 1870, quoted in A. L. White, *Ellen G. White,* vol. II, p. 294]
1870	"I have been a great sufferer from disease, having had five shocks of paralysis. I have been with my left arm bound to my side for months, because the pain in my heart was so great." [*Testimonies,* vol. II, p. 371]
1871	"On the night of April 30, 1871, I retired to rest much depressed in spirits. For three months I had been in a state of great discouragement. I had frequently prayed in anguish of spirit for relief." [*Testimonies,* vol. II, p. 604]
1871	James White describes his wife's recovery from cancer: "For two years past she has, most of the time, suffered from painful and discouraging evidence of a growing cancer in the breast. . . . [As a result of reconsecrating their lives to the Lord] Mrs. White is free and happy, and has the best of evidence that the growing cancerous swelling, which had become large, and was very painful, is entirely removed." [Quoted in A. L. White, *Ellen G. White,* vol. II, p. 329]
1872	Continued poor health, described in a letter to her son and daughter-in-law from the Rockies: "This trip among the mountains is doing much for my health. None of you were aware of my miserable state of health. I knew it would not make home better to complain. . . ." [Letter 12, 1872, quoted in A. L. White, *Ellen G. White,* vol. II, p. 347]
1872	Letter to her sons, Edson and Willie, regarding a spiritual experience in San Francisco: "The blessing and power of God rested upon your Father and Mother. We both fell to the floor. Your Father, as he rose up on his feet to praise God, could not stand. The blessing of God rested upon him with such remarkable power. The angels of God seemed all around us. . . . We shouted the high praises of God. . . . Streams of light seemed to come upon us from our heavenly Father and the room seemed to be illuminated with the presence of the Lord." [W-20-1872, White Estate]
1874	Marital difficulties, including temporary separations from her husband, described in letters to James: "When

APPENDIX 1

we can work the best together we will do so. If God says it is for His glory we work apart occasionally, we will do that. But God is willing to show me my work and my duty, and I shall look to Him in faith and trust Him fully to lead me." "I can say I know you view things in a perverted light. I have in the past felt so depressed and saddened with the thought that it might always be so, that life has seemed a burden. . . . If we have to walk apart the rest of the way, do let us not seek to pull each other down. I believe it is best for our labors to be disconnected and we each lean upon God for ourselves." "I cannot have you take the life and soul out of me by your blaming and censuring me. . . . I must be free in God. He wants me to be free and not suffering under a load of depressing discouragements that unfit me for any position." [Letters 38, 40, and 40a, 1874, quoted in A. L. White, *Ellen G. White,* vol. II, pp. 434-38]

1875 Early in January she went into vision as church leaders and family members prayed for her recovery from a severe case of influenza. As described in the *Review and Herald,* "the Lord, in answer to prayer, visited her in mercy and in power, and to the great joy of all present she was enabled [that night] to give a powerful exhortation and cheering testimony." [Quoted in A. L. White, *Ellen G. White,* vol. II, p. 461]

1876 Writing a life of Christ: "I want this summer, the whole of it, to do this work in. I must stop a day or two in the week and go somewhere or my head will break down. I begrudge every moment that I feel compelled to rest. These intensely interesting subjects weary me far more to write them out than to speak upon them." [Letter 9, 1876, in A. L. White, *Ellen G. White,* vol. III, p. 29]

1877 Speaking in Danvers, Mass.: ". . . I realized that I was sick, and had but little strength; yet the cars were fast bearing us on to my appointment in Danvers. Here I must stand before entire strangers, whose minds had been prejudiced by false reports and wicked slander. . . . I was too weary to arrange my thoughts in connected words; but I felt that I must have help, and asked for it with my whole heart.... As the time for the meeting drew on, my spirit wrestled in an agony of prayer for strength and power from God. While the last hymn was being sung, I went to the stand. I stood up in great weakness, knowing that if any degree of success attended my labors it would be through the strength of the Mighty One. The Spirit of the Lord rested upon me as I attempted to speak. Like a shock of electricity I felt it upon my heart, and all pain was instantly removed. I had suffered great pain in the nerves centering in the brain; this also was entirely removed. My irritated throat and sore lungs were relieved. My left arm and hand had become nearly useless in consequence of pain in my heart; but natural feeling was now restored. My mind was clear; my soul was full of the light and love of God. Angels of God seemed to be on every side, like a wall of fire." [*Testimonies,* vol. IV, pp. 280-81]

1877 Writing to her children after a falling-out with her niece and literary assistant, Mary Clough, during James's illness: "My trouble with Mary and her mother has told upon me severely. I am unable to write because of my hand and heart troubles. And Father is the last person in the world to whom I should go with any expectancy that he could get beyond himself sufficiently to appreciate my feelings. I must think and act all for myself. I so much long to have an interested God-fearing friend that I can talk and counsel with." [Letter 40, 1877, in A. L. White, *Ellen G. White,* vol. III, p. 78]

1878 "Sunday, June 10, ... I was prostrated with heart disease.... [In September] I had much difficulty in breathing, and my heart pained me continually.... [Once again I took] treatment at the Sanitarium." [*Testimonies,* vol. IV, pp. 286-301]

1878 At a large camp meeting in Michigan: "... although much worn, and suffering with heart difficulty, the Lord gave me strength to speak to the people nearly every day, and sometimes twice a day.... I did not think I should have strength to speak more than twice or three times during the meeting; but as the meeting progressed, my strength

APPENDIX 1

increased. Upon several occasions I stood on my feet four hours, inviting the people forward for prayers. I never felt the special help of God more sensibly than during this meeting. Notwithstanding these labors, I steadily increased in strength. And to the praise of God I here record the fact that I was far better in health at the close of that meeting than I had been for six months." [*Testimonies,* vol. IV, p. 302]

1879 — On the road with James, who had been behaving erratically: ". . . I have been sick the entire journey. Lost twelve pounds. . . . I have spoken every Sabbath to our camp because no one else seemed to feel the burden, and every Sabbath evening or Sunday in towns and villages. I am worn and feel as though I was about 100 years old. . . . My ambition is gone; my strength is gone, but this will not last. [Letter 20, 1879, in A. L. White, *Ellen G. White,* vol. III, pp. 116-17]

Late 1870s — Her daytime visions ceased, but inspired dreams — "visions of the night" — continued. According to one account, "Mrs. White experienced only about a dozen [visions] during the 1860's, only three in the 1870's, and none thereafter." Even she could not always distinguish between dreams and visions: in one letter she mentioned "a dream or vision of the night — I cannot tell certainly which." [R. D. Graybill, "The Power of Prophecy," pp. 97, 108]

1880 — At a General Conference she fell ill but was miraculously healed: "I spoke about twenty minutes when strength came to me and also upon the congregation. This was a great victory. I called them forward and hundreds came seeking the Lord. I am a new woman. God has indeed wrought for me." [Quoted in A. L. White, *Ellen G. White,* vol. III, p. 148]

1881 — During a discouraging period: "Up to the time I had commenced this work I was sick, but the Lord gave me strength. I did not get to rest until near midnight, and labored all through the day, writing. Wednesday night I felt I must have rest. A nervous twitching seized my thumb and I could have no control over it. It jerked continually. I feared paralysis.... I have felt crushed and heartbroken for months, but I have laid my burden on my Saviour and I shall no longer be like a bruised reed." [Letter 8a, 1881, in A. L. White, *Ellen G. White,* vol. III, pp. 165-67]

1881 Following her husband's death in August: "The shock of my husband's death — so sudden, so unexpected — fell upon me with crushing weight. In my feeble condition I had summoned strength to remain at his bedside to the last; but when I saw his eyes closed in death, exhausted nature gave way, and I was completely prostrated. For some time I seemed balancing between life and death. The vital flame burned so low that a breath might extinguish it. At night my pulse would grow feeble, and my breathing fainter and fainter till it seemed about to cease." [*Life Sketches,* p. 252]

1881 Regarding criticism that she was unnecessarily harsh in reproving her followers: "Some of the brethren have taken the responsibility of criticising my work, and proposing an easier way to correct wrongs. To these persons I would say, I take God's way, and not yours.... Within a few weeks past, standing face to face with death, I have had a near look into eternity. If the Lord is pleased to raise me from my present state of feebleness, I hope, in the grace and strength that comes from above, to speak with fidelity the words which he gives me to speak. All through my life, it has been terribly hard for me to hurt the feelings of any, or disturb their self-deception, as I deliver the testimonies given me of God. It is contrary to my nature. It costs me great pain, and many sleepless nights. To those who have taken the responsibility to reprove me, and in their finite judgment, to propose a way which appears wiser to them, I repeat, I do not accept your efforts. Leave me with God, and let him teach me. I will take the words from the Lord, and speak them to the people." [*Testimonies,* vol. V, pp. 19-20]

1882 "While visiting Healdsburg [Calif.] last winter, I was much in prayer, and burdened with anxiety and grief. But

Appendix 1

the Lord swept back the darkness at one time while I was in prayer, and a great light filled the room. An angel of God was by my side, and I seemed to be in Battle Creek. I was in your councils; I heard words uttered, I saw and heard things that, if God willed, I wish could be forever blotted from my memory. My soul was so wounded, I knew not what to do or what to say.... I had also several most striking dreams.... In the testimonies sent to Battle Creek, I have given you the light God has given me. In no case have I given my own judgment or opinion. I have enough to write of what has been shown me, without falling back on my own opinions." [*Testimony for the Battle Creek Church,* in A. L. White, *Ellen G. White,* vol. III, pp. 199-200]

1882 During the summer she fell seriously ill after being chilled. While still in a weakened condition, she asked to be taken to a nearby camp meeting, where she was placed on a sofa near the speaker's stand. At the close of the sermon, "I decided to rise to my feet, hoping that if I thus ventured out by faith, doing all in my power, God would help me to say a few words to the people. As I began to speak, the power of God came upon me, and my strength was instantly restored.... The instantaneous work wrought for me was unexpected. It cannot be attributed to imagination. The people saw me in my feebleness, and many remarked that to all appearance I was a candidate for the grave. Nearly all present marked the change which took place in me while I was addressing them. They stated that my countenance changed, and the deathlike paleness gave place to a healthy color." [*Life Sketches,* p. 264] In a letter she described the incident as follows: "All at once I felt a power come upon me, like a shock of electricity. It passed through my body and up to my head. The people said that they plainly saw the blood mounting to my lips, my ears, my cheeks, my forehead.... It was as if one had been raised from the dead.... This sight the people in Healdsburg were to have as a witness for the truth." [Letter 82, 1906, in A. L. White, *Ellen G. White,* vol. III, pp. 204-5]

1883	"For forty years, Satan has made the most determined efforts to cut off this testimony from the church; but it has continued from year to year to warn the erring, to unmask the deceiver, to encourage the desponding. My trust is in God. I have learned not to be surprised at opposition in any form or from almost any source. I expect to be betrayed, as was my Master, by professed friends." [Quoted in A. L. White, *Ellen G. White,* vol. III, p. 229]
1884	"I have been unable to sleep nights, thinking of the important things to take place [in the last days of earth's history]. Three hours' sleep, and sometimes five, is the most I get. My mind is stirred so deeply I cannot rest. Write, write, write, I feel that I must, and not delay." [Letter 11a, 1884, in A. L. White, *Ellen G. White,* vol. III, p. 242]
1884	She visited the scene of her childhood accident, which "made me a lifelong invalid." [Quoted in A. L. White, *Ellen G. White,* vol. III, p. 261]
1886	Five years earlier she had fallen on the ice, injuring her ankle and forcing her to use crutches for more than four months. Writing from Europe she complained: "I am now quite a cripple from the broken ankle. I was injured five years ago in Battle Creek. I cannot walk at times without a cane.... My hip remains afflicted more severely now than for some time, but I am thankful that I am improving in health." [Letter 18, 1886, in A. L. White, *Ellen G. White,* vol. III, pp. 340-41]
1886	In Europe during the summer she suffered an apparent attack of pleurisy: "Every breath was painful. It seemed impossible for me to travel, especially at night." [Quoted in A. L. White, *Ellen G. White,* vol. III, p. 344]
1886	While preaching in Scandinavia in a poorly ventilated auditorium: "I knew the moment I attempted to speak that our brethren had forgotten to ventilate the hall, and the outdoor air had not been introduced into the hall after the last meeting had been held. I got through the discourse wearied out.... I could not sleep that night, and the next morning I looked haggard and felt two years older than I did before I made the attempt to speak. I be-

APPENDIX 1

came very sick with nervous prostration. . . . I was suffering much with inflammation of head, stomach, and lungs." [Letter 114, 1886, in A. L. White, *Ellen G. White,* vol. III, p. 353]

1888 Chastising a congregation for singing too listlessly: "I have heard the angels sing. They do not sing as you are singing tonight. They sing with reverence, with meaning. Their hearts are in their expressions of song. Now, let us try again and see if we can put our hearts into the singing of this song." [Quoted in A. L. White, *Ellen G. White,* vol. III, p. 384]

1888 Discouraged by criticism and resistance to her work, she fell ill: "I felt no desire to recover. I had no power even to pray, and no desire to live. Rest, only rest, was my desire, quiet and rest. As I lay for two weeks in nervous prostration, I had hope that no one would beseech the throne of grace in my behalf. When the crisis came, it was the impression that I would die. This was my thought. But it was not the will of my heavenly Father. My work was not yet done." [MS 2, 1888, in A. L. White, *Ellen G. White,* vol. III, p. 386]

1888 During a period of theological controversy: "I was able to sleep but a few hours. I was writing all hours of the morning, frequently rising at 2:00 and at 3:00 a.m. and relieving my mind by writing upon the subjects that were presented before me. My heart was pained to see the spirit that controlled some of our ministering brethren, and this spirit seemed to be contagious." [MS 24, 1888, in A. L. White, *Ellen G. White,* vol. III, pp. 404-5]

1889 Returned from a camp meeting in New York "worn and exhausted . . . and was obliged to refrain from speaking for a time. Attended camp meeting in Wexford, Michigan, and the Lord strengthened me to speak to the people. After the meeting I was again prostrated through over labor. Attended the camp meeting in Kalamazoo, and the Lord strengthened me to speak and labor for the people. Returning home to Battle Creek, I was again prostrated, but the Lord helped me. I attended the meeting in Saginaw, and to the praise of God He raised me above my feebleness, and I was made strong when before the people. After the meeting I was again greatly prostrated but started on my journey to attend camp meeting in Colorado.... I then continued my journey to California.... Attended Oakland meeting and was very sick, but the Lord raised me up and strengthened me with His Spirit and power, and I spoke to the people eight times and several times before committees and ministers and in morning meetings." [MS 25, 1889, in A. L. White, *Ellen G. White,* vol. III, p. 418]

1889   On a trip to a camp meeting in Pennsylvania flooding made train travel impossible: "We were obliged to walk miles on this journey, and it seemed marvelous that I could endure to travel as I did. Both of my ankles were broken years ago, and ever since they have been weak. Before leaving Battle Creek for Kansas, I sprained one of my ankles, and was confined to crutches for some time; but in this emergency I felt no weakness or inconvenience, and traveled safely over the rough, sliding rocks." [Quoted in A. L. White, *Ellen G. White,* vol. III, p. 430]

1890   Regarding questions about her testimonies: "I take no credit of ability in myself to write the articles in the paper or to write the books which I publish. Certainly I could not originate them. I have been receiving light for the last forty-five years and I have been communicating the light given me of heaven to our people as well as to all whom I could reach. I am seeking to do the will of my heavenly Father.... This has been the hardest long and persistent resistance I have ever had." [Letter 60, 1890, in A. L. White, *Ellen G. White,* vol. III, p. 458]

1890   Caught a severe cold while traveling and debated whether she should continue her trip: "I knelt by my chair to pray, feeling disheartened in reference to my journeying. Many appointments were before me. I had not uttered a word when the whole room seemed filled with a soft, silvery light, and my pain and disappointment and discouragement were removed. I was filled with comfort and hope and the peace of Christ.... The presence of Jesus was in

Appendix 1

the room.... Indeed, heaven seemed very near to me, and my heart well filled with joy and gladness. I had no inclination to sleep. I wanted to feast upon the heavenly manna, that Bread of Life that if we eat thereof, we shall live forever. What a night that was to my soul!... I had a very marked experience which I hope never to forget. Through the night season I was in communion with God. I was taken out and away from myself, and was in different states and assemblies, bearing a decided testimony of reproof and warning." [MS 44, 1890, in A. L. White, *Ellen G. White,* vol. III, pp. 466-67]

1890 — Response to criticism: "My brethren have trifled and caviled and criticized and commented and demerited, and picked and chosen a little and refused much until the testimonies mean nothing to them. They put whatever interpretation upon them that they choose in their own finite judgment and are satisfied. I would, if I had dared [have] given up this field of conflict long ago, but some thing has held me.... I feel cut loose from many of my brethren; they do not understand me or my mission or my work, for if they did they could never have pursued the course they have done." [Letter 40, 1890, in A. L. White, *Ellen G. White,* vol. III, p. 471]

1891 — Sailed for Australia in November: "I have not been able to walk on deck without an assistant, but my limbs are now growing stronger. I was almost completely exhausted in mind and body when I came on board the vessel." [Letter 32a, 1891, in A. L. White, *Ellen G. White,* vol. IV, p. 21]

1892 — Shortly after arriving in Australia, "I was stricken with a severe illness. For eleven months I suffered from malarial fever and inflammatory rheumatism. During this period I experienced the most terrible suffering of my whole life. I was unable to lift my feet from the floor without suffering great pain. My right arm, from the elbow down, was the only part of my body that was free from pain. My hips and my spine were in constant pain. I could not lie on my cot for more than two hours at a time, though I had rubber cushions under me. I would drag myself to a similar bed to change my position. Thus the nights passed.... Physicians said I would never be able to walk again, and I had fears that my life was to be a perpetual conflict with suffering. But I would not give up, and the constant effort that I made, because of my faith that I could still be the Lord's messenger to the people, accomplished a great change in my health. Some of the meetings that I attended at this time were from four to twelve miles from home. On some of these occasions I was enabled to speak for a full hour at a time. The fact that I could speak in public in spite of my crippled condition was an encouragement to my brethren and sisters." [MS 75, 1893, in A. L. White, *Ellen G. White,* vol. IV, pp. 31-32]

1893   Regarding Anna Phillips, a rival prophet: "The Lord has not laid upon her the work of accusing, of judging, or reproving, of condemning and flattering others.... there will be, I have been shown, many who will claim to be especially taught of God, and will attempt to lead others, and they will undertake a work from mistaken ideas of duty that God has never laid upon them; and confusion will be the result." [Letter 54, 1893, in A. L. White, *Ellen G. White,* vol. IV, pp. 126-27] "It is a terrible mistake to present before the people that which we have not had unmistakable evidence is the revelation of God." [Letter 4, 1893, ibid., p. 130]

1893-95   When one of her literary assistants, Fannie Bolton, raised embarrassing questions about the sources of White's inspired writings, White received a vision: "A voice spoke to me, 'Beware and not place your dependence upon Fannie to prepare articles or to make books.... She is your adversary.... She is not true to her duty, yet flatters herself she is doing a very important work." [Letter 59, 1894, in A. L. White, *Ellen G. White,* vol. IV, p. 241] Later, writing to her son, she said that she "could not possibly relate the suffering of mind" this episode was causing her. [Letter 123a, 1895, ibid., p. 237]

1894   Reaction to articles criticizing the Adventist pioneers: "That night, in agony of distress both of soul and body, I

Appendix 1

	groaned in spirit; I feared I should not live.... All the next day my feelings were so intense that I could not write; all the next day I could not do anything.... The second night was one of sorrow and unspeakable grief. I felt crushed as a cart beneath the sheaves." [MS 27, 1894, in A. L. White, *Ellen G. White,* vol. IV, pp. 133-34] She recovered after Jesus consoled her in a dream.
1895	Despite mental and physical exhaustion, she determined to fulfill a speaking engagement: "The way was long, but I went trusting in God, and while speaking I received special strength. A change came to nerve and muscle, and to my soul." [Letter 114, 1895, in A. L. White, *Ellen G. White,* vol. IV, pp. 228-29]
1896	An unusual vision in which she remained fully conscious: "Friday, March 20, I arose early, about half past three o'clock in the morning. While [I was] writing upon the fifteenth chapter of John, suddenly a wonderful peace came upon me. The whole room seemed to be filled with the atmosphere of heaven. A holy, sacred presence seemed to be in my room. I laid down my pen and was in a waiting attitude to see what the Spirit would say unto me. I saw no person. I heard no audible voice, but a heavenly watcher seemed close beside me. I felt that I was in the presence of Jesus. The sweet peace and light which seemed to be in my room ... is impossible for me to explain or describe. A sacred, holy atmosphere surrounded me, and there was presented to my mind and understanding matters of intense interest and importance." [MS 12c, 1896, in A. L. White, *Ellen G. White,* vol. IV, pp. 245-46]
1897	After reproving some Adventist leaders, she wrote in her diary: "This duty was done at great cost to myself. I returned to my room and for some hours my heartache was so intense it seemed to me I could not live. But the Lord mercifully gave me rest and relief in my efforts to lay my burden upon Him. I was afflicted with physical suffering throughout the day." She hesitated to talk with others lest Satan gain an advantage over her. [MS 177, 1897, in A. L. White, *Ellen G. White,* vol. IV, pp. 337-38]

1898	Experience at a camp meeting in October: "On the last Sunday of the meetings the Lord gave me a great victory. I was much exhausted.... I seemed to have no strength at all, but at 3:00 p.m. I went on the platform. I had a portion of Scripture to speak upon, but I could not remember what I meant to bring before the people. I stood up, and another portion of Scripture came into my mind. I had been a little hoarse, but I felt that the angel of the Lord was by my side, for my voice was clear and full and distinct.... I felt that it was not Ellen G. White who had spoken, but that the Lord had spoken through the frail instrument." [MS 153, 1898, in A. L. White, *Ellen G. White*, vol. IV, p. 368]
1900	On the return voyage from Australia to America, she was awakened by a voice speaking to her: "The room was filled with a sweet fragrance, as of beautiful flowers." She fell asleep again only to be reawakened: "Words were spoken to me, assuring me that the Lord would protect me, that He had a work for me to do. Comfort, encouragement, and direction were given to me, and I was greatly blessed." [MS 29, 1901, in A. L. White, *Ellen G. White*, vol. V, p. 24]
1900	Back in the United States, she wrestled with deciding whether or not to attend meetings in Battle Creek: "For a week before I fully consented to go to Battle Creek, I did not sleep past one o'clock. Some nights I was up at eleven o'clock and many nights at twelve." [Letter 159, 1900, in A. L. White, *Ellen G. White*, vol. V, p. 45] Later she recalled: "I was afraid the burdens I would have to bear would cost my life." [Quoted ibid., p. 74]
1900	In December she refused to speak in a church that was over-heated and poorly ventilated: "So greatly did I feel the effects of the poison in the air that although I stayed in the church only fifteen minutes, I feared that it would cost me my life." She rescheduled her talk for the afternoon. [Letter 2, 1901, in A. L. White, *Ellen G. White*, vol. V, pp. 50-51]
1901	In February she was debating whether to stay with the controversial Dr. John Harvey Kellogg while visiting Battle

Appendix 1

Creek: "while I was praying and was sending up my petition, there was, as has been a hundred times or more, a soft light circling around in the room, and a fragrance like the fragrance of flowers, of a beautiful scent of flowers." [MS 43a, 1901, in A. L. White, *Ellen G. White,* vol. V, p. 53] A voice said: "'Respect the courtesy of My servant, John Kellogg, the physician by My appointment. . . .'" [Letter 33, 1901, ibid., pp. 53-54] In publicly recounting the incident, she explained: "Though none of the family saw what I saw, or heard what I heard, yet they felt the influence of the Spirit, and were weeping and praising God." [Quoted ibid., p. 54]

1901 The meetings at Battle Creek left her exhausted. The night before a promised visit to one ailing member she slept only an hour. The next day, however, "While praying at his bedside, the Lord came very near, and I was blessed indeed. After that I left renewed, soul and body. . . . The peace of Christ filled my heart. I did not feel at all weary." [Letter 70, 1901, in A. L. White, *Ellen G. White,* vol. V, p. 111]

1901 While traveling in the East during the winter, she fell ill: "I have been having a severe test of my faith. Overdoing is not profitable. I have been shorn of my strength, quite feeble, nearly voiceless, too weak to see or converse with anyone except it was positively essential. I have not dared to go from the rooms assigned me in the sanitarium, dared not to go home to California, which I so much desired to do in my weakness." [Letter 184, 1901, in A. L. White, *Ellen G. White,* vol. V, p. 142]

1902 Responding to allegations that her testimonies reflected her own views: "My personality is not my own, and I have no right to use it for selfish purposes. I can stand before the throne of God and be perfectly clear at this point, for I have never used my personality selfishly. My husband used to tell me that I was more in danger of going to the other extreme." [MS 123, 1902, in A. L. White, *Ellen G. White,* vol. V, p. 189]

1905 Writing at age 78: "Since the accident that happened to me when I was 9 years old, I have seldom been perfectly free from all pain. But I do not remember when I have been more free from pain than I am at present." [MS 142, 1905, in A. L. White, *Ellen G. White,* vol. VI, p. 54]

1907 "I was suffering with rheumatism in my left side, and could get no rest because of the pain. I turned from side to side, trying to find ease from the suffering. There was a pain in my heart that portended no good for me. At last I fell asleep. About half-past nine I attempted to turn myself, and as I did so, I became aware that my body was entirely free from pain. As I turned from side to side, and moved my hands, I experienced an extraordinary freedom and lightness that I cannot describe. The room was filled with light, a most beautiful, soft, azure light, and I seemed to be in the arms of heavenly beings. This peculiar light I have experienced in the past in times of special blessing, but this time it was more distinct, more impressive, and I felt such peace, peace so full and abundant no words can express it. I raised myself into a sitting posture, and I saw that I was surrounded by a bright cloud, white as snow, the edges of which were tinged with a deep pink. The softest, sweetest music was filling the air, and I recognized the music as the singing of the angels. Then a Voice spoke to me, saying, 'Fear not; I am your Saviour. Holy angels are all about you.' . . . After a time the light passed away, but the peace remained. After a while I fell asleep again." [*Testimonies,* vol. IX, pp. 65-66]

1907 Sleepless nights: "Now I am up in the morning, you know, before anyone else is up — at one o'clock, two o'clock, three o'clock, and seldom ever after four — more often by three. Recently, for nights and nights and nights, I have seldom been able to sleep after two o'clock, but have been up writing." [MS 109, 1907, in A. L. White, *Ellen G. White,* vol. VI, p. 156]

1910 "One day . . . the burden that was upon my soul continued to press upon me after I returned to my room. I was in distress of mind. That night I could not seem to lose myself in sleep. It seemed as if evil angels were right in the room where I was. And while I was suffering in mind, it seemed

APPENDIX 1

as if I was suffering great bodily pain. My right arm, which through the years has nearly always been preserved from disease and suffering, seemed powerless. I could not lift it. Then I had a most severe, excruciating pain in the ear; then the most terrible suffering in the jaw. It seemed as if I must scream. But I kept saying, 'Lord, You know all about it.' I was in perfect agony. It seemed that my brain and every part of my body was suffering. . . . The suffering continued, at times in the jaw, then in the brain, and then in other members of the body, until nearly daylight. Just before the break of day I fell asleep for about an hour. . . . Legions of evil angels were in that room, and if I had not clung by faith to the Lord, I do not know what might have become of me. I would not call anyone. I said, 'This must be between me and these evil spirits.' . . . no relief from pain and suffering came to me, until I stood here upon this platform with a manuscript in my hand, and began to read what I had to read to you. As soon as I stood up here with that manuscript in my hand, every pain left me. My right side was just as strong as it had been before. I shall never be able to give you a description of the satanic forces that were at work in that room. I shall never be able to tell it in a way that will enable you to comprehend it." [MS 25, 1910, in A. L. White, *Ellen G. White,* vol. VI, pp. 283-84]

1910 — An invitation to speak came while she was sick in bed, but she accepted and felt better: "I have my sick and suffering times, but whenever a call is made I get right up. I saw the Lord knows; He will strengthen me for the work. I am not feeling well, but when any calls come like this one, I shall be on my feet ready to speak." [Letter 151, 1910, in A. L. White, *Ellen G. White,* vol. VI, p. 296]

1911 — Treatment for suspected skin cancer: "For several weeks I took treatment with the X-ray for the black spot that was on my forehead. In all I took twenty-three treatments, and these succeeded in entirely removing the mark. For this I am very grateful." [Letter 30, 1911, in A. L. White, *Ellen G. White,* vol. VI, p. 344]

1914	In early summer she suffered a slight stroke, which affected the right side of her body. [A. L. White, *Ellen G. White,* vol. VI, p. 405] Later in the year those caring for her reported that she spent "a good deal of time, nights, in prayer, evidently mostly in her sleep. Sometimes she seems to be holding prayer meetings. The other night she preached for an hour, and as she was using her voice in full strength, Miss Walling at last thought to suggest that she had preached long enough, and that now she should rest and sleep, which she did." [Ibid., p. 411]
1915	Died in Napa County, California, from "chronic myocarditis," complicated by "asthenia resulting from intra capsular fracture of the left femur" and "arterio-sclerosis." [Death certificate]

References

Graybill, Ronald D. "The Power of Prophecy: Ellen G. White and the Women Religious Founders of the Nineteenth Century." Ph.D. dissertation, Johns Hopkins University, 1983.

White, Arthur L. *Ellen G. White.* 6 vols. Washington: Review and Herald Publishing Association, 1981-1986.

White, Ellen G. *Life Sketches of Ellen G. White.* Mountain View, Calif.: Pacific Press, 1915.

———. *Selected Messages: From the Writings of Ellen G. White.* 2 vols. Washington: Review and Herald Publishing Association, 1958.

———. *Spiritual Gifts.* 4 vols. Battle Creek: James White/SDA Publishing Association, 1858-64.

———. *Testimonies for the Church.* 9 vols. Mountain View, Calif.: Pacific Press, 1885-1909.

APPENDIX 2

The 1864 Dansville Visit

Ellen G. White to Bro. and Sister Lockwood, September 14, 1864, from "Our Home," Dansville, N.Y. (L-6-1864, White Estate.)

Dear Bro. and Sister Lockwood:

I have been trying to find time to write you for some days but there is so much to be done I cannot do half I wish to do.

Adelia and the children have been examined today. The doctor pronounces Adelia sick. We shall leave their written prescriptions this week, then you can know more in regard to them. I think Dr. Jackson gave an accurate account of the disposition and organization of our children. He pronounces Willie's head to be one of the best that has ever come under his observation. He gave a good description of Edson's character and peculiarities. I think this examination will be worth everything to Edson.

They have all styles of dress here. Some are very becoming, if not so short. We shall get patterns from this place, and I think we can get out a style of dress more healthful than we now wear, and yet not be bloomer or the American costume. Our dresses according to my idea, should be from four to six inches shorter than now worn, and should in no case reach lower than the top of the heel of the shoe, and could be a little shorter even than this with all modesty. I am going to get up a style of dress on my own hook which will accord perfectly with that which has been shown me. Health demands it. Our feeble women must dispense with heavy skirts and tight waists if they value health.

Brother Lockwood, don't groan now. I am not going to extremes, but conscience and health requires a reform.

We shall never imitate Miss Dr. Austin or Mrs. Dr. York. They dress very much like men. We shall imitate or follow no fashion we have ever yet seen. We shall institute a fashion which will be both economical and healthy.

You may ask what I think of this institution. Some things are excellent. Some things are not good. Their views and teachings in regard to health are, I think, correct. But Dr. Jackson mixes up his theology too much with health question [sic] which theology to us is certainly objectionable. He deems it necessary for the health of his patients to let them have pleasureable excitement to keep their spirits up. They play cards for amusement, have a dance once a week and seem to mix these things up with religion. These things of course, we should not countenance, yet, when I view the matter from another standpoint, I am led to inquire, What better can be done for the feeble sick who have no hope of heaven, no consolation received by the Christian. Their source of enjoyment must be derived from a different source, while the Christian has the elevating influence of the power of grace, the sinner must draw from another source his enjoyments. If I ever prize Christ and the Christian hope, it is here, while looking upon poor invalids with but little prospect before them of ever recovering their health and have no hope for a better life.

Dr. Jackson carries out his principles in regard to diet to the letter. He places no butter or salt upon his table, no meat or any kind of grease. But he sets a liberal table. Waiters are constantly in attendance and if a dish is getting low, they remove it and replenish. The food I call liberal and good. All the difficulty is, there is danger of eating too much. All our food is eaten with a keen relish. If any one requires a little salt they have it supplied for the asking. A little bell sits by their plate which they use to call the waiter who provides them what they ask.

From 12 o'clock to quarter before two are resting hours. Everything is quiet. All undress and go to bed. But I forgot to state at half past ten comes the taking of baths. All patients who take treatment enter a large carpeted room with stove in it. All around the room are hooks. Upon these hooks are the sheets of the patients. Each has their [sic] particular hook and their number over the hook.

Appendix 2

Upon entering this room, the one who undresses first, wraps a sheet about her and signifies her readiness for a bath. By removing a tin from a hook painted on the back side with brown paint, they hold that tin until the bath tending women ask, What does No. 1 want? She then tells them either sitz bath, half bath or dry rubbing according to their prescription. They say, All ready. Then the patient turns this tin brown side out and goes to her bath. This saves all confusion for it is known when all are served.

The bath women put on old duds reaching to the knees, are barefooted and bare-legged and look bad. Yet their manner of dress is according to their work.

I do think we should have an institution in Mich. to which our Sabbath keeping invalids can resort. Dr. Lay is doing well. He is in the very best place he could be in to learn. He is studying all his leisure moments and is coming out a thorough convert. His wife is doing well. She is gaining, walks well for her. She is one hundred per cent better than when she came here. Dr. Lay is respected in this institution. He ranks among their physicians. I think they [would] be unwilling to have him leave them. Dr. Lay thinks some of going to N. York City to Dr. Trall's college and attend lectures, obtain a diploma and come out a regular M.D. I believe the Lord's hand is in our coming to this place. We shall learn all we can and try to make a right use of it.

Yesterday we attended the celebration of a wedding conducted in a style, worthy of imitation. Dr.'s only son James was married to Miss Katie Johnson. They were married in their father's cottage and then came to the hall where all the patients were congregated and all the members of the household, also sick patients confined to their rooms were brought out, laid upon sofas and placed in rocking chairs upon the large platform occupied by those who lecture. Some were cripples, some diseased in various ways. The hall was decorated in tasteful style, nothing superfluous or silly. After the bridegroom and bride walked in, then Mrs. Dr. York conducted us to them and gave all who desired an introduction to them. There was a long table arranged with food which was placed upon the plates and passed around to each one. The waiters were constantly passing around with a supply if any more was required. Grapes were passed around in abundance. Everything was liberal, yet plain. They did not even on this occasion depart from their principles of diet which made the thing consistent and admirable. They had extras, graham pudding with dates in it, gems mixed with raisins, custard, apple pie and baked apples, a few other simple things, nothing like fine flour was seen, even upon this extra occasion.

I am afraid as a people we should not carry out our principles as well. After we had eaten Mr. Clark a great musician, sung and played upon an instrument of music, cabinet organ. His song was very amusing, but enough of this.

I don't know when you will get another letter. I meant to send the price of those shoes so if any wanted cheap shoes they could get them for their children. But there are so many hands and so many different prices and kinds of shoes that I think it would be impossible to tell you so that you could understand in regard [to] them. They had better remain until we return, I think.

We hope you will enjoy yourselves well in our absence. Be cheerful, above all things be happy. Look on the bright side and may the blessing of God rest upon you in rich abundance.

In love,
Ellen G. White

Description of Character of Willie C. White, by James C. Jackson, M.D., Our Home, Dansville, N.Y., September 14, 1864 (DF 783, White Estate).

This boy is of the nervous-bilious constitution and gets his peculiarities almost entirely from his father or from his father's mother's side. He is of good stock and good blood — he is "thorough bred." He has got a woman's temperament, and will be kind, loving and courteous. He has an excellent head, and will make a kind, good, true man. He will always make friends wherever he goes. He has a fine physical build throughout, with the exception of his bowels which are too large. He is of scrofulous habit and decidedly predisposed to enlargement of the mesenteric glands, and is in danger, under bad habits of living, of having them so increase in size as to break down his nutritive capacity. He should live upon the simplest food, making fruit an essential or staple of his aliment. He should not be pushed in school, but be permitted to learn largely from out of door things or inductively, cultivating his special senses rather than his abstract capacity for learning until he is twelve or fifteen years of age. If he is cared for with proper heed and propriety, there is no reason why he may not live, but he is liable to diseases of the glandular system, and bad habits of living (indicated by gross food and the use of stimulants and spices) would, in the long run, be very prejudicial to his health.

He has a very fine organization. His bone and brain, muscle and sinew and blood are all of fine quality. If he can be reared to manhood, he will take rank as a lover of whatever is good and true in any community where he may be. He naturally takes to the right and true. Of his own accord he would sustain loving relations to those of his own age or more advanced in years.

His education we could hardly speak of at present until he is older. That needs to be decided by what he will, in years to come, exhibit. He should eat but twice a day have his body kept clean, be brought up to industrious habits, and taught to regularity in their exhibition.

Adelia P. Patten to Sister Lockwood, September 15, 1864, from "Our Home" on the Side of a Mountain (DF 127b, White Estate).

Dear Sister Lockwood:

I don't think it would be serving you very pretty not to write you a letter as soon as opportunity presents itself. I wrote about half a letter to Anna, and now as I have got through with what I had to do on the Instructor I take time to tell you how I stand Cure life. I must say I am interested in hearing Dr. Jackson lecture, but he combines his theology, his medical instruction, his comical nonsense and his theatrical gestures all into his discourses. He flies about like a young man, and will come into the lecture hall with an old blue woolen cap on, which he takes off and puts under his arm and walks along and mounts the rostrum with all the firmness of an experienced lecturer.

We passed examination a day or two ago. As my turn came he set me [in] a chair, and said "My dear, you are sick ain't you." Bro. White gave him a little sketch of our Graham life during the past summer and of what my cares and labors had been. He said that I had evidently overworked, that I must make a decided change, and take a rest or it would tell seriously by and by. He gave advice &c. and said when I got thoroughly initiated to their style of living if I took proper exercise and rest I would enjoy better health than ever before. I have their system about one half of it practically learned.

We have the crackers, they don't furnish "gems" only in case of a wedding or some other extra occasion. They don't have salt. The pudding is thin and fresh squash and cabbage without salt or vinegar and oh such times. I had a little salt dish this noon and wanted to pocket the salt that was left and as none of our company had an envelope so had Bro. W[hite] tip it onto his passbook.

Yours in haste and love,
Adelia P. Patten

APPENDIX 3

The Trial of Elder I. Dammon

In February 1845, less than four months after the Great Disappointment, Israel Dammon, a Millerite elder, went on trial in Piscataquis County, Maine, for vagrancy and disturbing the peace. During the trial some three dozen witnesses testified about the activities of Dammon and his Millerite friends, which included kissing, touching, crawling, and shouting. Ellen G. White later condemned such post-Disappointment "fanaticism," but the trial record portrays Ellen Harmon and her future husband, James White, as enthusiastic participants. Ellen appears as a young trance medium called "Imitation of Christ," who for hours lay on the floor with a pillow under her head, receiving and relating her visions. Although stories about the trial appeared in a number of newspapers, and thus no doubt contributed to the public's association of Millerism with fanaticism, knowledge of the trial had long faded from memory when Frederick W. Hoyt discovered the following account in the *Piscataquis Farmer* for March 7, 1845:

IN OFFERING THE PUBLIC the following report I feel it due to them as well as myself, to make a few remarks. When I volunteered to do it, I had no doubt but that the examination would have been gone through within the course of a few hours. Judge then, what must be my surprise on finding the Court House filled to overflowing, and having it occupy such a length of time. To the witnesses I will say, I have abridged your testimony as much as possible, and have omitted much of the most unimportant part, in order to shorten the work, but have endeavored in no case to misrepresent you, and if you find an error, I beg you to impute it to my head, instead of heart. — To the reader I will remark, that much of the testimony was drawn out by questions, and I have omitted the questions in all cases where it could be dispensed with and shorten the work. To all, I, offer it as an imperfect and impartial report. In consequence of my total inexperience, being but a laboring man, I should shrink from publishing it, but from the urgent solicitation of others. Thanking the Court for the favor of a seat, by them, and the Court and Counsel for the use of their minutes, I sign myself this once THE REPORTER.

N.B. I have preserved the language of the witnesses as much as possible.

Monday, Feb. 17, 1845

STATE OF MAINE
vs.
ISRAEL DAMMON.

Prisoner arraigned before Moses Swett, Esq. of Foxcroft, associated by Seth Lee, Esq. of Atkinson, on the following complaint, to wit.

To Charles P. Chandler, Esq. one of the Justices of the Peace within and for the County of Piscataquis.

"HARTFORD J. ROWE, of Dover, in the Co. of Piscataquis, Yeoman, upon his oath complains, that Israel Dammon, Commorant of Atkinson, in said County, Idler, is, and for several days last past, has been a vagabond and idle person, going about in the town of Atkinson, aforesaid, in the county aforesaid, from place to place, begging: — that he the said Israel Dammon is a common railer or brawler, neglecting his calling, or employment, misspending his earnings, and does not provide for the support of himself [or] family & against the peace of the State of Maine, and contrary to form of Statute in such cases made and provided.

He therefore prays that the said I. Dammon, may be apprehended and held to answer to said complaint and dealt with relative to the same as law and justice may require."

Appendix 3

Plead Not Guilty.

Court adjourned to one o'clock, P.M.

Opened agreeably to adjournment.

C. P. Chandler, H. G. O. Morison, for State. J. S. Holmes, for Respondent.

Opened by Chandler. Cited chap. 178, sec. 9, Revised Statutes. Adjourned to Court House.

Ebenezer Blethen sworn. Have been in the house three times, saw nothing out of the way in elder Dammon. Have seen others. Objected to by Holmes. Confine your remarks to prisoner, he can in no ways be accountable for the conduct of others, and I object to any testimony except what goes to show what respondent has said or done, as wholly irrelevant.

Question by Chandler. Who was the presiding elder at the meeting?

Ans. Elder Dammon presided and took the lead of the meetings that I attended.

Chandler and Morison. The meetings appear to be elder Dammon's meetings — he took the lead and guided them, and is accountable for any public misconduct, and ought to check it: we propose to show the character of his meetings, to show the character of the man.

By the Court. You may relate any thing that took place at the meetings, where the respondent was presiding elder.

Witness. The first meeting I attended was two weeks ago yesterday — saw people setting on the floor, and laying on the floor; Dammon setting on floor; they were leaning on each other. It did not have the appearance of a religious meeting.

Cross examination. Saw nothing like licentiousness — there was exhortation and prayer each evening. Was there last time after part of my family.

J. W. E. Harvey, sworn. Have attended their meetings two days and four evenings. First meeting lasted eight days — have known Dammon six weeks — Dammon, White and Hall were leaders. Dammon said the sinners were going to hell in two days. They were hugging and kissing each other — Dammon would lay on the floor, then jump up — they would frequently go into another room. Dammon has no means to support himself that I know of. The meeting appeared very irreligious — have seen him sit on the floor with a woman between his legs and his arms around her. Cross examined. The room they went into was a back room; dont know what was in it — I was in two rooms where there was a fire. In the back room they said the world's people must not go. Dammon said the meeting was to be a private meeting and they wanted no one to come unless they believed as he did in the Advent doctrine. I did go considerably — if the meetings were religious ones I thought I had a right to go to them — I went to satisfy myself what was done. I had no hostile feeling against them. I think they held the first meeting a fortnight. Dammon said he wanted no one to attend their meetings unless they believed in the advent doctrine.

Wm. C. Crosby, Esq. sworn. I was at the meeting last Saturday night, from about 7 o'clock to 9. There was a woman on the floor who lay on her back with a pillow under her head; she would occasionally arouse up and tell a vision which she said was revealed to her. They would at times all be talking at once, halloing at the top of their voices; some of them said there was too much sin there. After the cessation of the noise, Dammon got up and was more coherent — he complained of those that came there who did not believe in the advent doctrine. At one time Dammon said there was hogs there not belonging to the band, and pointed at me, and said, I mean you, Sir. Subsequently he addressed me again — said, you can't drive us out of town; he stared me in the face and said, I am an honest man, or I could not look you in the face, and you have hell's brass or you could not look me in the face. Dammon said if he was owner of the house he would compel all unbelievers to leave it — they were setting and laying on the floor promiscuously and were exceedingly noisy. Cross examined. Did he not say if there was any there who did not come for instruction he did not want them there. Ans. That is not what he said — he pointed to me and said he meant you — I never was more pointedly addressed in my life — we stood 5 or 6 feet apart, most of the men were on the floor — most of the women in chairs — Do not know how long Dammon has been in town.

Thomas Proctor sworn. Saw the prisoner last Saturday — was present when he was taken; know nothing of the meetings myself.

Moses Gerrish, sworn. I have never attended any of their meetings, when the prisoner was present.

Appendix 3

Loton Lambert, sworn. They were singing when I arrived — after singing they sat down on the floor — Dammon said a sister had a vision to relate — a woman on the floor then related her vision. Dammon said all other denominations were wicked — they were liars, whoremasters, murderers, etc. — he also run upon all such as were not believers with him. He ordered us off — we did not go. The woman that lay on the floor relating visions, was called by Elder Dammon and others, imitation of Christ. Dammon called us hogs and devils, and said if he was the owner of the house he would drive us off — the one that they called imitation of Christ, told Mrs. Woodbury and others, that they must forsake all their friends or go to hell. Imitation of Christ, as they called her, would lay on the floor a while, then rise up and call upon some one and say she had a vision to relate to them, which she would relate; there was one girl that they said must be baptised that night or she must go to hell; she wept bitterly and wanted to see her mother first; they told her she must leave her mother or go to hell — one voice said, let her go to hell. She finally concluded to be baptised. Imitation of Christ told her vision to a cousin of mine, that she must be baptised that night or go to hell — she objected, because she had once been baptised. Imitation of Christ was said to be a woman from Portland. A woman that they called Miss Baker, said the devil was here, and she wanted to see him — she selected me and said, you are the devil, and will go to hell. I told her she wasn't my judge. Mr. Ayer then clinched me and tried to put me out door. I told him we had not come to disturb the meeting. The vision woman called Joel Doore, said he had doubted, and would not be baptised again — she said Br. Doore don't go to hell. Doore kneeled to her feet and prayed. Miss Baker and a man went into the bed room — subsequently heard a voice in the room hallo Oh! the door was opened — I saw into the room — she was on the bed — he was hold of her; they came out of the bed room hugging each other, she jumping up and would throw her legs between his. Miss Baker went to Mr. Doore and said, you have refused me before, he said he had — they then kissed each other — she said "that feels good" — just before they went to the water to baptise, Miss Baker went into the bed room with a man they called elder White — saw him help her on to the bed — the light was brought out and door closed. I did not see either of them afterwards. Once I was in the other room talking with my cousin. Dammon and others came into the room and stopped our discourse, and called her sister and me the devil. Imitation of Christ lay on the floor during the time they went down to the water to baptise, and she continued on the floor until I left, which was between the hours of 12 and 1 o'clock at night.

Cross examined. Answer. The visionist lay down on the floor I should think about 7 o'clock — she lay there from that time until I left. Dammon and others called her Imitation of Christ. Part of the time Dammon was down on the floor on his back — can't say certainly who first said she was Imitation of Christ, but can say Dammon repeatedly said so — Dammon said Christ revealed to her and she to others. I am not acquainted with elder White. They called him Eld. White. They said if the Almighty had any thing to say he revealed it to her, and she acted as mediator.

Wm. Ricker, sworn. Know elder Dammon — I went to attend their meeting once: they told me there would be none — I asked them where it would be on the next Sabbath? they told me they know not where; but they did not admit any but the advent band. I asked Dammon if that was Christ's religion? he said it is ours.

Leonard Downes, sworn. — Went to meeting with Loten Lambert, and kept with him; heard him testify, and know what he has related to be true. He omitted one thing. I saw Dammon kiss other people's wives. Witness underwent a severe cross examination, in which his testimony was so near a repetition of Mr. Lambert's, that it is by me, considered useless to copy it.

Wm. C. Crosby re-examined. I saw no kissing, but heard about it. I did not stay late, went about 7, left about 9 o'clock. After the visionist called them up she told them they doubted. Her object seemed to be to convince them they must not doubt. — Dammon called the churches whoremasters, liars, thieves, scoundrels, wolves in sheep's clothing, murderers, etc. He said read the Star. By spells it was the most noisy assembly I ever attended — there was no order or regularity, nor any thing that resembled any other meeting I ever attended — Dammon seemed to have the lead and the most art. I don't say Dammon shouted the loudest; I think some others stronger in the lungs than he.

Dea. James Rowe, sworn. I was at Ayer's a short time last Saturday evening — Elder Dammon found fault with us for coming to his

Appendix 3

meeting — he spoke of other denominations as Esq. Crosby has just testified — said the church members were the worst people in the world. I have been young, and now am old, and of all the places I ever was in, I never saw such a confusion, not even in a drunken frolic. Dammon stood up on the floor and said, I am going to stand here — and while I stand here, they can't hurt you, neither men nor devils can't hurt you. Cross examined. He said all churches, made no distinction. I put no meaning to what he said, I only state what he did say. I have been acquainted with the prisoner 20 or 30 years; his character was good until recently.

Jeremiah B. Green, sworn. I attended an afternoon meeting a fortnight ago yesterday — they had an exhortation and prayer in the evening — saw men wash men's feet, and women wash women's feet — they had dishes of water — elder Dammon was the presiding elder — I saw Dammon kiss Mrs. Osborn.

Ebenezer Trundy, sworn. I was at meeting week before last, — I heard Dammon say "God's a coming! God's a coming!!" Mr. Boobar was telling of going into the woods to labor — Dammon said he ought not to go. Boobar said he had a family to support and was poor. Dammon told him he must live on them that had property, and if God did not come then we must all go to work together.

Joseph Moulton, sworn. When I went to arrest prisoner, they shut the door against me. Finding I could not gain access to him without, I burst open the door. I went to the prisoner and took him by the hand and told him my business. A number of women jumped on to him — he clung to them, and they to him. So great was the resistance, that I with three assistants, could not get him out. I remained in the house and sent for more help; after they arrived we made a second attempt with the same result — I again sent for more help — after they arrived we overpowered them and got him out door in custody. We were resisted by both men and women. Can't describe the place — it was one continued shout.

Wm. C. Crosby, Esq. — called again.

Prisoner has been reported to have been there about a fortnight with no visible means of support.

J. W. E. Harvey, re-examined.

Prisoner has been there considerable. I know of no means he has of support, other than to live on his followers.

T. Proctor, re-examined —

Prisoner has been reported as a man who has no means of support — I do not know of his having any.

Jacob Martin sworn: It is the common report that the prisoner is living upon his followers. I have attended no meetings of theirs. Have seen a number of sleighs there, and fifteen or twenty strangers.

Benjamin Smith, Esq., Selectman of Atkinson sworn: I have been called upon by the citizens of Atkinson to interfere and put a stop to these meetings — they gave us a reason, that the defendant and others were living upon certain citizens of said town — and that they were liable to become town charge. I started to-day to go there, but learned that the prisoner had been arrested and that the others had dispersed.

Here the government stopped. Court adjourned to half past six o'clock.

Evening — Respondent's witnesses.

James Ayer, Jr., affirmed: The most of the meetings were at my house. I have generally attended them — sometimes I was out. I have heard the testimony on the part of the State. Some things stated I do not recollect. I was there last Saturday evening — saw no kissing. I agree with Crosby and Lambert substantially. I understood prisoner to say there were members of the churches who he referred to instead of the whole. Saw the woman with a pillow under her head — her name is Miss Ellen Harmon, of Portland. I heard nothing said by her or others about imitation of Christ. I saw Miss Baker laying on the floor. I saw her fall. Saw Miss Baker and sister Osborn go into the bed-room — sister Osborn helped her on to the bed, came out and shut the door. There was no man in the bed-room that evening. I heard the noise in the bed-room — brother Wood of Orrington and I went in; asked her what was the matter, she made no reply, and I went out. Brother Wood assisted her off of the bed, and helped her out — she appeared in distress. She told brother Doore she was distressed on his account — was afraid he would loose his soul, and advised him to be baptised. Did not see them kiss each other. It is a part of our faith to kiss each other — brothers kiss sisters and sisters kiss brothers, I think we have bible authority for that. I understood the prisoner to say, there was an account in the Star of a Deacon who had killed seven men. The reason of our kneeling, I consider an object of humiliation.

Appendix 3

Cross examined. — I know nothing about Miss Harmon's character. I did not say there was no kissing — I saw none. Did not hear her called imitation of Christ. Elder Dammon has had no other business, but to attend meetings. He and another man from Exeter, came with a young girl. Dammon said he had a spiritual wife and he was glad of it. I went to Mr. Lambert and said if he disturbed the meeting, he must go out door. We went to the water after eleven o'clock — brother Dammon baptized two. I know nothing about sister Baker's character — seen her at meeting in Orrington. I understood sister Harmon had a vision at Portland, and was travelling through the country relating it.

Job Moody affirmed: I was at meeting Saturday evening. Brother Dammon said in relation to other churches they were bad enough; said they were corrupt; he spoke of the Star — he did say they were thieves, etc. I am not certain, but think he said that evening there was exceptions. Sister Harmon would lay on the floor in a trance, and the Lord would reveal their cases to her, and she to them.

By the Court.

Answer. Mr. Dammon repeatedly urged upon us the necessity of quitting all labor. Kissing is a salutation of love; I greet them so — we have got positive scripture for it — I reside in Exeter.

Here the witness was told he might take his seat. He said I have some testimony in relation to brother Dammon's character, if I am not a going to be called again. He then stated that he had been acquainted with brother Dammon five or six years, and his character was good. He works part of the time, and preaches a part of the time. I have been serving the Lord and hammering against the devil of late.

Isley Osborn affirmed: I know nothing bad in brother Dammon's character. He believes there is good, bad and indifferent in all churches — he thinks it best to come out from them, because there is so many that has fallen from their holy position. — Do not recollect hearing him use the expressions about churches they have sworn to, but have heard him use as strong language against them. Do not call sister Harmon imitation of Christ. They lose their strength and fall on the floor. The Lord communicates to them through a vision, so we call it the Lord. Brother White did not go into the bed-room, nor any other man.

Cross-examined: She told them their cases had been made known to her by the Lord, and if they were not baptized that evening, they would go to hell. We believed her, and brother Dammon and I advised them to be baptised. Brother Dammon thought it best to keep the meetings secret, so they would not crowd in. Hold to kissing — have scripture exhortation for that. Sister Baker has a good character — the wickedest man in Orrington says she has a good character, and that's enough to establish any character, when the worst man admits it. (roar of laughter) We wish to go through the ordnance of washing feet in secret. Did not see any kissing, but presume their was, as it is a part of our faith. Think Esq. Crosby's testimony correct. By Court: —

Answer. Elder Dammon does advise us to quit all work.

Abraham Pease, affirmed. Reside in Exeter, prisoner's character is as good as any man in Exeter. He has a small farm, and small family. He is a reformation preacher — reformation has followed his preaching.

Gardner Farmer, affirmed: Reside in Exeter — prisoner provides well for his family. He has been to my house, and I to his — he always behaves well. I saw him in Atkinson a fortnight ago last Tuesday.

Court adjourned to Tuesday morning 9 o'clock.

Tuesday, 18.

Jacob Mason, affirmed: Reside in Garland. Brother Dammon said the churches were of that description — said they were lyers, rogues, &c. I did not understand him to include all, but individuals. Sister Baker's character is good. Do not recollect of brother Gallison using any compulsion, to make his daughter go forward in baptism. I saw elder White after sister Baker went into the bed-room, near sister Harmon in a trance — some of the time he held her head. She was in a vision, part of the time insensible. Saw nothing improper in brother Dammon that evening. I never knew him a beggar, or wasting his time.

Cross-examined: Do not know who it was that went into the bed-room with sister Baker — he was a stranger to me; he soon came out. Can't say how soon he went in again. I have heard Crosby testify, and think him correct. I thought her visions were from God — she would describe out their cases correct. She described mine correct. I saw kissing out door, but not in the house. A part of the time we sat on the floor — both men and women promiscuously. I saw no man go into the bed-room. They wash feet in the evening. It is a practice in our order to kiss, on our meeting each other. Sister Harmon was not called imitation of Christ to my knowledge. I think I should have heard it if she was. I believe in visions. Sister Harmon is 18 or 19 years of age; she is from Portland.

Joel Doore, affirmed: Reside in Atkinson — elder Dammon said there was bad characters in the churches; I did not understand him to say all. He preaches louder than most people; no more noisy than common preachers of this faith. The vision woman would lay looking up when she came out of her trance — she would point to some one, and tell them their cases, which she said was from the Lord. She told a number of visions that evening. Brother Gallison's daughter wanted to see her mother before she was baptised, but finally concluded to be baptised without seeing her. Sister Baker got up off the floor, and went to Lambert to talk with him. I saw no more of her, until I heard a noise in the bedroom — they went and got her out, as the other witnesses have stated. After she came out, she said she had a message to me. She said I had thought hard of her, (I acknowledged I had) but I became satisfied of my error, and fellowshiped her. We kissed each other with the holy kiss — I think elder White was not in the bed-room that evening; but I don't know how many, nor who were there. The girls that was baptised were 17 years old, one of them had been baptised before. We have scripture enough for every thing that was done. There was not one tenth part of the noise Saturday evening, that there generally is at the meetings I attend. As far as I am acquainted with elder Dammon, I consider him a moral good man.

Cross examined. When she kissed me, she said there was light ahead. We believe her (Miss Baker's) visions genuine. We believe Miss Harmon's genuine — t'was our understanding that their visions were from God. Miss Hammond [sic] told five visions Saturday night. I did not tell any person yesterday that it was necessary to have anyone in the room with her to bring out her trances. I did engage counsel in this case to defend the prisoner.

John H. Doore, sworn. I was not at meeting Saturday evening. I belong to the society, and have seen nothing out of character in anyone. Don't consider elder Dammon a bad man — he a man I highly esteem. My daughter was baptised Saturday evening — she has been baptised before. I have seen both men and women crawl across the floor on their hands and knees.

George S. Woodbury, sworn. I am a believer in the Advent doctrine — I have attended every one of the meetings in Atkinson.

[This witness was very lengthy in his testimony, both on examination and cross examination. It amounts to the same as the preceding witnesses for the defence with the following additions.]

He thinks elder White was not in the bed room, but others were in. We don't acknowledge any leaders, but speak according to the impulse. The elders baptise. I believe in Miss Harmon's visions, because she told my wife's feelings correctly. It is my impression that prisoner kissed my wife. I believe the world will come to an end within two months — prisoner preaches so. I believe this is the faith of the band. It was said, and I believe, that sisters Harmon and Baker's revelations as much as though they came from God. Sister Harmon said to my wife and the girls if they did not do as she said, they would go to hell. My wife and Dammon passed across the floor on their hands and knees. Some man did go into the bed room. Heard brother Dammon say the gift of healing the sick lay in the church.

By the Court.

Ans. Elder Dammon advises us not to work, because there is enough to live on until the end of the world.

John Gallison, affirmed. [Chandler observed that he had thought of objecting to this witness on the ground of insanity, but upon reflection, he would let him proceed, as he believed it would sufficiently appear in the course of the examination.]

I have been acquainted with elder Dammon as a Freewill elder a number of years. He asked Dammon how long it was. D. answered 6 years. I have been at his house frequently — every thing was in order and in its proper place. I have attended every meeting. I have seen some laying on the floor, two or more at a time — have seen nothing bad in the meetings. [Witness here described the position Miss Harmon lay in on the floor, when she was in a trance, and offered to lay down and show the Court if they wished to see. Court waived it.]

Witness related the visions similar to the other witnesses, but more unintelligible.

Did not hear her called Imitation of Christ. I know she won't, for we don't worship idols.

Cross examined. I believe in visions, and perfectly understand that, but suppose we are not before an Ecclesiastical Council. — Elder Dammon does not believe as he used to. [Witness read from the Bible.] We do wash each other's feet — do creep on the floor very decently. I think he has baptised about eleven, but can't say certain how many — I have the privilege of knowing how they behave as well as anyone else. I have no doubt sister Harmon's visions were from God — she told my daughter so. I expect the end of the world every day. I was in favor of my daughter being baptised — I could not see ahead to see the devil's rabble coming, but since they have come, I am certain we did just right.

Abel S. Boobar, affirmed. [Most of the testimony of this witness was a repetition of what others have testified to, of which the reader I think must be weary]

I did not see White go into the bed room and Miss Baker — heard the noise in the bed room. Others did go in. Elder D said the churches were in a fallen state, and he had rather risk himself in the hands of the Almighty as a nonprofessor, than to be in the place of some of the churches. I believe fully in the faith. [Witness affirmed the story of kissing, rolling on the floor, and washing of feet.]

Joshua Burnham, sworn. I have known Miss Dorinda Baker from five years of age — her character is good — she is now 23 or 24 yrs of age. She is a sickly girl, her father has expended $1000 in doctoring her. I was at the meeting Saturday night — it was appointed for the lady to tell her visions.

Adjourned to half past one o'clock.

Levi M. Doore, sworn. I have attended more than half of the meetings — my brother's testimony is correct — agree also with Mr. Boobar.

Question by Respondent. Answer. Elder Dammon's mode of worship now is similar to what it used to be.

Cross examined by Morison. Did they use to sit on the floor?

Ans. No. Did they use to lay or crawl on the floor? Ans. No. Did they use to kiss each other? Ans. No. Did they use to go into the bed room? Ans. No. Did they use to tell visions? Ans. No.

By Morison. Why do you say that his mode of worship is similar to what it used to be? Because he preaches similar. Did he use to preach that the end of the world was at hand, and baptise in the dead hours of night? Ans. No. The reason we sit on the floor is to convene more people — sometimes we take some in our laps, but not male and female. Don't know of br. D. spending money uselessly. I am a believer. Sometimes we sit on the floor for formality. Our faith don't hold it to be essential. [Witness repeated the mode of kissing, visions, etc. similar to the others] I never heard br. Dammon say he wished to destroy the marriage covenant. [Respondent here re-examined a number of witnesses, all of whom testified that he used his wife well, and appeared to love her.]

Stephen Fish, Exeter, sworn. I attended the meetings at Atkinson, last summer — have attended most all of the Quarterly Meetings for seven years — have been to elder Dammon's house, and he to mine — he provides well in his house — he has always opposed the mode of paying the ministry by regular salary. [Here the defence closed.]

WITNESSES FOR STATE.

Ebenezer Lambert, Esq. sworn. Last Sunday evening Loton Lambert told me the story of the meeting the evening before — he related as he testified yesterday almost verbatim.

John Bartlett, of Garland, sworn. I have heard the respondent say that one of their band was as near to him as another — he considered them all alike. It is the general opinion in our town that the prisoner is a disturber of the peace, and ought to be taken care of. I have been acquainted with Elder Dammon seven years — his character was always good until within about 6 weeks.

Loten Lambert re-examined. He affirmed all his former testimony — does not know elder White, but Joel Doore told me it was White that was in the bed room with Miss Baker.

Cross examined. There was nothing to obstruct my views — the man had on a dark colored short jacket, and I think light pantaloons.

Leonard Downes re-examined. Did see Miss Baker come out of the bed room with a man he had his arm around her — see her go in

Appendix 3

with a man and shut the door. He had on a short jacket, dark colored, and light colored pantaloons — saw her kiss Mr. Doore — she said "that feels good."

Thomas Proctor re examined. Prisoner stated to me that Miss Baker had an exercise in the bed room, and he went in and helped her out. Cross examined. I have said I wished they were broken up, and wished somebody would go and do it. I have said elder Hall ought to be tarred and feathered if he was such a character as I heard he was. I was at one meeting, but as to divine worship there was none. They told us they allowed none there but believers.

A. S. Bartlett, Esq. sworn. Yesterday I saw Mr Joel Doore and Loton Lambert conversing together. I went to them — I heard Doore say to him, it was Elder White that was in the bed room with Miss Baker — Lambert said that was what I wanted to know. I so understood, and think I am not mistaken. I also heard Doore say there was a noise in the bed room.

Elder Flavel Bartlett, sworn. I think Prisoner does not belong to the Free Will Baptist Church. He is not in fellowship with them.

Joseph Knights of Garland, sworn. I attended one of Dammon's meetings in Garland, he behaved well until meeting was over. After meeting was over I saw him hugging and kissing a girl. It is the common report in Garland, that he is a disturber of the peace.

Plyn Clark, sworn. I attended their meeting a week ago last Wednesday or Thursday night. [This witness gave a general character of the meeting as described by others.]

I heard one hallo out "I feel better" — others said "good enough." I think the whole character of the meeting was demoralizing.

J. W. E. Harvey, called. I have attended the meetings a number of times — I have seen prisoner on the floor with a woman between his legs — I have seen them in groups hugging and kissing one another. I went there once on an errand — Dam[mon] halloed out "Good God Almighty, drive the Devil away." I once saw elder Hall with his boots off, and the women would go and kiss his feet. One girl made a smack, but did not hit his foot with her lips. Hall said "he that is ashamed of me before men, him will I be ashamed of before my father and the holy angels." She then gave his feet a number of kisses.

Joel Doore, Jr. called for the defence. I have heard brother

The Trial of Elder I. Dammon

Dammon preach that the day of grace was over with sinners. Respondent said "that is my belief."

Levi M. Doore, called. Br. Wood was dressed in light pants and dark jacket.

Joel Doore, Jr. called. Br. Wood had light pants and dark jacket.

Abel Ayer called. Brother Wood went to the baptism and was about all the evening.

James Boobar called. Sister Baker and br. Wood were about all the evening. Elder White had a frock coat and dark pants.

Prisoner opened his defence & cited Luke 7 chapter 36 verse — John 13 chapter — Last chapter in Romans — Philippians 4th chapter — 1st Thessalonians 5th chapter. Holmes followed with the defence. Court adjourned one hour. [Holmes closed the defence with signal ability. Chandler commenced in behalf of the State. Cited 178 chapter 9th and 10th sections Revised Statutes; he dwelt upon the law; after which

Morison summoned up the testimony and closed with a few brief and appropriate remarks.

Elder Dammon again rose for further defence. Court indulged him to speak. He read 126th Psalm, and the 50th Psalm. He argued that the day of grace had gone by, that the believers were reduced; but that there was too many yet, and that the end of the world would come within a week.

The Court after consultation sentenced the prisoner to the House of Correction for the space of Ten Days, From this judgment Respondent appealed.

Tuesday morning the prisoner having taken his seat, rose just as the Court came in, and shouted Glory to the strength of his lungs.

Tuesday afternoon, after the Court had come in and were waiting for the counsel, the prisoner and his witnesses asked permission, and sung as follows:

"COME OUT OF HER, MY PEOPLE."
See Rev. 18th Ch. 4th V.
By JOHN CRAIG.

While I was down in Egypt's land,
I heard my Saviour was at hand;

Appendix 3

The midnight cry was sounding,
And I wanted to be free,
So I left my former brethren
To sound the jubilee.

They said that I had better stay
And go with them in their old way;
But they scoff at my Lord's coming
With them I could not agree,
And I left their painted synagogue
To sound the jubilee.

Then soon I joined the Advent Band,
Who just came out from Egypt's land;
They were on the road to Canaan,
A blest praying company,
And with them I am proclaiming
That this year's the jubilee.

They call us now a noisy crew,
And say they hope we'll soon fall thro';
But we now are growing stronger,
Both in love and unity,
Since we left old mystic Babylon
To sound the jubilee.

We're now united in one band,
Believing Christ is just at hand
To reward his faithful children
Who are glad their Lord to see;
Bless the Lord our souls are happy
While we sound the jubilee.

Though opposition waxes strong,
Yet still the battle won't be long;
Our blessed Lord is coming,
"His glory we shall see;"
Keep up good courage brethren —
This year's the jubilee.

The Trial of Elder I. Dammon

If Satan comes to tempt your mind,
Then meet him with these blessed lines,
Saying, "Get behind me, Satan,"
I have naught to do with thee;
I have got my soul converted,
And I'll sound the jubilee.

The battle is not to the strong,
The weak may sing the conqueror's song;
I've been through the fiery furnace,
And no harm was done to me,
I came out with stronger evidence
This year's the jubilee.

A little longer here below,
And home to glory we will go
I believe it! I believe it!
Hallelujah, I am free
From all sectarian prejudice —
This year's the jubilee.

We'll soon remove to that blest shore,
And shout and sing forever more,
Where the wicked cannot enter
To disturb our harmony;
But we'll wear the crowns of glory
With our God eternally.

APPENDIX 4

The Secret 1919 Bible Conferences

Four years after Ellen White died, a select group of about sixty-five Seventh-day Adventist church officers, editors, and educators — not including Mrs. White's son Willie — gathered in closed session in Takoma Park, Maryland, for a special Bible Conference, held July 1-19, 1919. Afterward many participants stayed on for a confidential Bible and History Teachers' Council, which lasted through August 1. Much of the discussion at the conferences focused on such prophetic topics as "The 1260 Years of Daniel 7" and "The Beast Power of Revelation." But during the last two days of the second conference delegates took up the "delicate question" of Ellen White's authority as an interpreter of the Bible and as a historian. Such open discussion of the prophetess was unprecedented. As General Conference President Arthur G. Daniells said during a mid-month evening lecture on "The Spirit of Prophecy," the widely used code for Mrs. White and her writings, "I do not take this up through the Review nor in camp-meetings, or in other public meetings,

---

Sources: Transcripts of the conferences are now available on the Web site of the Office of Archives and Statistics, General Conference of Seventh-day Adventists. Additional documentation comes from two unpublished manuscripts, also available through the Office of Archives and Statistics: Robert W. Olson, "The 1919 Bible Conference and Bible and History Teachers' Council," September 24, 1979; and Bert Haloviak, "In the Shadow of the 'Daily': Background and Aftermath of the 1919 Bible and History Teachers' Conference," November 14, 1979.

or personally with individuals unless something arises that calls for it. But on this occasion I have the privilege of speaking from the heart to the members of the General Conference Committee and the men connected with our schools. . . ." Unfortunately, after reminiscing briefly about his close association with James and Ellen White, he instructed the stenographer not to transcribe the rest of his talk. Two weeks later, however, he freely joined in a two-day airing of questions related to the nature of Mrs. White's inspiration. The candid dialog left some attendees shaken. One worried minister described the "secret Bible Council" as "the most unfortunate thing our people ever did." Some frustrated delegates, including three from Washington Missionary College, soon severed their connection with the church. Despite impassioned calls to educate church members on the subject, the stenographic record of the conference remained, as Daniells had recommended, locked up in a vault — forgotten until the mid-1970s, when the church archivist discovered and released it.

"The Use of the Spirit of Prophecy in Our Teaching of Bible and History"

July 30, 1919

W. E. Howell [secretary, General Conference Department of Education]: Our topic for this hour, as arranged in the program, is "The Use of the Spirit of Prophecy in our Teaching of Bible and History." Elder Daniells is here with us this morning to fulfill his promise to our teachers that he would give us a talk along this line, and I am sure the opportunity of considering this question further will be greatly appreciated.

A. G. Daniells [president, General Conference]: I have been a little uncertain in my own mind as to just what line it would be best to follow. There is so much in this that it can not be fully presented in one talk, and I would regret missing the mark and taking up that which would not be of most interest to you; and so I finally decided that I

Appendix 4

would prefer to have a round-table talk. I would prefer to have you question me and then I would try to answer such points as are of most interest to you. I may not be able to give another talk here, and you probably would not have the time, and so I would like to make this hour most profitable. I will present one or two points as briefly as I can to start with, and then I will just open the way for questions.

First of all I want to reiterate what I stated in the talk I gave some evenings ago on this subject, — that I do not want to say one word that will destroy confidence in this gift to this people. I do not want to create doubts. I do not want to in any way depreciate the value of the writings of the spirit of prophecy. I have no doubt in my own mind. I do not know whether every man can say that or not, but I can say it with all honesty. I have had perplexities through the forty years I have been in the ministry. I have found things similar to that to which Peter referred in Paul's writings, — hard to be understood. You know Peter said that, and I have had personal testimonies come to me that I could not understand. That is a remarkable thing, isn't it, for a man to get such a message as that? But that is what nearly all doubters hark back to when they get away from us, — they got a testimony they could not understand and believe. I could not understand then, but time has helped me to understand; and I have concluded that we do not see from the Lord's standpoint, and we do not know as much as the Lord knows about ourselves and so when He reveals things to us that we do not understand, it is because He knows more about us and our tendency and dangers than we do, ourselves.

The first one I got that threw me into confusion charged me very strongly with sort of — well, I will put it in the worst form — a tendency to domineer over my brethren in administrative matters, not giving them the freedom of mind and thought that they were entitled to. I did not understand that. It did not seem so. I asked some of my good friends, and they said they never had felt it, and that threw me into worse trouble. Even some members of the Committee had never seen that. What was I to do? They were not the right men for me to get my information from. I soon found that there were some men who believed that the message was right. Inside of a year or so I found a very strong tendency, under a bit of nervousness and weariness, to do that very thing; so I got the message out and reread it prayerfully, and acknowledged it to the Lord, and I am trying all the time to guard against any domineering spirit, for I think it is a most abominable thing for a man in office to begin to lord it over people who are not in office; but it is in human nature. You have heard the story of the Irishman who was promoted to the position of foreman of a section gang. The next morning he went out and said to one of the men: "Timothy O'Brien, come here." When the man came, he said to him: "I discharge ye this morning, not because I have anything agin ye, but to show me authority." [Laughter] He had been put in office, and the very first thing he wanted to do was to show his authority. That is human nature, but it is not Christianity; and it is to be abominated and avoided by everyone who gets office, whether president of the General Conference, or principal of a school, or head of a department in a school. All should avoid that and give every man his rights and freedom and liberty.

As I said, I have met things that were hard to be understood, but time has helped me to understand them, and I can honestly say this morning that I go along in this movement without any doubts in my mind. When I take positions differing from other men, that is not proof that I am a doubter. I may be a doubter of their views or their interpretation, but that does not make me a doubter of the spirit of prophecy. I may differ with a man about his interpretation of the Bible, but that does not make me a doubter of the Bible. But there are men who just hold me right up as a doubter of the Testimonies because I take the position that the Testimonies are not verbally inspired, and that they have been worked up by the secretaries and put in proper grammatical shape. A few years ago a man came onto the nominating committee and wanted me kept out of the presidency because I did not believe the Testimonies were verbally inspired. That was because I differed with him on theory and interpretation; but I am the one to say whether I doubt the Testimonies, am I not? [Voices: Yes, yes!] And so are you. I want to leave the impression that I am not trying in any way to put any doubts in your mind. And O, I would feel terribly to have this denomination lose its true, genuine, proper faith in this gift that God gave to this church in these messages that have come to us. I want that we shall stay by this clear through to the end. [Amens]

Now with reference to the evidences: I differ with some of the brethren who have put together proofs or evidences of the genuineness of this gift, in this respect, — I believe that the strongest proof is found in the fruits of this gift to the church, not in physical and outward demonstrations. For instance, I have heard some ministers preach, and have seen it in writing, that Sister White once carried a heavy Bible — I believe they said it weighed forty pounds — on her outstretched hand, and looking up toward the heavens quoted texts and turned the leaves over and pointed to the texts, with her eyes toward the heavens. I do not know whether that was ever done or not. I am not sure. I did not see it, and I do not know that I ever talked with anybody that did see it. But, brethren, I do not count that sort of thing as a very great proof. I do not think that is the best kind of evidence. If I were a stranger in an audience, and heard a preacher enlarging on that, I would have my doubts. That is, I would want to know if he saw it. He would have to say, No, he never did. Then I would ask, "Did you ever see the man that did see it?" And he would have to answer, "No, I never did."

Well, just how much of that is genuine, and how much has crawled into the story? I do not know. But I do not think that is the kind of proof we want to use. It has been a long time since I have brought forward this sort of thing, — no breath in the body, and the eyes wide open. That may have accompanied the exercise of this gift in the early days, but it surely did not in the latter days, and yet I believe this gift was just as genuine and exercised just the same through these later years as in the early years.

C. P. Bollman [managing editor, *Liberty*]: Isn't the same thing true of the Bible? Can't you size it up and believe it because of its fruit, what it does, and not because of the supernatural things related in it?

A. G. Daniells: Yes. For instance, I would not take the story of David killing a lion and a bear, or of Samson killing a lion, and herald that to unbelievers or strangers as proof that the Bible was inspired, especially about Samson. Here is the way I would want to teach the boys and girls: I would want to begin with the beginning of this movement. At that time here was a gift given to this person; and with that gift to that individual, at the same time, came this movement of the three-fold message. They came right together in the same year.

That gift was exercised steadily and powerfully in the development of this movement. The two were inseparably connected, and there was instruction given regarding this movement in all its phases through this gift, clear through for seventy years.

Then, in my own mind, I look the phases over. We will take one on the Bible. What shall be the attitude of the people in this movement toward the Bible? We know that that should be our authority without a creed and without the higher criticism. This is the Book. The position we hold today is the right position, we believe, — to magnify this Book, to get our instruction from this Book, and to preach this Book. The whole plan of redemption, everything that is necessary to salvation, is in this Book, and we do not have to go to anything outside of the Book to be saved. That has been the attitude of the spirit of prophecy toward this book from the beginning, hasn't it? [Voices: Yes.] And I suppose we can give credit to that gift for our attitude toward the Book as much as to any influence that anybody has exercised.

Now take the doctrines of the Bible: In all the other reformations that came up, the leaders were unable to rightly distinguish between all error and truth, — the Sabbath day, Baptism, the nature of man, etc., — and so they openly taught errors from this book. But now, when we come to this movement, we find the wonderful power of discrimination on the part of the spirit of prophecy, and I do not know of a single truth in this Book that is set aside by the spirit of prophecy, nor a single biblical or theological error that came down through the dark ages that has been fostered by the spirit of prophecy and pressed upon the people that we have to discredit when we come to this Book. The doctrines of baptism, the law, the place and value and dignity of the Holy Spirit in the church, and all the other teachings that we have, have been magnified by this gift among us. Take another line, — the activities of the church. Here is our attitude toward foreign missions or world evangelism. Who among us has ever exercised greater influence than this gift in behalf of world evangelism? Take the question of liberal, unselfish support of the work. When you go to those writings, you find them full of exhortations, and if we would live them out better than we do our gifts would be greater, and our progress would be more rapid.

Then take our attitude on our service that we are to render to our fellowmen, Christian help work, — all those activities where a Christian should be a real blessing, an unselfish individual in the community to help people in their sorrows and misfortunes, their poverty and sickness, and every way that they need help. We find that the writings of the spirit of prophecy abound with exhortations to an unselfish life in living among our fellowmen.

Take the question of health and the medical missionary work, and all these activities, and take the service that should be put forth in behalf of the young. Where do you find in any movement that we read about where better instruction has been given as to the attention that should be given to the young people. Take the question of education: Why, brethren, none of our teachers ever have stood in advance of the counsel, that good wholesome instruction, that we find in the spirit of prophecy.

Those things I point to as really the convincing evidence of the origin of this gift, and the genuineness of it, — not to some ocular demonstrations that a few people have seen. I have no objections to persons speaking of those; but in close work with students I certainly would take the time to note down all these actual facts and hold them before the students, and show that from the beginning of this movement there has been inseparably and intimately and forcefully and aggressively connected with it this gift that has magnified everything good and has discounted, I think, everything bad. And if that is not evidence of the source of this gift among us, then I do not know what would be evidence.

W. E. Howell: I am sure the teachers would like to have some suggestions on the use of the spirit of prophecy and its writings in their teaching work.

A. G. Daniells: Well, give me a question that will be definite, in a particular way.

C. L. Taylor [Bible teacher, Canadian Junior College]: I would like to ask you to discuss for us the exegetical value of the Testimonies. Of course I think it is generally understood by us that there are many texts to which she makes no reference. There are many texts that she explains, and there may be other explanations that are equally true that she does not touch. But my question is really this: May we accept the explanations of scripture that she gives? Are those dependable?

A. G. Daniells: I have always felt that they were. It may be that in some very critical matters there may be some difficulties; but I have used the writings for years in a way to clarify or elucidate the thought in the texts of scripture. Take "Desire of Ages" and "Patriarchs and Prophets." In reading them through I have found many instances of good illumination.

Does that answer your question? Do you mean whether students should resort to the writings for their interpretation of the Bible, or to get additional light? That is to say, is it necessary to have these writings in order to understand the Bible? must we go to her explanations to get our meaning of the Bible? Is that the question or is that involved in it?

C. L. Taylor: Not directly, but possibly indirectly. But I will give a more concrete example. We will suppose that a student comes for help on a certain scripture, and wants to know what it means. Is it proper for the teacher to explain that scripture, with perhaps other scriptures illuminating the text, and then bring in the spirit of prophecy also as additional light on the text? Or suppose two students differ on the meaning of a text, and they come to the teacher to find out what it means: Should the teacher explain the text and then use the Testimonies to support the position he takes? Or take still a third case: Suppose that two brethren, both of them believers in the Testimonies, and of course believers in the Bible primarily, have a difference of opinion on a certain text: Is it right for them in their study of that text to bring in the spirit of prophecy to aid in their understanding of it, or should they leave that out of the question entirely?

A. G. Daniells: On that first point, I think this, that we are to get our interpretation from this Book, primarily. I think that the Book explains itself, and I think we can understand the Book, fundamentally, through the Book, without resorting to the Testimonies to prove up on it.

Appendix 4

W. E. Howell: The spirit of prophecy says the Bible is its own expositor.

A. G. Daniells: Yes, but I have heard ministers say that the spirit of prophecy is the interpreter of the Bible. I heard it preached at the General Conference some years ago, when it was said that the only way we could understand the Bible was through the writings of the spirit of prophecy.

J. N. Anderson [teacher of biblical languages and missions, Union College]: And he also said "infallible interpreter."

C. M. Sorenson [dean of theology, Washington Missionary College]: That expression has been canceled. That is not our position.

A. G. Daniells: It is not our position, and it is not right that the spirit of prophecy is the only safe interpreter of the Bible. That is a false doctrine, a false view. It will not stand. Why, my friends what would all the people have done from John's day down to the present if there were no way to understand the Bible except through the writings of the spirit of prophecy! It is a terrible position to take! That is false, it is error. It is positively dangerous! What do those people do over in Roumania? We have hundreds of Sabbath-keepers there who have not seen a book on the spirit of prophecy? What do those people in China do? Can't they understand this Book only as we get the interpretation through the spirit of prophecy and then take it to them? That is heathenish!

L. L. Caviness [associate editor, *Review and Herald*]: Do you understand that the early believers got their understanding from the Bible, or did it come through the spirit of prophecy?

A. G. Daniells: They got their knowledge of the Scriptures as they went along through the Scriptures themselves. It pains me to hear the way some people talk, that the spirit of prophecy led out and gave all the instruction, all the doctrines, to the pioneers, and they accepted them right along. That is not according to the writings themselves, "Early Writings." We are told how they did; they searched these scriptures together and studied and prayed over them until they got together on them. Sister White says in her works that for a long time she could not understand, that her mind was locked over these things, and the brethren worked their way along. She did not bring to this movement the Sabbath truth. She opposed the Sabbath truth. It did not seem right to her when Brother [Joseph] Bates presented it to her. But she had help from the Lord and when that clear knowledge was given her in that way, she was a weak child, and could not understand theology, but she had a clear outline given to her, and from that day to her death she never wavered a minute. But the Lord did not by revelation give to another all that He had given in this Book. He gave this Book, and He gave men brains and thinking power to study the Book.

I would not, in my class work, give out the idea at all to students that they can not understand this book only through the writings of Sister White. I would hold out to students, as I do to preachers, and in ministerial meetings, the necessity of getting our understanding of the Bible from the Bible itself, and using the spirit of prophecy to enlarge our view. I tell them not to be lazy about studying the Book, and not to rummage around first for something that has been written on a point that they can just swallow without study. I think that would be a very dangerous thing for our ministers to get into that habit. And there are some, I must confess, who will hunt around to find a statement in the Testimonies and spend no time in deep study of the Book. They do not have a taste for it, and if they can look around and find something that is already made out, they are glad to pick that up and go along without studying the Bible. The earnest study of the Bible is the security, the safety of a man. He must come to the book itself and get it by careful study, and then whatever he finds in the spirit of prophecy or any other writings that will help him and throw light and clarify his vision on it, — that is alright. Does that cover your point?

C. L. Taylor: It does to a certain extent; and yet when you take the case of those two brethren who accept the Bible and the Testimonies, but still have a difference of interpretation that they want help on, — is it right for them to use the Testimonies in their study of that text, as well as the Bible?

APPENDIX 4

A. G. Daniells: I think it is right to take the whole trend of teaching and thought that is put through the Testimonies on that subject. If I am perplexed about a text, and in my study of the spirit of prophecy I find something that makes it clear, I take that. I think Brother [William W.] Prescott illustrates that in this matter of Matthew 24, of which there is a clear outline in the spirit of prophecy.

W. W. Prescott [field secretary, General Conference, and former president of several Adventist colleges]: For two or three years I spent a lot of time in the study of the 8th chapter of Daniel, to get what I thought to be the proper interpretation of that chapter. I got up to the point one time where I felt that I must get that clearer, where I could use it, and I made it the special subject of prayer. I was over in England, stopping at the home of a brother there. It came to me just like a voice, "Read what it says in 'Patriarchs and Prophets' on that subject." I turned right around to a book case back of me, and took up "Patriarchs and Prophets" and began to look through it. I came right to the chapter that dealt with the subject, and I found exactly the thing I wanted to clarify my mind on that subject. It greatly helped me. That, Brother Daniells, is my own personal experience over this matter that Brother Taylor raises.

In connection with what Brother Taylor has asked, I would like to suggest this, Whether a comment on the spirit of prophecy upon the Authorized Version establishes that version as the correct version against the Revised Version, where the reading is changed; and if one accepted the Revised Version, it would throw out the comment made in the spirit of prophecy. I have a definite case in mind.

* * *

F. M. Wilcox [editor, *Review and Herald*]: I have a paragraph here I would like to read. This is so completely in harmony with what Brother Daniells has expressed that I thought I would like to read it. James White, in the *Review* of 1851, wrote this and it was republished again four year later, as expressing what he considered the denominational view with respect to the Testimonies back there:

"GIFTS OF THE GOSPEL CHURCH"

"The gifts of the Spirit should all have their proper places. The Bible is an everlasting rock. It is our rule of faith and practice. In it the man of God is 'thoroughly furnished unto all good works.' If every member of the church of Christ was holy, harmless, and separate from sinners, and searched the Holy Scriptures diligently and with much prayer for duty, with the aid of the Holy Spirit, we think, they would be able to learn their whole duty in 'all good works.' Thus 'the man of God may be perfect.' But as the reverse exists, and ever has existed, God in much mercy has pitied the weakness of his people, and has set the gifts in the gospel church to correct our errors, and to lead us to his living Word. Paul says that they are for the 'perfecting of the saints,' 'till we all come in the unity of the faith.' The extreme necessity of the church in its imperfect state is God's opportunity to manifest the Spirit.

"Every Christian is therefore in duty bound to take the Bible as a perfect rule of faith and duty. He should pray fervently to be aided by the Holy Spirit in searching the Scriptures for the whole truth, and for his whole duty. He is not at liberty to turn from them to learn his duty through any of the gifts. We say that the very moment he does, he places the gifts in a wrong place, and takes an extremely dangerous position. The Word should be in front, the eye of the church should be placed upon it, as wisdom, from which to learn duty in 'all good works.' But if a portion of the church err from the truths of the Bible, and become weak and sickly, and the flock become scattered, so that it seems necessary for God to employ the gifts of the Spirit to correct, revive, and heal the erring, we should let him work. Yea, more, we should pray for him to work, and plead earnestly that he would work by the Spirit's power, and bring the scattered sheep to his fold. Praise the Lord, he will work. Amen." — *Review and Herald* of April 21, 1851.

"We wrote the above article on the gifts of the gospel church four years since. It was published in the first volume of the *Review*. One object in republishing it is that our readers may see for themselves what our position has ever been on this subject, that they may be better prepared to dispose of the statements of those who seek to injure us.

"The position that the Bible, and the Bible alone, is the rule of faith and duty, does not shut out the gifts which God set in the church. To reject them is shutting out that part of the Bible which presents them. We say, Let us have a whole Bible, and let that, and that alone, be our rule of faith and duty. Place the gifts where they belong, and all is harmony." — *Review and Herald* of October 3, 1854.

W. W. Prescott: How should we use the writings of the spirit of prophecy as an authority by which to settle historical questions?

A. G. Daniells: Well, now, as I understand it, Sister White never claimed to be an authority on history, and never claimed to be a dogmatic teacher on theology. She never outlined a course of theology, like Mrs. [Mary Baker] Eddy's book on teaching. She just gave out fragmentary statements, but left the pastors and evangelists and preachers to work out all these problems of scripture and of theology and of history. She never claimed to be an authority on history; and as I have understood it, where the history that related to the interpretation of prophecy was clear and expressive, she wove it into her writings; but I have always understood that, as far as she was concerned, she was ready to correct in revision such statements as she thought should be corrected. I have never gone to her writings, and taken the history that I found in her writings, as the positive statement of history regarding the fulfillment of prophecy. I do not know how others may view that, but I have felt that I should deal with history in the same way that I am exhorted to deal with the Bible, — prove it all carefully and thoroughly, and then let her go on and make such revisions from time to time as seem best.

Just one more thought: Now you know something about that little book, "The Life of Paul" [written by Ellen White]. You know the difficulty we got into about that. We could never claim inspiration in the whole thought and makeup of the book, because it has been thrown aside because it was badly put together. Credits were not given to the proper authorities, and some of that crept into "The Great Controversy," — the lack of credits; and in the revision of that book those things were carefully run down and made right. Personally that has never shaken my faith, but there are men who have been greatly hurt by it, and I think it is because they claimed too much for these writings. Just as Brother White says, there is a danger in going away from the Book, and claiming too much. Let it have its full weight, just as God has fixed it, and then I think we will stand without being shaken when some of these things do appear that we can not harmonize with our theory.

W. W. Prescott: There is another experience that you know of that applies to what Brother Taylor has brought up. Some of the brethren here remember very well a serious controversy over the interpretation of the 8th chapter of Daniel, and there were some of the brethren who ranged themselves against what was called the new view, and they took her writings to uphold their position. She wrote to those brethren and instructed them not to use her writings to settle that controversy. I think that ought to be remembered as being her own counsel when brethren that did claim to believe the Bible and the spirit of prophecy were divided over an interpretation, and it was a matter of public controversy.

J. N. Anderson: How far would you take that word from Sister White to be a general statement about her writings?

A. G. Daniells: I think it was especially on the case then, but I think we have to use the same judgment about using her writings in other cases.

C. A. Shull [history teacher, Lancaster Junior College]: Just how shall we use the Testimonies in the class room? What shall be our attitude toward them in the line of history, especially? Before I knew that there was any statement in the spirit of prophecy regarding the experience of John, I stated to the class that there was a tradition that John had been thrown into a caldron of boiling oil, and a student immediately produced that statement in the Testimonies that John was thrown into the boiling oil. Now, I want to know, was she given a divine revelation that John was thrown into a vat of boiling oil?

Now another question, on the taking of Babylon. Mrs. White in the spirit of prophecy mentions that Babylon was taken according to the historian, by the turning aside of the waters. Modern scholarship says it was not taken that way. What should be our attitude in regard to such things?

Appendix 4

Mrs. Flora Lampson Williams [educational superintendent, East Michigan Conference]: We have that question to meet every year.

E. F. Albertsworth [history teacher, Washington Missionary College]: I have been confronted in my classes by students who come with the Testimonies and endeavor to settle a question by quoting where she says, "I have been shown." They said that of all things that must settle the matter. I have wanted to know what attitude we should take on a question of that kind.

C. P. Bollman: Wouldn't that latter question require a concrete example?

A. G. Daniells: Yes, I think it would.

E. F. Albertsworth: I do not recall the example; but some of the students would say that meant she had a direct revelation, and others would say that meant that she was shown by people around her.

A. G. Daniells: I do not think that is what she means when she says that. When she was shown, it was by the angel or the revelation that was made to her. I feel sure that was her meaning.

E. F. Albertsworth: I have found students who had doubts about that.

W. G. Wirth [Bible teacher, Pacific Union College]: Suppose we do have a conflict between the authorized and revised versions?

A. G. Daniells: That question was up before. You must not count me an authority for I am just like you in the matter. I have to form my own opinions. I do not think Sister White meant at all to establish the certainty of a translation. I do not think she had that in mind, or had anything to do with putting her seal of approval on the authorized version or on the revised version when she quoted that. She uses whichever version helps to bring out the thought she has most clearly. With reference to this historical matter, I cannot say anything more than I have said, that I never have understood that Sister

White undertook to settle historical questions. I visited her once over this matter of the "daily," and I took along with me that old chart, — as early a chart as we have access to.

C. P. Bollman: The same chart that Elder Haskell sells?

A. G. Daniells: Yes, it was that same chart. I took that and laid it on her lap, and I took "Early Writings" and read it to her, and then I told her of the controversy. I spent a long time with her. It was one of her days when she was feeling cheery and rested, and so I explained it to her quite fully. I said, "Now here you say that you were shown that the view of the 'daily' that the brethren held was correct. Now," I said, "there are two parts here in this 'daily' that you quote. One is this period of time, the 2300 years, and the other is what the 'daily' itself was."

I went over that with her, and every time, as quick as I would come to that time, she would say, "Why, I know what was shown me, that that period of 2300 days was fixed, and that there would be no definite time after that. The brethren were right when they reached that 1844 date."

And I believe it was, brethren. You might just as well try to move me out of the world as to try to move me on that question, — not because she says it, but I believe it was clearly shown to her by the Lord. But on this other, when she says she was not shown what the "daily" was, I believe that, and I take "Early Writings" 100% on that question of the "daily," fixing that period. That is the thing she talks about, and I take the Bible with it, and I take the Bible as to what the "daily" itself is.

So when it comes to those historical questions about the taking of Babylon, I think this, brethren, we ought not to let every little statement in history that we find lead us away from the spirit of prophecy. You know historians contradict each other, don't you? Of course your work is to get back, get back, get back to the fountain head, the original thing; and when you get back there, and get it perfectly clear, I do not believe that if Sister White were here to speak to you today, she would authorize you to take a historical fact, supposed to be a fact, that she had incorporated in the book, and put it up against an actual thing in history. We talked with her about that when "Great Controversy" was being revised, and I have letters in my file in the vault there where we were warned against using Sister White as a historian. She never claimed to be that. We were warned against setting up statements found in her writings against the various history that there is on a fact. That is where I stand. I do not have to meet it with students, and I do not have to explain myself in a congregation. I suppose I have it easier than you teachers do.

W. W. Prescott: On that very point you mention as to the capture of Babylon, one of the most recent editions of the Bible (?) takes the position of Herodotus against the ———, and he says: "Why should we discount the writings on parchment in favor of the writings on clay?"

A. G. Daniells: That is what I mean, that we should not allow every historical statement that we find that contradicts the Testimonies to set us wild. If there are two authorities of equal value on that point, bring up the authority that is in harmony with what we have.

C. A. Shull: We teachers have a great responsibility on us to take the right attitude. If we say that a certain thing in the Testimonies is not correct, students are likely to carry away the impression that we do not have faith in the Testimonies.

A. G. Daniells: There are two ways to hurt students in this matter. One way is to discount the Testimonies and cast a little bit of question and doubt on them. I would never do that, brethren, in the school room. No matter how much I was perplexed, I would never cast a doubt in the mind of a student. I would take hours to explain matters to ground the student in it. Casting doubts and reflections is one way to hurt a student. Another way is to take an extreme and unwarranted position. You can do that and pass it over; but when that student gets out and gets in contact with things, he may be shaken, and perhaps shaken clear out and away. I think we should be candid and honest and never put a claim forth that is not well founded simply to appear to believe. You will have to be careful in giving this instruction, because many of the students have heard from their parents things that are not so, and they hear from preachers things that are not so, and so their foundation is false.

I must refer again to the attitude of A. T. Jones. In his heyday you know he just drank the whole thing in, and he would hang a man on a word. I have seen him take just a word in the Testimonies and hang to it, and that would settle everything, — just a word. I was with him when he made a discovery, — or, if he didn't make it, he appeared to make it, and that was that there were words in the Testimonies and writings of Sister White that God did not order her to put in there, that there were words which she did not put in by divine inspiration, the Lord picking the words, but that somebody had helped to fix that up. And so he took two testimonies and compared them, and he got into great trouble. He went on with Dr. [John Harvey] Kellogg, where he could just pick things to pieces.

F. M. Wilcox: Back in the 60's or 70's a General Conference in session passed this resolution, — they said, we recognize that the Testimonies have been prepared under great pressure and stress of circumstances, and that the wording is not always the happiest, and we recommend their republication with such changes as will bring them to a standard.

A. G. Daniells: I would like to get hold of that resolution. Now, brethren, I want to ask you honestly if there is a man here who has had doubt created in your mind from my attitude and the positions I have taken? [VOICES: No! No!] Or is there one of you that thinks I am shaky on the Testimonies? I will not say [is there anyone] that thinks my position is not just right, for you might not agree with me, but from what I have said, is there a tendency to lead you to believe that I am shaky, and that some time I will help to get you away from the Testimonies? [Several decided no's were heard.]

C. L. Taylor: In your talk a few evenings ago I agreed 100% in everything you said. Today there is just one question in my mind.

A. G. Daniells: Let us have it.

C. L. Taylor: That is regarding those outward manifestations, those things of perhaps a miraculous nature. I do not know whether you intend to carry the impression that you discredit those or that you simply would not teach them. If it is that you would not hold them up as proof that the work is inspired, I am heartily in agreement with that. On the other hand, if you take the position that those things are not to be relied on, that [the early Adventist historian] Elder [John] Loughborough and others are mistaken about these things, I should have to disagree with you.

A. G. Daniells: No, I do not discount them nor disbelieve them; but they are not the kind of evidence I would use with students or with unbelievers.

C. L. Taylor: I agree with that.

A. G. Daniells: I do not question them, but I do not think they are the best kind of evidence to produce. For instance, I do not think the best kind of proof for me to give an audience on the Sabbath question or the nature of man or baptism, is to go and read Sister White's writings to them. I believe the best proof I can give is the Bible. Perhaps you will remember that it fell to me to preach Sister White's funeral sermon; and if you will remember, I took that occasion to give evidence of her high calling. I did not give a long list of fruits and miraculous evidences. I knew the matter would be published to the world in hundreds of papers, and I wanted to give them something that would be a high authority, and this is what I gave: First, that she stood with the word of God from Genesis to Revelation in all its teaching. Then, she stood with mankind in his highest endeavors to help mankind, — elaborating on those points. That is what I mean, Brother Taylor; but I do not discount those other things.

What I want to know is this, brethren: Does my position appear to be of such a character that you would be led to think I am shaky? [VOICES: No!] If you think it, just say it right out! I do not want to do that, but I have to be honest, — I can not camouflage in a thing like this. I have stood through it about forty years unshaken, and I think it is a safe position; but if I were driven to take the position that some do on the Testimonies, I would be shaken. [VOICE: That's right!] I would not know where to stand, for I can not say that white is black and black is white.

H. C. Lacey [teacher of sacred languages and literature, Washington Missionary College]: To us there is no doubt that you believe the Testimonies, but will you mind my adding another personal note to it?

A. G. Daniells: No.

H. C. Lacey: It is this: Those who have not heard you, as we have here, and are taking the other side of the question, — some of them are deliberately saying that neither you nor Professor Prescott believe the Testimonies. For instance, I went out to Mt. Vernon [Academy] and I met the graduating class there, and when the exercises were over, I had a private talk with three or four of those young people, and they told me that they certainly understood that our General Conference men down here — they did not mean me or Brother [C. M.] Sorenson — did not believe the Testimonies.

W. W. Prescott: You are not telling us news.

H. C. Lacey: We as teachers are in a terribly hard position. We have got nearly down to bed-rock in the questions that have been asked here; but the students do get right down to bed-rock on some of these things, and we need to get a little deeper here. There are people here at these meetings who do not dare to ask certain questions that have come up in their minds or in private talks. But you know that the teacher is in a very difficult position.

On that matter of the capture of Babylon, I have felt free to say that I thought the evidence was that Cyrus did not capture it that way, but we would hold the matter in abeyance and simply study it. Suppose now that further tablets would come to light, and other evidence would be brought in to prove indisputably that Cyrus did not capture Babylon that way, would it be right to say that if there is a revision of that book, — "Patriarchs and Prophets," which indorses, in one casual sentence, that old view, — the revision would be brought into harmony with recently discovered facts?

A. G. Daniells: I think that is the position Sister White occupies. I think that is what she has done. I never understood that she put infallibility into the historical quotations.

APPENDIX 4

H. C. Lacey: But there are some who do understand it.

W. W. Prescott: It is interesting to know that even a higher critic like George Adams Smith agrees with Herodotus (?) on that.

Brother Daniells was speaking about this question of physical outward evidences. One of those evidences has been that the eyes were open, as you will remember, and this scripture in the 24th chapter of Numbers is always referred to, showing that it is in harmony with that. But you read the Revised Version, and you find it reads, "And he took up his parable, and said, Balaam the son of Beor saith, And the man whose eye was closed saith." In this text it puts it just the other way. Then I would not want to use that as an argument, that the prophet's eyes were open.

A. G. Daniells: That is what I mean by referring to secondary matters.

H. C. Lacey: In our estimate of the spirit of prophecy, isn't its value to us more in the spiritual light it throws into our own hearts and lives than in the intellectual accuracy in historical and theological matters? Ought we not to take those writings as the voice of the Spirit of our hearts, instead of as the voice of the teacher to our heads? And isn't the final proof of the spirit of prophecy its spiritual value rather than its historical accuracy?

A. G. Daniells: Yes, I think so.

J. N. Anderson: Would you set about to explain things as you have this morning? Would you explain that you do not think the Testimonies are to be taken as final in the matter of historical data, etc., so as to justify a position?

A. G. Daniells: Who gives the teaching in the school on the spirit of prophecy? Is it the Bible teacher? How do you get that question before the students?

C. L. Taylor: Both Bible and history teachers catch it.

W. H. Wakeham [dean of the school of theology, Emmanuel Missionary College]: It comes up in every Bible class.

H. C. Lacey: Wouldn't it be a splendid thing if a little pamphlet were written setting forth in plain, simple, straight-forward style the facts as we have them, — simple, sacred facts, — so that we could put them into the hands of inquiring students?

Voice: Our enemies would publish it.

Voice: Our enemies would publish it everywhere.

C. L. Benson [education secretary, Central Union]: I think it would be a splendid thing if our brethren were a little conservative on these things. We had a man come to our Union and spend an hour and a half on the evidences of the spirit of prophecy through Sister White. The impression was conveyed that practically every word that she spoke, and every letter she wrote, whether personal or otherwise, was a divine inspiration. Those things make it awfully hard for our teachers and ministers.

W. G. Wirth: I want to second what Professor Lacey has brought out. I wish you general men would get out something for us, because we are the ones that suffer.

W. W. Prescott: To my certain knowledge, a most earnest appeal was made for that from her office to issue such a statement, and they would not do it.

C. P. Bollman: It wasn't made to her, though.

W. W. Prescott: No, but it was made to those who were handling her manuscripts.

A. G. Daniells: Some of those statements like what Brother Wilcox read here this morning have been up a number of times, and Brother [James] White always took a good sensible position.

APPENDIX 4

W. W. Prescott: Brother Wilcox had a letter from Sister White herself that he read.

A. G. Daniells: When these things were under pretty sharp controversy, W. C. White, for his mother, sent out things that we had in our vaults here that greatly modified this, and helped to smooth out these wrinkles and get a reasonable ground on which to stand. I do not know but what perhaps the General Conference Committee might appoint a committee to do this, and have reliable, responsible men that the people do not question at all take hold of that and bring out these facts. It does seem to me that in our schools there ought to be an agreement among the teachers. The history and Bible teachers and others that have to do with these things should get together and have their stories and their teaching alike, if possible. The truth should be given to those students, and when you give the truth to them you will have them founded and established on this without trouble. But when these erroneous views are given them, they get a false idea and then there is danger when an honest man takes the true side and states his position.

W. E. Howell: It seems to me that the point is of very great importance. I have been somewhat perplexed on this matter. We have talked over things very freely and frankly here at the other meeting and at this, and I think the teachers here at [sic] all satisfied as to the place that is to be given to the spirit of prophecy in its relation to their work. But these teachers, when they get back to their places of work, will have all kinds of questions put to them, and it has been a question with me as to how far a teacher ought to go with a class of young people or with an indiscriminate body to deal with and attempt to bring out the things that they have heard here and have received and believed for themselves. I think there is where the difficulty is going to be. We have only two teachers here out of an entire faculty. Some other member of the faculty might not be cleared up on these things. There may be teachers who are endeavoring to teach science out of the spirit of prophecy; or another teacher who has not had the benefit of this discussion, may have some other viewpoint. And it really puts these teachers in a very hard situation. If there is anything that can be done by way of putting something in the hands of the teachers so that they could give the true representation in the matter, I think it would be a very great help.

W. W. Prescott: Can you explain how it is that two brethren can disagree on the inspiration of the Bible, one holding to the verbal inspiration and the other opposed to it, and yet no disturbance be created in the denomination whatever? That situation is right here before us. But if two brethren take the same attitude on the spirit of prophecy, one holding to verbal inspiration and the other discrediting it, he that does not hold to the verbal inspiration is discredited.

F. M. Wilcox: Do you believe that a man who doesn't believe in the verbal inspiration of the Bible believes the Bible?

W. W. Prescott: I do not have any trouble over it at all. I have a different view myself. If a man does not believe in the verbal inspiration of the Bible, he is still in good standing; but if he says he does not believe in the verbal inspiration of the Testimonies, he is discounted right away. I think it is an unhealthful situation. It puts the spirit of prophecy above the Bible.

W. G. Wirth: Really that is my biggest problem. I shall certainly be discredited if I go back and give this view. I would like to see some published statement given out by those who lead this work so that if that thing should come up there would be some authority back of it, because I am in for a lot of trouble on that thing. I would like to see something done, because that education is going right on, and our students are being sent out with the idea that the Testimonies are verbally inspired, and woe be to the man out where I am that does not line up to that.

Now as to health reform: Frequently a student will come to me and quote what Sister White says about butter. But we serve butter on our tables right along. And they will bring up about meat, how under no consideration is that to be eaten. And I know that that is unreasonable, and there are times when it is necessary to eat meat. What shall we do about that? I would like a little light on some of those details, as to whether we ought to take them at full value.

Appendix 4

A. G. Daniells: I am willing to answer part of that, for I have had it about a thousand times. Take this question of health reform. It is well known from the writings themselves and from personal contact with Sister White, and from common sense, that in traveling and in knowledge of different parts of the world, that the instruction set forth in the Testimonies was never intended to be one great wholesale blanket regulation for peoples' eating and drinking, and it applies to various individuals according to their physical condition and according to the situation in which they find themselves. I have always explained it that way to our ministers in ministers' meetings. We had a ministers' meeting over in Scandinavia, and we had one man there from the "land of the midnight sun," up in Hammerfest where you never grow a banana or an apple or a peach, and hardly even a green thing. It is snow and cold there nearly all the time, and the people live to a large extent on fish and various animal foods that they get there. We had sent a nurse from Christiania [Oslo] up there as a missionary. He had the strict idea of the diet according to the Testimonies, and he would not touch a fish or a bit of reindeer, nor any kind of animal food, and he was getting poor; because missionaries that are sent out do not have much money, and they cannot import fresh fruits; and it was in the days when even canned goods were not shipped much. The fellow nearly starved to death. He came down to attend that meeting, and he was nearly as white as your dress [speaking to Sister Williams]. He had hardly any blood in his body. I talked to him, and I said, "Brother Olson, what is the matter with you? We will have to bring you away from up there if you do not get better. You have no red blood corpuscles in your blood." I talked with him a while, and finally asked him, "What do you live on?"

"Well," he said, "I live a good deal on the north wind."

I said, "You look like it, sure enough."

We went on talking, and I found out that the man wasn't eating much but potatoes and starchy foods, — just a limited dietary. I went at him with all the terror I could inspire for such foolishness.

Voice: Did you make any impression?

A. G. Daniells: Yes, I did. And I got other brethren to join me. We told that man he would be buried up there if he tried to live that way. We talked with him straight about it. When I got back to this country I talked with Sister White about it, and she said, "Why don't the people use common sense? Why don't they know that we are to be governed by the places we are located?" You will find in a little testimony a caution thrown out, modifying the extreme statements that were made.

F. M. Wilcox: Sister White says in a copy of the [*Youth's*] *Instructor* that there are some classes that she would not say should not eat some meat.

A. G. Daniells: There are very conscientious men and ministers who are very much afraid they will eat something they ought not to. On that very point Paul says that the kingdom of God is not meat or drink, but righteousness and peace; and we are working and trying to get through to the kingdom just as much on the ground of works by eating or not eating as by any other thing in this world. You never can put down vegetarianism as the way to heaven. I have been over in India where they are mighty strict about their eating, but they do not get righteousness that way.

C. L. Taylor: It is true of all works, isn't it?

A. G. Daniells: Certainly. You take men who have never allowed a piece of animal food to pass their lips, and some of them are the most tyrannical, brutal men; and when we try to reach them with the gospel, we have to tell them that is not the way to God, that they will have to come and believe in the Lord Jesus Christ and have His righteousness imputed to them on confession, forgiveness, and all of that. We have people among us that are just as much in danger of trying to establish this righteousness by works in the matter of the dietary as the world has seen in any thing. You know from what Sister White brought out on the matter of righteousness that it was not her purpose to put down eating and drinking as the way to heaven. It has its place. It is important, and I would not want to see this denomination swing away over to the position of other denominations; but I do not like to hear of teaching that would lead this people to fall back on eating and drinking for righteousness, for Paul said that is not the way. I do not think proper caution was used in putting out some of these things, and I have told Sister White so.

Mrs. Williams: You mean in publishing them?

A. G. Daniells: Yes, when they were written. I told Sister White that it seems to me that if conditions in the arctic regions and in the heart of China and other places had been taken into account, some of those things would have been modified. "Why," she said, "yes, if the people are not going to use their judgment, then of course we will have to fix it for them." It seemed so sensible to me. Sister White was never a fanatic, she was never an extremist. She was a level-headed woman. She was well-balanced. I found that so during a period of 40 years of association with her. When we were down in Texas, and old Brother White was breaking down, that woman just got the most beautiful venison every day to eat, and my wife cooked it; and he would sit down and eat some of that and say, "O, Ellen, that is just the thing!" She did not hold him up and make him live on a diet of starch! I always found her well-balanced. There are some people who are extremists, who are fanatical; but I do not think we should allow those people to fix the platform and guide this denomination. I do not propose to do it, for one. And yet I believe that we should use all the caution and all the care that is set out for the maintenance of health. And brethren, I have tried to do it, but I have not lived all my life on the strictest dietary set down there. I have had to go all over this world, and as you know, I have had to be exposed to all the disease germs. I have had to live on a very spare dietary in places in my travel, and I have lived on wheels, and under great pressure, and it was prophesied when I went into this in 1901 that a decade would finish me, and I would either be a broken down old man on the shelf or in the grave. That is the way my friends talked, and they sympathized with me, and regretted that I ever took this position; but I said to myself, "By the grace of God, I will live in every possible way just right as far as I know it, to conserve my strength." This is my 19th year, and I am not broken down, and I am not on the shelf or in the grave. I am strong and well. I am weary, but I can get rested. I have tried to be honest and to be true to my sense of what was the right thing to do, and it has kept me well and strong. That is the basis on which I propose to work. I do not propose to have any extremist lay down the law to me as to what I shall eat up in the heart of China. I propose to use my sense as to what I ought to eat in those places where you can not get a green thing, hardly.

Mrs. Williams: In the interior of Africa, we had to cook everything we ate, so as to kill the germs.

A. G. Daniells: Why, yes, in China you must sterilize your hands and your knife, and if you eat an apple, it must be sterilized after it is peeled, and even then it is not always safe. I do not think we have to take an extreme position on the question of the diet for all classes. We are not all alike. What is good for one man is not good for another. I have seen Elder [George A.] Irwin [former president of the General Conference] sit down and eat two or three raw apples at night just before going to bed; but one apple at night would upset me so that my tongue would be covered with fur and my head all swelled up. I would not eat one if you would give me five dollars. I count that health reform, to reject that which I know injures me and take that which I know strengthens me and maintains me in the strongest physical trim for service and hard work. That is my health reform. Raw apples are good for people that have the right digestion for them; but if a person hasn't that sort of digestion, he must lay down the law, No raw apples for him. That is the way a lot of things got into the Testimonies. They were many of them written for individuals in various states of health, and then they were hurried into the Testimonies without proper modification. That is not to say that they are false things, but it is to say that they do not apply to every individual the world over alike. And you can not put a health-reform regime or rule down for the whole world alike, because of the different physical conditions that maintain. That is what I tell in ministers' meetings and I do not think I destroy the force of the message at all, only to the extremist.

N. J. Waldorf [Bible teacher, College of Medical Evangelists]: I have had no trouble for over twenty years with the spirit of prophecy or with the Bible. The more I have studied both the more firmly I have become convinced on this platform. I have read the whole of higher criticism right through, and the other side of it. There are 50,000 different readings in the Bible. There are many mistakes that were made in transcribing. Now in the matter of historical complication, I take the Bible and the spirit of prophecy exactly alike.

A. G. Daniells: Here is one illustration of a mistake in the Bible: In Samuel it says a man lifted up his hand against 800 men whom he slew; then in Chronicles this same thing is spoken of, and it says that he lifted up his hand against 300 men, whom he slew.

N. J. Waldorf: I have never held up the spirit of prophecy as being infallible. But students come to me from different teachers, having different views. One comes and says Professor Lacey taught me this way, and another comes from Professor Johnson [possibly fellow participant H. A. Johnston, history teacher at Southern Junior College] who taught him some other way. There are lots of them coming to the medical college that way from different teachers. They do not know whether every word of the spirit of prophecy is inspired or not. I teach them this way: That when this message was first started, God brought this gift of prophecy into the church, and through this gift God has approved of the major doctrines that we hold right down from 1844. I for one hold that the gift of the spirit of prophecy was given to us in order to get the mold, lest we should trust human reasoning and modern scholarship, for I believe that modern scholarship has gone bankrupt when it comes to Greek and Hebrew.

As for meat eating, I haven't touched meat for twenty-one years; but I buy meat for my wife. I often go into a butcher shop and get the very best they have in order to keep her in life. I never will use the Testimonies as a sledge hammer on my brother.

A. G. Daniells: I will tell you one thing, a great victory will be gained if we get a liberal spirit so that we will treat brethren who differ with us on the interpretation of the Testimonies in the same Christian way we treat them when they differ on the interpretation of the Bible. That will be a good deal gained, and it is worth gaining, I want to tell you, for I have been under criticism ever since the controversy started in Battle Creek. Isn't it a strange thing that when I and some of my associates fought that heresy year after year, and we got message after message from the spirit of prophecy — some of them very comforting and uplifting messages — and all that time we were counted as heretics on the spirit of prophecy? How do you account for that? Why didn't the spirit of prophecy get after us? I claim that I know as well as any man whether I believe in the spirit of prophecy or not. I do not ask people to accept my views, but I would like the confidence of brothers where we differ in interpretation. If we can engender that spirit, it will be a great help; and I believe we have to teach it right in our schools.

Suppose students come to you with questions about the Bible that you do not know what to do with, — or do you always know? I would like to go to a teacher for a year that would tell me everything in here that puzzles me! What do you do when students come to you with such questions?

W. H. Wakeham: I tell them I do not know, and I do not lose their confidence, either.

A. G. Daniells: Well, when they come to you with something in the spirit of prophecy that is puzzling, why not say, as Peter did, that there are some things hard to be understood. I do not think that destroys the confidence of the people. But we have got the idea that we have got to just assume full and complete knowledge of everything about the spirit of prophecy and take an extreme position in order to be loyal and to be true to it.

W. E. Howell: I just want to remark two things. One is on the question Professor Prescott raised on our previous meeting as to why people take these different attitudes toward a man on the Bible and on the Testimonies. I am not philosopher enough to explain an attitude of that sort, but I do think that the cause of it lies primarily in the making of extreme and radical positions. I think that is where the root of the difficulty lies, especially with reference to the spirit of prophecy.

Brother Daniells and Brother Prescott and others have come in here with us and have talked very frankly with us, and I am sure every man here will say that they have not covered up anything. They have not withheld from you anything that you have asked for that they

Appendix 4

could give you in reference to this matter. I do not doubt that it is your experience as it is mine, when I go out from Washington, to hear it said that Brother Daniells or Brother Prescott does not believe the spirit of prophecy.

A. G. Daniells: Brother [William A.] Spicer [secretary of the General Conference, who three years later replaced Daniells as president of the General Conference], too.

W. E. Howell: Yes, and Brother Spicer. I feel confident of this, that as you go out from this council you can be a great help in setting people straight on these things, and I believe it is our privilege to do it, brethren, to help the people on these points. Many of them are sincere and honest in that position, from what they have heard. I think it is our duty to help such persons all we can as we meet them.

C. L. Benson: Is this subject going to be dropped here? From what Brother Daniells has said, I know what it is going to mean to some of our schools and to our General Conference men. I feel it would be unfair to us as teachers to go back and make any statement. Letters have already come in, asking about the general men with reference to interpreting the spirit of prophecy. I do not think it is fair for us to go out and try to state the position of our General Conference men. On the other hand, I know the feeling and doctrine as taught in our conferences, and they are the Bible teachers of the people; and if our Bible and history teachers take these liberal positions on the spirit of prophecy, our schools are going to be at variance entirely with the field. Our people are beginning to wonder about the condition our schools are in. They say they read in the *Review* of this spirit of paganism, and they say those articles surely would not have been published in the *Review* if these conditions did not exist in our own schools. Why, what would they be putting it in the *Review* for if that were not the case? That is a fact, many of our people take the position that those articles were written because of conditions existing in our own schools. I think we ought to get down to a solution of this thing if we can, and start some kind of a campaign of education. Out in the field we have stressed the importance of the spirit of prophecy more than the Bible, and many of our men are doing it right along.

They tell of the wonderful phenomena, and many times they get their entire sermon from the spirit of prophecy instead of the Bible. If a break comes between our schools and the field we are in a serious place.

T. M. French [teacher of homiletics and missions, Emmanuel Missionary College]: I believe it would help us a great deal if some general statement were issued, and if some of this matter that has been brought up could be given, showing that we are not shifting our position, that we are viewing the spirit of prophecy as it has been viewed all along. I believe it would help to settle the situation in our conferences, and would be a great help both to the conferences and to the schools. I am sure from what has been read here of letters and resolutions of the past that we have not shifted our position, but the matter is just up again; and if we could get out statements as to our attitude all along, and restate the matter, I believe it would do much good.

W. E. Howell: The next topic we have is a consideration of how to teach the spirit of prophecy in our schools. In our recent general educational convention we provided for a semester's work in the curriculum in this subject. I think we ought to take ten minutes' intermission, and then take up this topic, which will give opportunity for further questions along this line.

Inspiration of the Spirit of Prophecy as Related to the Inspiration of the Bible

August 1, 1919

W. E. Howell, Chairman: The topic for this hour, as arranged for on Wednesday, is a continuation, in a measure, of our consideration of the spirit of prophecy, and the subject of inspiration connected with that, as related to the inspiration of the Bible. This hour is not intended to be a formal discourse, occupying the whole period, but Brother Daniells will lead in the topic, and then he has expressed a wish that it might be a kind of round-table in which we will study things together.

Appendix 4

A. G. Daniells: Brother Chairman, I think there has been a misunderstanding among us. I protested against taking such a heavy topic the other day, under the circumstances, and I dismissed it from my mind, and have been thinking along another line, that of pastoral training, and a further discussion of the question we had before us. I would not feel free, under the circumstances, to give a talk on the subject that I understand was looked for.

As you know, there are two views held by eminent men regarding the verbal inspiration of the Bible. You read their views in the books they have put out. One man, — scholarly, devout, earnest, a full believer in the Bible in every sense of the word, — believes that it was a revelation of truth to the writers, and they were allowed to state that truth as best they could. Another man — equally scholarly and pious and earnest in his faith — believes that it was a word-for-word inspiration or revelation, that the actual words were given, — that every word in the original, as it was written by the prophets down from Moses to Malachi, was given to them by the Lord. These men differ, and differ honestly and sincerely; and they have their followers among us, right here at the conference, both of them; and I see nothing to be gained by a man in my position, with my knowledge of these things, attempting to prove up on this. I do not wish to do it. We would all remain of the same opinion, I think, as we are now; so I want to beg you to allow me to dismiss that part of it, and either go directly into the other question of pastoral training or open the way for further questions and discussions of the matter we had before us. I feel more at home in that, for all these years since the Battle Creek controversy began I have been face to face with this question of the Testimonies. I have met all the doubters, the chief ones, and have dealt with it in ministerial institutes, and have talked it over and over until I am thoroughly familiar with it, whether I am straight or not. I do not know that there is a crook or a kink in it that I have not heard brought up by these men that have fallen away from us. I would be willing to hear further questions and further discussion, if it is the wish of the convention.

W. E. Howell: I am sure I do not want Brother Daniells to feel that he is disappointing us in any real sense this morning; and if I understand the wishes of the teachers, it has not been that he should discuss so much the rather technical question of the verbal or truth-revealed inspiration of the Bible, but rather that he will give us some further instruction along the line of the inspiration of the spirit of prophecy and its relation to that of the Bible. I have nothing further to press along that line, but as teachers have expressed themselves to me, I have felt that it might be well to consider some aspects of that question a little further, particularly the use of unpublished writings, letters, talks, etc., in the light of what was referred to here the other day. Sister White herself said that if we wanted to know what the spirit of prophecy said on a thing, we should read her published writings. That is one question I think the teachers have in mind, Brother Daniells.

F. M. Wilcox: I have enjoyed these discussions very much. I enjoyed the evening of last week when the question of the spirit of prophecy was considered. I enjoyed very much the talk Elder Daniells gave on the question, and I think the view he took of the question very fully agrees with my own view. I have known for long years the way in which Sister White's works were brought together and her books compiled. I have never believed in the verbal inspiration of the Testimonies. I must say, however, that last Wednesday evening and also since then, some remarks have been made without proper safeguarding, and I should question the effect of those statements and positions out in the field. I know that there is considerable talk around Takoma Park over positions that have been taken here, and there will be that same situation out in the field. As Brother Wakeham suggested the other day, I think we have to deal with a very delicate question, and I would hate terribly to see an influence sweep over the field and into any of our schools that the Testimonies were discounted. There is great danger of a reaction, and I do feel concerned.

I have heard questions raised here that have left the impression on my mind that if the same questions are raised in our classes when we get back to our schools, we are going to have serious difficulty. I believe there are a great many questions that we should hold back, and not discuss. I am not a teacher in a school, although I did teach the Bible 13 years in a nurses' training school, where I had a large number of young people; but I can not conceive that it is necessary for us to answer every question that is put to us by students or others, or be driven into a place where we will take a position that will lessen faith. I think the Testimonies of the Spirit of God are a great asset to this denomination, and I think if we destroy faith in them, we are going to destroy faith in the very foundation of our work. I must say that I do view with a great deal of concern the influence that will go out from this meeting, and from questions that I have seen raised here. And unless these questions can be dealt with most diplomatically, I think we are going to have serious trouble. I surely hope the Lord will give us wisdom so that we shall know what to say and do in meeting these things in the future.

C. L. Benson: I have felt very much concerned along the same line; and the question that has raised itself in my own mind goes a little further than has been brought up here; but it seems to me it is almost a logical step. That is this: If there are such uncertainties with reference to our historical position, and if the Testimonies are not to be relied on to throw a great deal of light upon our historical positions, and if the same is true with reference to our theological interpretation of texts, then how can we consistently place implicit confidence in the direction that is given with reference to our educational problems, and our medical school, and even our denominational organization? If there is a definite spiritual leadership in these things, then how can we consistently lay aside the Testimonies or partially lay them aside when it comes to the prophetic and historic side of the message and place these things on the basis of research work? That question is in my mind, and I am confident that it is in the minds of others.

N. J. Waldorf: That is in my mind. That is why I brought out that illustration on the blackboard this morning, — those three rivers, history, spirit of prophecy, and the Bible.

J. N. Anderson: I thought when we dismissed [discussed?] the subject the other day the main question was how we as teachers should deal with this question when we stand before our students. I think we have come to quite a unanimous opinion about this matter among ourselves here, and we stand pretty well together, I should say, as to what position the Testimonies occupy, — their authority and their relation to the Bible, and so on, — but the question in my mind, and in the mind of some others, too, I think, is What shall we as teachers do when we stand before our classes and some historical question comes up, such as we have spoken of here, where we have decided that Sister White's writings are not final? We say there are many historical facts that we believe scholarship must decide, that Sister White never claimed to be final on the historical matters that appear in her writings. Are we safe to tell that to our students? Or shall we hold it in abeyance? And can we hold something in the back of our head that we are absolutely sure about, and that most of the brethren stand with us on? — can we hold those things back and be true to ourselves? And furthermore, are we safe in doing it? Is it well to let our people in general go on holding to the verbal inspiration of the Testimonies? When we do that, aren't we preparing for a crisis that will be very serious some day? It seems to me that the best thing for us to do is to cautiously and very carefully educate our people to see just where we really should stand to be consistent protestants, to be consistent with the Testimonies themselves, and to be consistent with what we know we must do, as intelligent men, as we have decided in these meetings.

Of course these are not such big questions, because I do not teach along this line. Still, they do sometimes arise in my classes. But personally I am not concerned about it. I am concerned about the faith of the young men and women that come into our schools. They are to be our leaders, and I think these are the days when they should be given the very best foundation we can give them. We should give them the most sincere and honest beliefs that we have in our own hearts.

I speak with some feeling because it does come close to my convictions that something should be done here in this place, — here is where it can be done — to safeguard our people, to educate them and to bring them back and cause them to stand upon the only foundation that can ever be secure as we advance and progress.

C. L. Taylor: With regard to the verbal inspiration of the Testimonies, I would say that I have heard more about it here in one day than ever before in my life. I think we have made a great big mountain of difficulty to go out and fight against. I do not believe that our people generally believe in the verbal inspiration of the Testimonies. I think that the general idea of our people is that the Testimonies are the writings of a sister who received light from God. As to verbal inspiration, I think they have a very ill-defined idea. I think they believe that in some way God gave her light, and she wrote it down, and they do not know what verbal inspiration means.

But I do see a great deal in the question Professor Benson raised, and that is if we must lay aside what Sister White has said interpreting history, or what we might call the philosophy of history, as unreliable, and also lay aside as unreliable expositions of scripture, the only natural conclusion for me, and probably for a great many others, would be that the same authorship is unreliable regarding organization, regarding pantheism, and every other subject that she ever treated on; — that she may have told the truth, but we had better get all the historical data we can to see whether she told the truth or not. That is something I would like to hear discussed. I do not believe we shall get to the foundation of the question unless we answer Professor Benson's question.

A. G. Daniells: Shall we consider some points as settled, and pass on? Take the matter of verbal inspiration. I think it is very much as Brother Taylor says, that among the most of our people there is no question. It is not agitated. They do not understand it, and they do not understand the technical features of the inspiration of the Bible, either. And the power of the Bible and its grip on the human race does not depend on a technical point as to their belief in it, whether it is verbally inspired or truth-inspired. The men who hold directly opposite positions have the same faith in the Bible. I will not allow a man who believes in the verbal inspiration of the Bible to depreciate my faith in the Bible because I do not hold with him, — I will not consent to that a moment. I know my own faith in it, I know that I have enough faith in it to get forgiveness of my sins and companionship with my Lord and the hope of heaven. I know that, and a man that holds a different view need not try to depreciate my faith because I do not hold the same view that he does. I do not depreciate another man's faith or standing with God at all because he holds a different view. I think we could argue about the inspiration of the Bible — I was going to say till doomsday — till the end, and not come to the same view, but all have the same confidence in it, and have the same experience, and all get to the same place at last.

But now with reference to the Testimonies: I think more mischief can be done with the Testimonies by claiming their verbal inspiration than can with the Bible. If you ask for the logic of it, it might take some time to bring it out, and I might not be able to satisfy every mind; but if you ask for practical experience, I can give it to you, plenty of it.

F. M. Wilcox: Because we know how the Testimonies were brought together, and we do not know anything about the Bible.

A. G. Daniells: Yes, that is one point. We do know, and it is no kind of use for anybody to stand up and talk about the verbal inspiration of the Testimonies, because everybody who has ever seen the work done knows better, and we might as well dismiss it.

M. E. Kern [secretary, Young People's Missionary Volunteer Department, and former president of the Foreign Mission Seminary]: I am not so sure that some of the brethren are right in saying that we are all agreed on this question. I came in here the other day for the first time to attend the Conference, and I would hear the same man in the same talk say that we could not depend on this historical data that was given in the spirit of prophecy, and then assert his absolute confidence in the spirit of prophecy and in the Testimonies. And then a little further along there would be something else that he would not agree with. For instance, the positive testimony against butter was mentioned, and he explained that there are exceptions to that. Later he would again say, "I have absolute confidence in the inspiration of the spirit of prophecy." The question is, What is the nature of inspiration? How can we feel, and believe and know that there is an inconsistency there, — something that is not right, and yet believe that the spirit of prophecy is inspired? Do you get the question?

A. G. Daniells: Yes, I get your question alright!

M. E. Kern: That is the difficulty we have in explaining this to young people. We may have confidence ourselves, but it is hard to make others believe it if we express this more liberal view. I can see how some might take advantage of this liberal view and go out and eat meat every meal, and say that part of the Testimonies is not reliable.

Question: Can't he do the same thing if he believes in the verbal inspiration?

M. E. Kern: Not quite so consistently. If he believed every word was inspired, he could not consistently sit down and eat meat.

A. G. Daniells: But I have seen them do it.

M. E. Kern: But not conscientiously. But now take a man who delves into the Scriptures, and he reads the Hebrew and the Greek, and he goes out and tells the people, If you understood the Greek, you would not get that meaning from the Bible, or If Sister White had understood the Greek, she would not have said that. Such a man can take a lot of license from this liberal view. Now, the question is running in my mind this way: In the very nature of the case, isn't there a human element in inspiration, because God had to speak through human instruments?

And can we, either in the Bible or the Testimonies, play upon a word and lay down the law and bind a man's conscience on a word instead of the general view of the whole scope of interpretation? I do not believe a man can believe in the general inspiration of the spirit of prophecy and still not believe that vegetarianism is the thing for mankind. I can understand how that testimony was written for individuals, and there are exceptions to it, and how Sister White in her human weakness could make a mistake in stating a truth, and still not destroy the inspiration of the spirit of prophecy; but the question is how to present these matters to the people. Brother Taylor may see no difficulty, but I see a lot of difficulty, not only in dealing with our students, but with our people in general.

A. G. Daniells: On the question of verbal inspiration?

M. E. Kern: Brother Benson's question is to the point. We had a council here a few weeks ago, and we laid down pretty straight some principles of education, and also some technicalities of education, and we based our conclusions on the authority of the spirit of prophecy, as it was written. Now we come to those historical questions, and we say, "Well, Sister White was mistaken about that, and that needs to be revised." The individual who did not quite see the points that we made at the educational council may say, "Well, possibly Sister White is wrong about the influence of universities," and it is hard to convince him that she was right, perhaps. I want, somehow, to get on a consistent basis myself.

Many years ago I was in a meeting where Dr. Kellogg and others were considering a business matter. Dr. Kellogg there took a position exactly contrary to something Sister White had said. When asked how he explained what she had said, he replied that she had been influenced to say it. He was running down the Testimonies there. A short time after that I read one of his articles in the paper, in which he was laying down the law on the basis of the Testimonies. That made me lose my confidence in Dr. Kellogg. On one point that he did not agree with, he said she had been influenced. Then he took this other thing that pleased him and he said it was from the Lord. Perhaps he thought one was from the Lord and the other was not. But we certainly do have difficulty in showing the people which is human and which is divinely inspired.

G. B. Thompson [secretary, North American Division]: Wouldn't that be true of the Bible?

M. E. Kern: That is why I propose that we discuss the nature of inspiration. I have a sort of feeling that Sister White was a prophet just as Jeremiah was, and that in time her work will show up like Jeremiah's. I wonder if Jeremiah, in his day, did not do a lot of talking and perhaps some writing which was, as Paul said, on his own authority. I wonder if, in those days, the people did not have difficulty in differentiating between what was from the Lord and what was not. But the people make it more difficult now because all of Sister White's articles and books are with us, and her letters, too, and many think that every word she has ever said or written is from the Lord. We have had sanitariums built on account of letters she has written from a depot somewhere. And undertakings involving great financial investments have been started because of a letter from her. There is no question but what many young people, and also ministers, have that idea, and it is a real problem with me. I wish we could get down to bedrock. I do not think we are there yet.

W. W. Prescott: I would like to ask if you think that, after his writings had been published a series of years, Jeremiah changed them because he was convinced that there were historical errors in them?

M. E. Kern: I can not answer that.

W. H. Wakeham: There is a real difficulty, and we will have it to meet. We may say that the people do not believe in the verbal inspiration of the Testimonies. Perhaps technically they do not know what it means. But that is not the question at all. They have accepted the Testimonies all over the country, and believe that every identical word that Sister White has written was to be received as infallible truth. We have that thing to meet when we get back, and it will be brought up in our classes just as sure as we stand here, because it has come to me over and over again in every class I have taught. It not only comes out in classes, but in the churches. I know we have a very delicate task before us if we meet the situation and do it in the way the Lord wants it done. I am praying very earnestly for help as I go back to meet some of the things I know I am going to meet.

W. E. Howell: Surely we are getting our difficulties aired well this morning, and that is perfectly proper; but we have only ten minutes left of the period in which to give some attention to the solution of those difficulties. We have invited men of much larger experience than we are to come in and help us and give us their counsel. It seems to me we ought to give them some time.

G. B. Thompson: It seems to me that if we are going to preach the Testimonies and establish confidence in them, it does not depend on whether they are verbally inspired or not. I think we are in this fix because of a wrong education that our people have had. [Voice: That is true.] If we had always taught the truth on this question, we would not have any trouble or shock in the denomination now. But the shock is because we have not taught the truth, and have put the Testimonies on a plane where she says they do not stand. We have claimed more for them than she did. My thought is this, that the evidence of the inspiration of the Testimonies is not in their verbal inspiration, but in their influence and power in the denomination. Now to illustrate: Brother Daniells and I were in Battle Creek at a special crisis, and word came to us that some special testimonies were on the way to us from Sister White, and for us to stay there until they came. When they came we found they were to be read to the people. They were of a very serious character. They had been written a year before and filed away. Brother Daniells and I prayed about it, and then we sent out the word to the people that a meeting was to be held at a certain time. When the time came, about 3,000 people came into the Tabernacle, and they filled it up, even away back up into the "peanut gallery." There were unbelievers and skeptics there, and all classes. Brother Daniells stood up there and read that matter to them, and I tell you there was a power went with it that gripped that whole congregation. And after the meeting was over, people came to us and told us that the Testimony described a meeting they had held the night before. I was convinced that there was more than ordinary power in that document. It was not whether it was verbally inspired or not, but it carried the power of the Spirit of God with it.

I think if we could get at it from that line, we would get along better. They are not verbally inspired, — we know that, — and what is the use of teaching that they are?

M. E. Kern: I would like to suggest that this question of verbal inspiration does not settle the difficulty.

C. M. Sorenson: Does Sister White use the word "inspiration" concerning her own writings, or is that merely a theory we have worked up ourselves? I ask for information. I have never seen that in her writings.

A. G. Daniells: I hardly know where to begin or what to say. I think I must repeat this, that our difficulty lies in two points, especially. One is on infallibility and the other is on verbal inspiration. I think Brother James White foresaw difficulties along this line away back at the beginning. He knew that he took Sister White's testimonies and helped to write them out and make them clear and grammatical and plain. He knew that he was doing that right along. And he knew that the secretaries they employed took them and put them into grammatical condition, transposed sentences, completed sentences, and used words that Sister White did not herself write in her original copy. He saw that, and yet he saw some brethren who did not know this, and who had great confidence in the Testimonies, just believing and teaching that these words were given to Sister White as well as the thought. And he tried to correct that idea. You will find those statements in the *Review and Herald,* like the one Brother Wilcox read the other day. If that explanation had been accepted and passed on down, we would have been free from a great many perplexities that we have now.

F. M. Wilcox: Articles were published in those early *Reviews* disclaiming that.

A. G. Daniells: Yes, but you know there are some brethren who go in all over. We could mention some old and some young who think they cannot believe the Testimonies without just putting them up as absolutely infallible and word-inspired, taking the whole thing as given verbally by the Lord. They do not see how to believe them and how to get good out of them except in that way; and I suppose some people would feel that if they did not believe in the verbal inspiration of the Bible, they could not have confidence in it, and take it as the great Book that they now see it to be. Some men are technical, and can hardly understand it in any other way. Some other men are not so technical in logic, but they have great faith and great confidence, and so they can go through on another line of thought. I am sure there has been advocated an idea of infallibility in Sister White and verbal inspiration in the Testimonies that has led people to expect too much and to make too great claims, and so we have gotten into difficulty.

Now, as I have studied it these years since I was thrown into the controversy at Battle Creek, I have endeavored to ascertain the truth and then be true to the truth. I do not know how to do except that way. It will never help me, or help the people, to make a false claim to evade some trouble. I know we have difficulties here, but let us dispose of some of the main things first. Brethren, are we going to evade difficulties or help out the difficulties by taking a false position? [Voices: No!] Well, then let us take an honest, true position, and reach our end somehow, because I never will put up a false claim to evade something that will come up a little later on. That is not honest and it is not Christian, and so I take my stand there.

In Australia I saw "The Desire of Ages" being made up, and I saw the rewriting of chapters, some of them written over and over and over again. I saw that, and when I talked with Sister [Marian] Davis about it, I tell you I had to square up to this thing and begin to settle things about the spirit of prophecy. If these false positions had never been taken, the thing would be much plainer than it is today. What was charged as plagiarism would all have been simplified, and I believe men would have been saved to the cause if from the start we had understood this thing as it should have been. With those false views held, we face difficulties in straightening up. We will not meet those difficulties by resorting to a false claim. We could meet them just for today by saying, "Brethren, I believe in the verbal inspiration of the Testimonies; I believe in the infallibility of the one through whom they came, and everything that is written there I will take and I will stand on that against all comers." If we did that, I would just take everything from A to Z, exactly as it was written, without making any explanations to anyone; and I would not eat butter or salt or eggs if I believed that the Lord gave the words in those Testimonies to Sister White for the whole body of people in this world. But I do not believe it.

M. E. Kern: You couldn't and keep your conscience clear.

A. G. Daniells: No, I couldn't; but I do not believe that; and I can enter upon an explanation of health reform that I think is consistent, and that she endeavored to bring in in later years when she saw people making a bad use of that. I have eaten pounds of butter at her table myself, and dozens of eggs. I could not explain that in her own family if I believed that she believed those were the Lord's own words to the world. But there are people who believe that and do not eat eggs or butter. I do not know that they use salt. I know plenty of people in the early days did not use salt, and it was in our church. I am sure that many children suffered from it.

There is no use of our claiming anything more on the verbal inspiration of the Testimonies, because she never claimed it, and James White never claimed it, and W. C. White never claimed it; and all the persons who helped to prepare those Testimonies knew they were not verbally inspired. I will say no more along that line.

D. A. Parsons [president, Eastern Pennsylvania Conference]: She not only did not claim it, but she denied it.

A. G. Daniells: Yes, she tried to correct the people.

Now on infallibility. I suppose Sister White used Paul's text, "We have this treasure in earthen vessels," as much as any other scripture. She used to repeat that often, "We have this treasure in earthen vessels," with the idea that she was a poor, feeble woman, a messenger of the Lord trying to do her duty and meet the mind of God in this work. When you take the position that she was not infallible, and that her writings were not verbally inspired, isn't there a chance for the manifestation of the human? If there isn't, then what is infallibility? And should we be surprised when we know that the instrument was fallible, and that the general truths, as she says, were revealed, then aren't we prepared to see mistakes?

M. E. Kern: She was an author and not merely a pen.

A. G. Daniells: Yes; and now take that "Life of Paul," — I suppose you all know about it and knew what claims were put up against her, charges made of plagiarism, even by the authors of the book, Conybeare and Howson, and were liable to make the denomination trouble because there was so much of their book put into "The Life of Paul" without any credit or quotation marks. Some people of strict logic might fly the track on that ground, but I am not built that way. I found it out, and I read it with Brother [E. R.] Palmer [general manager of the Review and Herald Publishing Association] when he found it, and we got Conybeare and Howson, and we got Wylie's "History of the Reformation," and we read word for word, page after page, and no quotations, no credit, and really I did not know the difference until I began to compare them. I supposed it was Sister White's own work. The poor sister said, "Why, I didn't know about quotations and credits. My secretary should have looked after that, and the publishing house should have looked after it."

She did not claim that that was all revealed to her and written word for word under the inspiration of the Lord. There I saw the manifestation of the human in these writings. Of course I could have said this, and I did say it, that I wished a different course had been taken in the compilation of the books. If proper care had been exercised, it would have saved a lot of people from being thrown off the track.

Mrs. Williams: The secretary would know that she ought not to quote a thing without using quotation marks.

A. G. Daniells: You would think so. I do not know who the secretary was. The book was set aside, and I have never learned who had a hand in fixing that up. It may be that some do know.

B. L. House [Bible teacher, Southwestern Junior College]: May I ask one question about that book? Did Sister White write any of it?

A. G. Daniells: O, yes!

B. L. House: But there are some things that are not in Conybeare and Howson that are not in the new book, either. Why are those striking statements not embodied in the new book?

A. G. Daniells: I cannot tell you. But if her writings were verbally inspired, why should she revise them?

B. L. House: My difficulty is not with the verbal inspiration. My difficulty is here: You take the nine volumes of the Testimonies, and as I understand it, Sister White wrote the original matter from which they were made up, except that they were corrected so far as grammar, capitalization and punctuation are concerned. But such books as "Sketches of the Life of Paul," "Desire of Ages," and "Great Controversy," were composed differently, it seems to me, even by her secretaries than the nine volumes of the Testimonies. Is there not a

Appendix 4

difference? I have felt that the Testimonies were not produced like those other books.

A. G. Daniells: I do not know how much revision she might have made in those personal Testimonies before she put them out.

B. L. House: Did anyone else ever write anything that is found in the nine volumes of the Testimonies?

A. G. Daniells: No, I do not know that there are any quotations in the Testimonies.

B. L. House: Isn't there a difference, then, between the nine volumes of the Testimonies and those other books for which her secretaries were authorized to collect valuable quotations from other books?

A. G. Daniells: You admit that she had the right to revise her work?

B. L. House: O, Yes.

A. G. Daniells: Then your question is, Why did she leave out of the revision some striking things that she wrote that it seems should have been put in?

B. L. House: Yes.

M. E. Kern: In the first volume of the spirit of prophecy there are some details given, if I am not mistaken, as to the height of Adam. It seems to me that when she went to prepare "Patriarchs and Prophets" for the public, even though that had been shown her, it did not seem wise to put that before the public.

A. G. Daniells: And she also left out of our books for the public that scene of Satan playing the game of life.

B. L. House: In that old edition of "Sketches of the Life of Paul," she is very clear about the ceremonial law. That is not in the new book, and I wondered why that was left out.

D. A. Parsons: I have an answer to that. I was in California when the book was compiled, and I took the old edition and talked with Brother Will White about this very question. He said the whole book, with the exception of that chapter, had been compiled for some time, and they had held it up until they could arrange that chapter in such a way as to prevent controversy arising. They did not desire the book to be used to settle any controversy, and therefore they eliminated most of these statements on the ceremonial law just to prevent a renewal of the great controversy over the ceremonial law in Galatians.

B. L. House: It is not a repudiation of what was written by her in the first volume, is it?

D. A. Parsons: No, not at all; but they just put in enough to satisfy the inquiring mind, but eliminated those striking statements to prevent a renewal of the controversy.

F. M. Wilcox: I would like to ask, Brother Daniells, if it could be accepted as a sort of rule that Sister White might be mistaken in details, but in the general policy and instruction she was an authority. For instance, I hear a man saying, I can not accept Sister White on this, when perhaps she has devoted pages to the discussion of it. A man said he could not accept what Sister White said about royalties on books, and yet she devotes pages to that subject, and emphasizes it again and again; and it is the same with policies for our schools and publishing houses and sanitariums. It seems to me I would have to accept what she says on some of those general policies or I would have to sweep away the whole thing. Either the Lord has spoken through her or He has not spoken through her; and if it is a matter of deciding in my own judgment whether He has or has not, then I regard her books the same as every other book published. I think it is one thing for a man to stultify his conscience, and it is another thing to stultify his judgment. It is one thing for me to lay aside my conscience, and it is another thing for me to change my judgment over some views that I hold.

A. G. Daniells: I think Brother Benson's question on historical and theological matters has not been dealt with yet, and I do not know

Appendix 4

that I am able to give any light. Perhaps some of you may know to what extent Sister White has revised some of her statements and references or quotations from historical writings. Have you ever gone through and made a list of them?

W. W. Prescott: I gave nearly an hour to that the other day, taking the old edition of "Great Controversy" and reading it and then reading the revised edition. But that did not cover all the ground.

A. G. Daniells: We did not create that difficulty, did we? We General Conference men did not create it, for we did not make the revision. We did not take any part in it. We had nothing whatever to do with it. It was all done under her supervision. If there is a difficulty there, she created it, did she not?

F. M. Wilcox: She assumed the whole responsibility for it.

M. E. Kern: But we have to meet it.

A. G. Daniells: Well, now, which statement shall we take, the original or the revised?

B. L. House: My real difficulty is just here: Sister White did not write either the old edition or the revised, as I understand it.

A. G. Daniells: What do you mean by saying that she did not write either edition?

B. L. House: As I understand it, Elder J. N. Anderson prepared those historical quotations for the old edition, and Brother [Dores E.] Robinson and Brother [Clarence C.] Crisler, Professor Prescott and others furnished the quotations for the new edition. Did she write the historical quotations in there?

A. G. Daniells: No.

B. L. House: Then there is a difference between the Testimonies and those books.

W. W. Prescott: Changes have been made in what was not historical extract at all.

A. G. Daniells: Shall we not confine ourselves just now to this question of Brother Benson's and lead our way up to the real difficulty, and then deal with it? Do you have a clear conception of the way the difficulty arose? — that in making the first edition of "Great Controversy" those who helped her prepare the copy were allowed to bring forward historical quotations that seemed to fit the case. She may have asked, "Now, what good history do you have for that?" I do not know just how she brought it in, but she never would allow us to claim anything for her as a historian. She did not put herself up as a corrector of history, — not only did not do that, but protested against it. Just how they dealt in bringing the history along, I could not say, but I suspect that she referred to this as she went along, and then allowed them to gather the very best historical statements they could and submit them to her, and she approved of them.

C. L. Benson: This is my query, and it underlies all of her writings: How did she determine upon the philosophy of history? If she endorsed our interpretation of history, without any details, do we dare to set that aside? I understand she never studied medical science; but she has laid down certain fundamental principles; and that she has done the same with education and organization.

A. G. Daniells: Sister White never has written anything on the philosophy of history.

C. L. Benson: No, but she has endorsed our 2300 day proposition, from 538 to 1798.

A. G. Daniells: You understand she did that by placing that in her writings?

C. L. Benson: Yes.

A. G. Daniells: Yes, I suppose she did.

Appendix 4

C. A. Shull: I think the book "Education" contains something along the line of the philosophy of history.

W. E. Howell: Yes, she outlines general principles.

C. M. Sorenson: Nobody has ever questioned Sister White's philosophy of history, so far as I know, — and I presume I have heard most of the questions raised about it, — along the line of the hand of God in human affairs and the way the hand of God has been manifested. The only question anybody has raised has been about minor details. Take this question as to whether 533 has some significance taken in connection with 538. She never set 533, but if there is a significance attached to it in human affairs, it certainly would not shut us out from using it, and that would not affect the 1260 years. Some people say antichrist is yet to come, and is to last for three and one-half literal years. If you change those positions, you will change the philosophy.

W. W. Prescott: Do I understand Brother Benson's view is that such a statement as that in "Great Controversy," that the 1260 years began in 538 and ended in 1798, settles the matter infallibly?

C. L. Benson: No, only on the preaching of doctrines in general. If she endorses the prophetic part of our interpretation, irrespective of details, then she endorses it.

W. W. Prescott: Then that settles it as being a part of that philosophy.

C. L. Benson: Yes, in this way: I do not see how we can do anything else but set up our individual judgment if we say we will discount that, because we have something else that we think is better evidence. It is the same with education and the medical science.

W. W. Prescott: You are touching exactly the experience through which I went, personally, because you all know that I contributed something toward the revision of "Great Controversy." I furnished considerable material bearing upon that question.

A. G. Daniells: By request.

W. W. Prescott: Yes, I was asked to do it, and at first I said, "No, I will not do it. I know what it means." But I was urged into it. When I had gone over it with W. C. White, then I said, "Here is my difficulty. I have gone over this and suggested changes that ought to be made in order to correct statements. These changes have been accepted. My personal difficulty will be to retain faith on those things that I can not deal with on that basis." But I did not throw up the spirit of prophecy, and have not yet; but I have had to adjust my view of things. I will say to you, as a matter of fact, that the relation of those writings to this movement and to our work, is clearer and more consistent in my mind than it was then. But still you know what I am charged with. I have gone through the personal experience myself over that very thing that you speak of. If we correct it here and correct it there, how are we going to stand with it in the other places?

F. M. Wilcox: Those things do not involve the general philosophy of the book.

W. W. Prescott: No, but they did involve quite large details. For instance, before "Great Controversy" was revised, I was unorthodox on a certain point, but after it was revised, I was perfectly orthodox.

C. M. Sorenson: On what point?

W. W. Prescott: My interpretation was, (and I taught it for years in *The Protestant Magazine*) that Babylon stood for the great apostasy against God, which headed up in the papacy, but which included all minor forms, and that before we come to the end, they would all come under one. That was not the teaching of "Great Controversy." "Great Controversy" said that Babylon could not mean the Romish church, and I had made it mean that largely and primarily. After the book was revised, although the whole argument remained the same, it said that it could not mean the Roman Church *alone,* just that one word added.

F. M. Wilcox: That helped you out.

W. W. Prescott: Yes, but I told W. C. White I did not think anybody had any right to do that. And I did not believe anybody had any right

Appendix 4

to use it against me before or afterward. I simply went right on with my teaching.

J. N. Anderson: Would you not claim other portions of the book as on the same basis?

W. W. Prescott: No, I would refuse to do that. I had to deal with A. R. Henry [the deceased head of the Seventh-day Adventist Publishing Association] over that question. He was determined to crush those men that took a wrong course concerning him. I spent hours with that man trying to help him. We were intimate in our work, and I used to go to his house and spend hours with him. He brought up this question about the authority of the spirit of prophecy and wanted me to draw the line between what was authoritative and what was not. I said, "Brother Henry, I will not attempt to do it, and I advise you not to do it. There is an authority in that gift here, and we must recognize it."

I have tried to maintain personal confidence in this gift in the church, and I use it and use it. I have gotten great help from those books, but I will tell you frankly that I held to that position on the question of Babylon for years when I knew it was exactly contrary to "Great Controversy," but I went on, and in due time I became orthodox. I did not enjoy that experience at all, and I hope you will not have to go through it. It means something.

C. L. Benson: That is the pivotal point. You had something that enabled you to take that position. What was it?

W. W. Prescott: I can not lay down any rule for anybody. What settled me to take that position was the Bible, not any secular authority.

J. N. Anderson: Your own findings must be your authority for believing and not believing.

W. W. Prescott: You can upset every thing by applying that as a general principle.

C. P. Bollman: Could you tell, in just a few words, how the Bible helped you?

W. W. Prescott: That would involve the whole question of the beast.

Voice: To your knowledge, has Sister White ever made a difference between her nine volumes and her other books?

W. W. Prescott: I have never talked with her about it. In my mind, there is a difference between the works she largely prepared herself and what was prepared by others for sale to the public.

A. G. Daniells: You might as well state that a little fuller, the difference in the way they were produced.

W. W. Prescott: If I should speak my mind frankly, I should say that I have felt for years that great mistakes were made in handling her writings for commercial purposes.

C. M. Sorenson: By whom?

W. W. Prescott: I do not want to charge anybody. But I do think great mistakes were made in that way. That is why I have made a distinction as I have. When I talked with W. C. White about it (and I do not know that he is an infallible authority), he told me frankly that when they got out "Great Controversy," if they did not find in her writings anything on certain chapters to make the historical connections, they took other books, like "Daniel and the Revelation," and used portions of them; and sometimes her secretaries, and sometimes she herself, would prepare a chapter that would fill the gap.

C. A. Shull: I would like to ask if Brother Prescott wishes to be understood that his attitude is that wherever his own judgment comes in conflict with any statement in the spirit of prophecy, he will follow his judgment rather than the spirit of prophecy?

W. W. Prescott: No, I do not want anybody to get that understanding. That is the very understanding that I do not want anybody to get.

C. A. Shull: Then that was an exceptional case?

Appendix 4

W. W. Prescott: Yes, I was forced to that from my study of the Bible. When I made up my mind to that, I did not parade it before the people and say, "Here is a mistake in 'Great Controversy,' and if you study the Bible you will find it to be so." I did not attack the spirit of prophecy. My attitude has been to avoid anything like opposition to the gift in this church, but I avoid such a misuse of it as to set aside the Bible. I do not want anybody to think for a moment that I set up my judgment against the spirit of prophecy.

A. G. Daniells: Let us remember that, brethren, and not say a word that will misrepresent Brother Prescott.

B. L. House: Did Sister White herself write that statement that the term Babylon could not apply to the Catholic Church, or was that copied from some other author?

W. W. Prescott: That was in the written statement.

B. L. House: Has she ever changed any of the nine volumes of the Testimonies?

W. W. Prescott: "Great Controversy" is the only book I know of that has been revised.

C. M. Sorenson: Hasn't "Early Writings" been revised? I understand some omissions have been made in the later editions.

W. W. Prescott: Perhaps some things have been left out, but I do not think the writing itself has been revised.

A. G. Daniells: You know there is a statement that the pope changed the Sabbath, and another one, that the papacy was abolished. What do you do with those?

B. L. House: There is no trouble with that.

A. G. Daniells: Why not? The pope did not change the Sabbath?

B. L. House: But the pope stands for the papacy.

A. G. Daniells: There are people that just believe there was a certain pope that changed the Sabbath, because of the way they follow the words. She never meant to say that a certain pope changed the Sabbath; but do you know, I have had that brought up to me a hundred times in ministers' meetings.

B. L. House: I have never had any trouble on that.

A. G. Daniells: But you are only one. There are about 2,000 others. I have had to work with men just gradually and carefully and all the time keep from giving out the idea that I was a doubter of the Testimonies.

I know it is reported around that some of us men here at Washington, in charge of the general administrative work, are very shaky and unbelieving, but I want to tell you that I know better. I know that my associates have confidence right down on the solid platform of this whole question; and I know that if many of you had gone at this thing and experienced what we have, you would have passed through an experience that would have given you solid ground. You would have shaken a bit, and you are beginning to shake now, and some of you do not know where you are going to land. These questions show it. But that is not to say there is not a foundation. It is to say that you have not gone through the toils yet and got your feet on solid ground.

I want to make this suggestion, because with all these questions we can not follow one line of thought logically: We must use good sense in dealing with this whole question, brethren. Do not be careless with your words. Do not be careless in reporting or representing men's views. I have had this thing to deal with for years and years, as you know, in every ministers' meeting; and I have been called into college classes over and over again, and have had to say things that those ministers and students never heard before about this; and I have prayed for wisdom and for the Spirit of the Lord to direct them and to give faith and to cover up those things that would leave doubt. And I have never had it come back on me that a careful, cautious statement made in the fear of God has upset a single person. It may

Appendix 4

have done it, but it has never come back to me. You take our ministers: This brother [meaning Brother Waldorf] knows how much this was brought up in our ministers' meetings over in Australia, and we dealt with it plainly. We did not try to pull the wool over the people's eyes, and I believe you will find the Australian preachers and churches as firm believers in the spirit of prophecy and in Sister White's call by the Lord as you will find any place on the face of the earth. Take New Zealand: I brought them up there, and I think it is well known that there is not a place in the world where the people stand truer to this gift than they do there.

I do not believe it is necessary to dissemble a bit, but I do believe, brethren, that we have got to use wisdom that God alone can give us in dealing with this until matters gradually work over. We have made a wonderful change in nineteen years, Brother Prescott. Fifteen years ago we could not have talked what we are talking here today. It would not have been safe. This matter has come along gradually, and yet people are not losing their confidence in the gift. Last year we sold 5,000 sets of the Testimonies, and they cost eight or nine dollars a set. In one year our brethren and sisters, under the influence of the General Conference, and the union conference and local conference men and our preachers, under their influence, without any compulsion, our brethren came along and spent forty or fifty thousand dollars for the Testimonies. What would you consider that an indication of?

Voice: Confidence.

A. G. Daniells: Yes, confidence, and a friendly attitude. They did not buy them as critics to tear them to pieces. We must be judged by our fruits. I want to tell you that the clearer view we get on the exact facts in the case, the stronger the position of our people will be in the whole thing.

Now, Brother Benson, I see the whole line running through there that you referred to. We can not correct that in a day. We must use great judgment and caution. I hope you Bible teachers will be exceedingly careful. I was called up here twice to speak on the spirit of prophecy to the Bible and pastoral training classes. They brought up this question of history. I simply said, "Now, boys, Sister White never claimed to be a historian nor a corrector of history. She used the best she knew for the matter she was writing on." I have never heard from a teacher that those boys buzzed around them and said, "Brother Daniells does not believe Sister White's writings are reliable." I believe the Lord will help us to take care of this if we will be careful and use good sense. I think that is all I can say in this sort of discussion.

Index

(**Boldface** numbers refer to pictures.)

Abolition, 93, 102, 103, 121
Advent Mirror, 56-57
Advent Review and Sabbath Herald, 71, 72-73, 86, 87, 93, 128-31, 136-37, 140, 149-50, 157-59, 162, 165-66, 171, 181, 220, 228, 231, 254, 258
Adventist Heritage, 15, 21
Albany Conference of 1845, 58, 71
Albertsworth, E. F., 358
Alcohol, 83, 84-85, 100, 102, 109, 219, 225, 227-29, 231, 236, 265. *See also* Temperance
Alcott, Bronson, 103
Alcott, Louisa May, 103
Alcott, William A., 103-5, **104**, 107, 110, 120, 207
Amadon, Martha Byington, 140
American Anti-Tobacco Society, 87
American costume, 123, 124, 130, 144, 185, **189**, 190, 191, 195-97, 320. *See also* Dress and dress reform; Bloomer costume
American Health and Temperance Association, 229-30
American Hydropathic Institute, 115, 117, 123
American Medical Association, 263

American Medical Missionary College, 253, 254, 261, 262
American Phrenological Journal, 120, 206
American Physiological Society, 105-6
American Vegetarian Society, 120
Anderson, Eric, 31
Anderson, J. N., 352, 357, 364, 378-79, 392
Andrews, Angeline Stevens, 141, 143
Andrews, Charles Melville, 141
Andrews, John N., 87, 131, 140-41, 143, 157, 164, 174, 244
Andrews University Bookstore, 30
Animal passions. *See* Sex
Animals, cruelty to, 221, 133, 135
Ann Arbor, Michigan, 252
Anthony, Susan B., 185
Anti-liquor and tobacco pledge, 229
Anti-meat pledge, 13, 134-35
An Appeal to Mothers (EGW), 14, 208-11, **209**, 212, 216, 221, 272
Arthur, Jesse, 255
Association of Adventist Forums, xii
Austin, Harriet N., 123-24, 144, **189**, 191, 196, 321

Index

Australia, 233, 235, 245-46, 247, 258

Baby Fae, xxvi
Baker, Miss, 330, 333, 335-41
Bangkok, Thailand, 266
Bangs, Elizabeth Harmon, 44, **46**, 52, 284
Barnes, John D., 145
Bartlett, Elisha, 113
Barton, Clara, 153
Basel, Switzerland, 244
Bates, Joseph, 57-58, 71, 84, 85, 128
Bathing, 99, 101, 102, 115, 129. *See also* Hydropathy
Battery, shocks from, 150
Battistone, Joseph J., 35-36
Battle Creek, Michigan, 75, 91, 92, 107, 129, 132, 138, 140, 144, 145-46, 150, 151, 153, 156, 171, 173, 215, 238, 240, 247, 254
Battle Creek College, 179, 243
Battle Creek Reform Club, 228
Battle Creek Sanitarium, 181, 232, 238, 243, 247, **248**, 261, 262; burning, 247; establishment of training programs, 251-53. *See also* Western Health Reform Institute
Battle Creek schism, 253-62
Beards, 101, 204
Beaumont, William, 100
The Beauties and Deformities of Tobacco-Using (Coles), 109-10, 135
Beethoven Hall (Portland), 54, 60
Belém, Brazil, 266
Bellevue Hospital Medical School, 179
Benson, C. L., 365, 374-75, 378, 393-96, 400
Bible Christian Church, 97
Bible Conferences of 1919, xii, 38-39, 344-401
Bigelow, Jacob, 182
Bloomer, Amelia, 185, **187**
Bloomer Costume, xxxi, 120, 121, 185, **187**, 188, 190, 320. *See also* American costume; Dress and dress reform
Bollman, C. P., 348, 358-59, 365, 396
Bolton, Frances, 258-59, 287-88, 313
Bonnets, 198
Boston, Massachusetts, 100, 103, 136, 249
Boston Medical and Surgical Journal, 109
Boston Medical Association, 108
Botanic remedies, 79, 111, 263. *See also* Thomsonianism
Boulder, Colorado, 241, 247
Bourdeau, D. T., 151-52, 158, 164
Bowling, 146
Brackett Street School, 44
Brand, Leonard, xxiv
Branson, Roy, xii, xviii, 5, 26, 40
Branson, W. H., 4
Bread, 99, 101, 121, 125, 137-38
Breast paddings, 203
Brigham, Amariah, 273
Brighton, Australia, 233, 273
Brodie, Fawn, 10, 29
Brook Farm, 103
Broussais, François J. V., 99, 211
Brown, Samuel E., 54-55
Brownsberger, Sidney, 179
Bull, Malcolm, 6
Butler, G. I., 182, 206
Butler, Jonathan M., xi, xviii-xix, xxvi, 36, 40
Butter, 100, 125, 138, 164, 219, 223, 224, 231, 236-37, 238, 256, 321, 387
Buxton, Maine, 51
Byington, John F., 91
Byington, John F., Jr., 162, 165

Cake, 236
California, 202, 228, 233, 235, 241, 246-47, 248-49
Calomel, 135, 165

Index

Cambell, David (or Campbell), 102, 106
Camden, New York, 80
Cancer, 86, 227, 235, 236. *See also* Cancerous humors
Cancerous humors, 134, 210, 237, 272. *See also* Cancer
Canright, Dudley M., 4, 9, 27
Card-playing, 145, 153, 321
Carlson, Clayton, 23-24
Carner, Vern, v, xi, xxxiv, 15, 19
Casco Street Christian Church (Portland), 50-51
Castleton Medical College, 108
Catalepsy, 63
"The Cause of Exhausted Vitality" (Miller), 216
Caviness, L. L., 352
Celibacy, 217-18
Centerport, New York, 78
Cereals, 250
Chamberlain, Josie, **199**
Chamberlain, Mary A., 162
Charcoal, 245
Charlotte, Michigan, 243
Cheese, 84, 100, 219, 223, 224, 231, 236, 238
Chestnut Street Methodist Church (Portland), 51, 53
Cheyne, George, 96
Chicago, 249, 253; alleged building in, 255-56
Chocolate, hot, 102
Cholera epidemic of 1832, 79, 97, 99
Christian Connection, 68, 84
Christian Science, xxx, 26, 67, 265, 290. *See also* Eddy, Mary Baker
Christian Temperance and Bible Hygiene (EGW), xxxii, 217, 233
Christiania (Oslo), Norway, 244
Church of God (Adventist), 150
Cider, 82
Circumcision, 217
Cities, 247

Civil War, 87, 93-94, 121, 145, 149
Clark, J. W., 129, 130
Clarke, Joseph, 130
Clemons, Sister, 60
Clough, Mary L., 207, 240, 241, 305
Coffee, 83, 84, 88, 95, 100, 102, 115, 125, 134, 219, 225-27, 229, 232, 235
Coles, Larkin B., xxxii, 34, 107, 108-10, 127, 134-35, 140, 146, 148-49, 164, 207, 211, 236, 265, 271
College of Medical Evangelists, 262-63, 264. *See also* Loma Linda University
Colorado, 231, 240-41, 247
Combe, Andrew, 96
Combe, George, 96, 117
Comet of 1843, 54
Complex partial seizures, 268, 278-79
Condiments, 100, 164
Conkin, Paul K., xvi
Conklin, William D., xxvii
The Constitution of Man (G. Combe), 96
Consumption, 65, 76, 137, 207, 212, 242
Consumption (Jackson), 137
Contraception, 216-17
Conybeare, William J., 257, 388-89
Cook, Marietta V., 130, 141, 190
Coon, Glenn, 4
Coon, Roger W., xxiii
Cooper, James Fenimore, 115
Cooranbong, Australia, 245
Copenhagen, Denmark, 247
Corn flakes, 251
Cornell, M. E., 87, 88
Corsets, 101, 102, 120, 184, 185
Cosmetics, 203
Cottrell, Roswell F., 128, 139
Counsels on Diets and Foods (EGW), 265
Country settings for sanitariums, 247-49
Couperus, Molleurus, xii, 268
Cranmer, Gilbert, 88
Cream, 138, 164, 224

Index

The Creationists (Numbers), xxvii
Crisler, Clarence C., 392
Curtis, Alva, 113
Curtis, Eli, 190

Dain, Norman, 270
Dairy products, 100, 164, 174-75, 220, 223-25, 231, 236, 237, 256. *See also* Butter; Milk
Dancing, 101, 145, 153, 321
Dammon, Israel, xii, 326-43
Daniel, prophecies of, 48, 55, 56
Daniells, A. G., 38, 234-35, 254, 259, 261; and the 1919 Bible conferences, xiii-xiv, 344-401
Dansville, 121, 124-25, 128, **129**, 130, 136, 140-45, 146, 150-54, 156, 157, 160, 185, 188, 191, 195-97, 206, 220, 225. *See also* Our Home on the Hillside
Darwin, Charles, 290
Davies, Marian, 387
Day-Star, 70
Defense of Elder James White and Wife, 172, 239-40
Demonic possession, 270
The Desire of Ages (EGW), 387, 389
Detroit Medical College, 160
Diagnostic and Statistical Manual of Mental Disorders, 278
Diet, 84, 86, 89-90, 95-101, 102, 103, 105, 125, 131, 133, 134, 137-38, 144, 145, 159, 162, 211, 219-38, 250-51, 156-57, 172, 321
Diphtheria, "Diphtheria, Its Causes, Treatment and Cure" (Jackson), 94, 126, 127, 130, 131, 136, 265
The Disappointed (Numbers and Butler), xxvi
Ditzion, Sidney, 120
Divorce, easy, 188
Dixboro Ghost, 190
Dixon, Jeane, 20
Dodge, Brother and Sister, 72

Douglass, Herbert E., xxiv-xxv
Dow, Neal, 83
Drake, Daniel, 112
Dress and dress reform, xxxi, 51-52, 90, 96, 101, 105, 115, 123, 131, 144, 145, 184-203, **186**, **187**, **189**, **194**, **199**, **201**, 320-21. *See also* American costume; Bloomer costume
Drugs, attitudes of health reformers to, 96, 101, 109, 125, 131, 133-35, 146, 156, 159, 164, 241, 249, 252, 263
Duck, wild, 13, 231
Durben, Sister, 60
Dyspepsia, 95, 207, 225
Dyspepsy Forestalled and Resisted (Hitchcock), 96

Early Writings (EGW), 398
East Kingston, New Hampshire, 49
Eclecticism, 111
Eddy, Mary Baker, xix-xx, xxi, xxvii, xxx, xxxiii, 3, 26, 67, 264-65, 290
Edersheim, Albert, 35
Edson, Hiram, 55, 56, 143
Education (EGW), 394
Eggs, 100, 219, 223-24, 231, 236, 237, 256, 387
Ellen G. White Estate, xvi-xvii, xxiv, xxviii, 268
Epilepsy, 110. *See also* Partial complex seizures
Exercise, 96, 99, 101, 105, 107, 109, 125, 153, 154, 162, 263
Exeter, Maine, 57, 60

Fairfield, Will, 183
Family Botanic Medicine (Thomson), 111
Fanaticism, 59-61, 202, 224, 237, 273-74, 326-43
Farrington, William F., 53
Finney, Charles G., 49, 103
Fitch, Charles, 127

INDEX

Flour, refined. *See* Bread
Ford, Desmond, 36-37, 40
Foss, Hazen, 61
Foss, Louisa, 61, 66
Foss, Mary Harmon, 61, 66, 67
Foss, Samuel, 61, 66
Fowler, Lorenzo N., 117, 120
Fowler, Lydia, 120
Fowler, Orson Squire, 120, 211, 216
Fox, Kate, 190
Fox, Margaret, 190
Foy, William, 60-61
Franklin Institute, 97
Free love movement, 117, 188
Free will, 271
French, T. M., 375
Fresh air, 115, 125, 131, 133, 135, 146, 263
Fruitlands, 103

Gage, William C., 174-75
Gall, Franz Joseph, 117
Germs, 237
Ginley, J. H., 162, 172
Gleason, Silas O., 121, 123
Glen Haven Water Cure, 123-24, 185
Glendale Sanitarium (California), 248
Goatees, 204
Gorham, Maine, 44, 69
Gospel of Health, 174
Gossip and stimulants, 226-27, 272
Gould, Abner, 53
Gove, Mary. *See* Mary Gove Nichols
Graham, Sylvester, xxxi, 49, 84, 86, 97-103, **98**, 105, 107, 110, 120, 125, 128, 145, 146, 148, 151, 207, 211, 216, 221, 224, 325
Graham boarding houses, 102, 103
Graham gems, 140, 144, 146, 149, 233, 325
Graham Journal of Health and Longevity, 102
Graham pudding, 46-48

Grahamism, 97-103, 113, 120, 125, 128, 137, 265, 325
Granola, 250
Granose flakes, 251
Graybill, Ronald, xv-xvii, xxviii, xxix, 14-17, 20, 23, 24-25, 37, 40
The Great Controversy (EGW), 34, 257, 286, 298, 389, 394-95, 397
The Great Controversy between God and Man (Hastings), 82
Great Disappointment (1844). *See* Millerite movement
The Great Visions of Ellen G. White (Coon), xxiii
Greeley, Horace, 103, 115
Greenville, Michigan, 154, 198
Grimké, Angelina, 185
Grimké, Sarah, 185
Grob, Gerald N., 32
Groveland, Massachusetts, 228
Guy, Fritz, 27-28

Hahnemann, Samuel, 112
Hair styles, 204-5
Hale, Apollos, 56
Hale, Ezekiel, Jr., 49, 127
Hall, Lucinda, xvi, 91
Hall, W. W., 131, 149
Hall's Journal of Health, 131
Harman, Ellen Beard, 188
Harmon, Elizabeth. *See* Elizabeth Harmon Bangs
Harmon, Ellen Gould. *See* Ellen G. White
Harmon, Eunice, 44, 53, 69, 79-80
Harmon, Mary. *See* Mary Harmon Foss
Harmon, Robert, 44, 47, 53, 65
Harmon, Robert, Jr., 53, 65
Harmon, Sarah, 66, 242
Harmon family, 44, 45, 53, 54, 69
Haskell, S. N., 182, 359
Hastings, H. L., 82
Hats, 198, 203; making of, 47
Haverhill Reform Club, 228-29

Index

"Health" (EGW), 134
Health foods, 250-51
Health; or, How to Live (EGW). *See How to Live* (EGW)
Health reform, 95-110, 114-15, 117, 120, 125-26, 127-40, 144-45, 146-49, 155, 156-83, 320-23, 324-25
"The Health Reform" (Cottrell), 139-40
Health Reformer, 162, 164-65, 174-76, 198, 205, 206, 220, 240
Henry, A. R., 396
Hilliard, Aaron, 132
Himes, John G. L., 128
Himes, Joshua V., 48, 49, 56, 59, 60, 68, 128, 136, 160
Hinsdale Sanitarium (Illinois), 249
Hinshaw, David, 18-19
History of the Sabbath (Andrews), 140
Histrionic personality style, 268, 279-90. *See also* Hysteria
Hitchcock, Edward, 96
Hobart, John, 51
Hodder, Delbert, 268
Holmes, Oliver Wendell, 95, 113, 182
Homeopathy, 107, 110, 112-13
Homosexuality, 208, 277
Hoop skirts, 90, 137, 185, 190
House, B. L., 389-92, 398-99
Houston (a black Millerite), 61
How to Live (EGW), 146-49, **147**, 191, 192, 193, 195, 215, 216, 257, 288
How to Live (Robinson), 146
"How to Rear Beautiful Children" (Jackson), 126
How to Treat the Sick without Medicine (Jackson), 125-26
"How to Use Graham Flour" (Amadon), 140
How You Can Live Six Extra Years, xxvi
Howell, W. E., 345, 350, 352, 366-67, 373-77, 384
Howland, Stockbridge, 69-70
Howson, John S., 257, 388-89
Hoyt, Frederick, xii, 37, 326

Hull, Moses, 130
Humors, disease-producing, 237. *See also* Cancerous humors
Hurd, Henry, 183
Hutchins, A. S., 89
Hutchinson, Anne, xx
Hydropathic Encyclopedia (Trall), 141
Hydropathy, 94, 95, 110, 113-17, 120, 121-26, 132, 140-41, 143, 145, 150-55, 157, 176-78, 182, 241, **248**, 263, 265, 321-22
Hygeio-Therapeutic College, 117, 160, 162, 172, 176-79, **178**, 322
Hygienic Institute Nursery, 175
Hypnotism, 9, 63
Hysteria, 9, 63, 81, 143, 144, 280. *See also* Histrionic personality style

Inheritance and mental health, 270-71
Imitation of Christ, Ellen White as, xii, 326, 329-31, 333-38
Insanity, 86, 110, 207, 208, 210, 267, 270-76; and Millerism, 54, 270, 273-74; and religion, 270
Intercourse, frequency of, 102, 216
Investigative judgment, 92
Iowa rebellion, 149-50
Irwin, Bernadette L., 269

Jackson, James C., 28, 63, 94, 95, 121-26, **122**, 135-37, 140, 141, 143, 144, 146, 149, 150, 173, 185, 207, 208, 211, 220, 224, 240, 242, 320-24
Jackson, James (Jr.), 179, 322
Jacobs, Enoch, 70
James 5:14-15, 76, 77
Jehovah's Witnesses, xxx
Jesus (illegitimate child), 240
Jewelry, 51, 188
Johnson, President Andrew, 157
Jones, A. T., 254, 361
Joy, Charlotte A., 196

Karachi, Pakistan, 266

INDEX

Kellogg, J. P., 128, 177
Kellogg, John Harvey, xxxii, 6, 7, 27, 63, 128, 148, 169, 176, 177-83, **180**, 202, 217, 229-30, 231, 232, 243, 247, 249, 260, 262, 316, 383; development of health foods, 250-51; disfellowshipped from Adventist church, 238, 253-62; establishment of a scientific sanitarium, 181-83; establishment of medical educational institutions, 251-53; leadership of Adventist health-reform movement, 230; renewal of health reform, 234
Kellogg, Merritt, xxix, 63, 128, 172-73, 177-78, 247, 258, 262
Kellogg, Will Keith, 128, 251
Kern, M. E., 381-85, 387-88, 390, 392
Kingston, Jamaica, 266
King, Sister S. H., 240
Koch, Robert, 237
Kohut, Thomas A., 277
Kress, Daniel, 257
Krohn, Alan, 280

Labor unions, 247-48
Lacey, H. C., 363-65
Lamson, Phoebe, 160, 162, **163**, 198
Land, Gary, 30
Laws of Life, 125, 135, 137, 141
Lay, Horatio S., 133, 143, 150, 159-60, **161**, 162, 165-66, 167, 171-72, 174, 322
A Lecture to Young Men on Chastity (Graham), 102, 207
Lectures on the Science of Human Life (Graham), 97, 99, 101, 224
Lee, Ann, xxi, 58, 217
Lehrer, Tom, 31
Leprosy, 134
Letter Box, 125
Lewis, Dioclesian (Dio), 106-7, 131, 140, 146, 149, 240

Life and Epistles of the Apostle Paul (Conybeare and Howson), 257
The Lily, 185
Lockhart, Keith, 6
Lockwood, Brother and Sister, 320, 324
Loma Linda Sanitarium, 248, 249, 262
Loma Linda University, xxvi, xxxi, 18-19, 263
Longfellow, Henry Wadsworth, 115
Los Angeles, California, 248, 250, 264
Los Angeles Times, 35
Loughborough, John, 43, 128, 149-53, 157, 158, 164, 166, 173-74, 212

McAdams, Donald, xii, 34, 40
McAndrew, William, 129
McArthur, Benjamin, 30-31
McMahon, Don S., xxiv
McPherson, Aimee Semple, xx
Madison Sanitarium (Tennessee), 249
Magan, Percy, 263
Maine Liquor Law, 83
Mann, Horace, 106-7, 120, 146, 149, 213
Marriage relationship, 102, 215-16
Marty, Martin E., xix, 6, 31
Masten, L. V., 78-79, 110
Masturbation, xxxi, 7-8, 102, 126, 207-12, 217, 270, 272, 288
Maxson, Sister M. F., 150
Maxwell, A. Graham, 19
Meals, frequency of, 100, 107, 125, 131, 137-38, 149, 164, 219-20, 231
Meat, clean and unclean, xxix. *See also* Vegetarianism
Meat substitutes, 250
Medicine, regular, in 19th-century America, 96, 110, 113, 121, 156, 165, 176; attitudes of health reformers to, 101, 109, 110, 114, 125, 127, 131, 132, 133, 134-35, 138, 164, 165, 241, 249, 252, 262
Melbourne, Australia, 245

Index

Melrose Sanitarium (Massachusetts), 249
Menopause and cessation of visions (EGW), 242
Mental illness. *See* Insanity
Mercury, 135; poisoning, 47
Merritt, M. Angelina, 188, 200
Mesmerism, 59, 66-68, 206, 270, 275, 281, 295
Messenger of the Lord (Douglass), xxiv
Metcalfe, William, 97, 120
Methodist Church, 45, 51, 52, 53-54, 83
Miasma, 147; poisonous, 134
Michigan State Normal College, 177
Milk, 100, 105, 138, 174-75, 220, 224, 236, 256
Millennialism, 49, 110. *See also* Second Coming of Christ
Miller, E. P., 216
Miller, Elizabeth Smith, 123, 185, **186**, 188
Miller, H. C., 130, 233
Miller, William, xix-xx, 6, 47-48, 50-51, 54, 55, 59, 68, 83, 102, 108, 117-19, 206
Millerite movement, 48-51, 53-60, 65, 66, 68, 70, 83, 108, 127, 270, 272-74; Great Disappointment (1844), 55, 56, 108, 172-73, 284
Mince pies, 164, 211, 236
Mind cure, 275
The Ministry of Healing (EGW), 217, 235, 265
Minneapolis, Minnesota, 238
Moral Reformer (Alcott), 105
Moral therapy, 274
Morantz, Regina Markell, 106
Mormonism, 59, 64, 270. *See also* Smith, Joseph
Moroni, 64
Morristown, Vermont, 87
Mustaches, 204

Nashville, Tennessee, 249
National Dress Reform Association, 123, 196
National Health Reform Association, 160
The Natural Method of Curing the Diseases of the Body (Cheyne), 96
Nature, as physician, 162, 179, 247
Nervous system, 214-15
Neurasthenia, 277
New Guide to Health (Thomson), 111
New York Hygeio-Therapeutic College, 117
New Zealand, 245
Nichols, Henry, 77
Nichols, Mary Gove, 114, 115, 117, 123, 211
Nichols, Thomas Low, 115, 117, 176
Nightingale, Florence, 290
Nissenbaum, Stephen, 102
Noorbergen, Rene, 20
Norway, 244
Norwood, Wm. Frederick, 27
Novel reading, 272
Numbers, Ernest R., 2
Numbers, Janet S., 37
Numbers, Raymond W., 1-2, 40-41
Numbers, Ronald L., 1-41

Oakland, California, 228, 241, 244
Oberlin College, 103, 128, 172
Olson, Robert, 20, 23, 30
"Opening Heavens" (Bates), 58
Opium, 135, 229, 271
Orion, 58
Oswego, New York, 70, 85
Otsego, Michigan, xxxi, 132
"Our Home on the Hillside," 121, 124-25, 128, **129**, 140-52, 154, 155, 157, 158, 160, 185, 188, 191, 192, 195-97, 206, 220, 225, 320-25. *See also* Dansville
Oysters, 231, 257

INDEX

Paradise Valley Sanitarium (California), 248, 249
Parallels between writings of EGW and other authors, xiv-xv, xxxii, 11-12, 34-35, 129, 134-35, 146, 148-49, 160, 200, 211, 212, 213-15, 216, 257-58, 261, 289-90. *See also* Plagiarism
Parsons, D. A., 388, 390-91
Parsons, William (Lord Rosse), 58
Pasteur, Louis, 237
Pastries, 84, 100, 219, 223
Pathology of the Reproductive Organs (Trall), 137
"Patriarchs and Prophets" (EGW), 363, 390
Patten, Adelia, 141-43, **142**, 320, 324-25
Peanut butter, 250
Penington, Isaac, 258
Pennsylvania Society for Discouraging the Use of Ardent Spirits, 97
Peterson, Donald I., 278
Peterson, William S., xii, xviii, xxviii, 13, 35, 40
Phelps, H. F., 130
Phillips, Anna, 313
Philosophy of Health (Coles), xxxii, 109, 148, 214, 221-22, 225-27, 257
Phrenology, 117-20, 143, 146, 205-7, 216, 221, 257, 320, 323-24
Physical education, 107
Physicians, attitudes of health reformers to regular, 77-82, 114, 126, 131, 134-35, 156. *See also* Medicine, attitudes . . .
Pickering, Sir George, 290
Pierson, Robert H., 29
Pies, 100, 146. *See also* Mince pies
Plagiarism, xiv-xv, 9, 12, 34-35, 257-59, 289. *See also* Parallels . . .
Plain Facts about Sexual Life (Kellogg), 217
Poland, Maine, 61-66, 67
Pork, 89-90, 134, 164, 224

Portland, Maine, 44, 45, 50-51, 54-55, 56, 60, 66, 83
Portland, Oregon, 247
Poyen, Charles, 66
Prayer for healing, 77-81, 150-54, 225, 241, 246, 275
Prenatal influences, 146, 207
Prescott, W. W., 254, 354, 356-57, 360, 363-67, 384, 392-98
Priessnitz, Vincent, 113-14
The Principles of Physiology Applied to the Preservation of Health (A. Combe), 96
Prior, Sister, 80
Prophets and visionaries, 58-61, 279, 281
Psychology, 206, 268
Pulte, J. E., 113
Purple, M. N., 82

Quimby, Phineas Parkhurst, 66-67, 265
Quinine, 135

Rational medicine, 182
Rea, Walter, xiv, xviii, 35, 40
Reform dress, 184-203, **199, 201**, 320-21. *See also* Dress and dress reform
Remmers, Carolyn Numbers, 2
Restaurants, vegetarian, 250
Review and Herald. *See Advent Review and Sabbath Herald*
Review and Herald "Extra," 72
Riverside, California, 248
Robinson, Dores E., 29, 392
Rochester, New York, 74-75, 81, 124, 141, 150-52, 154, 192
Roosevelt, New York, 74
Rosenberg, Charles E., 127
Rosse, Lord. *See* Parsons, William
Rum, 82
Rural Health Retreat, 247
Russell, Charles Taze, xxx

410

Index

Russell, William, 63, 162, 179

Sabbath Readings for the Home Circle (EGW), 229
Sadler, William S., 254-57, 261
St. Albans Academy, 68
St. Helena, California, 246, 247
St. Martin, Alexis, 100
Salt, 100, 107, 138, 144, 174-75, 219, 224, 225, 236, 325, 387-88
San Diego, California, 248
San Francisco, California, 241, 250
Sanborn, Isaac, 88, 164
Sandeen, Ernest, 1, 26
Sanitation, 95
Sanitariums, 246, 264. *See also* Battle Creek Sanitarium
Santa Rosa, California, 241
Satan, 64, 67, 69, 82, 154, 203, 206, 218, 247, 275, 285
Sawyer, Hannah, **199**
Schoepflin, Rennie B., xxvii
Schools, public, 107
Schwarz, Richard W., 24-25, 27-28
Science, 112
Scrofula, 134
Second Coming of Christ, 43-44, 47-49, 51, 54, 55, 66, 69, 71, 84, 85, 90, 145, 158, 233, 250
Sectarian medicine, 110-17, 121-26, 127, 177-79, 241, 263. *See also* Eclecticism; Homeopathy; Hydropathy; Thomsonianism
Self-Abuse. *See* Masturbation
Seneca Falls, New York, 185
Seventh-day Adventists: doctrines, 92; during Civil War, 93-94; Millerite origins, 58; organization, 90-92; selection of a name, 91; size in 1860s, 90; visions as a test of fellowship, 73-74, 261, 262
Seventh-day Sabbath, 58, 71, 89
Sex, 101-2, 105, 109, 120, 126, 184, 207-18; and diet, 221-22, 235

Sexual disorders, treatment of, 126, 216
The Sexual Organism (Jackson), 137
Shakers, 58-59, 70, 103
Shapiro, David, 289
Shaving, 101, 204
Shawls, 198
Shew, Joel, 114-15, 120
Shock therapy, 150
Shull, C. A., 357, 360, 394, 397
Shut door, 56, 57, 60, 70, 72
Shyrock, Richard H., 114
Les Signes des Tempes, 244
Signs of the Times, 108, 241
A Sketch of the Christian Experience and Views of Ellen G. White, 72, 80
Sketches from the Life of Paul (EGW), 257, 356, 388-89, 390-91
Sleep, 99, 101, 102, 105, 125, 131, 159, 162
Smith, Annie, 130, 257
Smith, Elizabeth Oakes, 83
Smith, Gerrit, 121, 123, 185
Smith, Joseph, xix-xx, xxx, xxxiii, 3, 10, 29, 59, 64
Smith, Timothy L., 15
Smith, Uriah, 74, 149-52, 157, 165, 167-68, 179, 231, 262
Smith-Rosenberg, Carroll, 63, 280
Snow, Samuel S., 55
Snuff, 86, 219, 236
Solemn Appeal (EGW), 216
Solitary vice. *See* Masturbation
Somatization disorder, 269, 279-80, 282
Sorrenson, C. M., 352, 363, 385, 394-98
Spectrum, xii, xxiii, xxvii, xxviii, 26-28, 29, 30, 40
Spicer, William A., 374
Spices, 100, 102, 138, 219, 223, 236
Spiritual Gifts, vol. II (EGW), 80
Spiritual Gifts, vol. IV (EGW), 133-34
Spiritualism, 66, 117, 190-91, 265, 270, 275, 281

Index

Spurzheim, Johann Gaspar, 117
Stanton, Elizabeth Cady, 185, 188, 273
Starkweather, John, 59
Starr, George B., 258-59
Stewart, Charles E., 254-57, 261
Stimulants, 99, 133, 139, 211, 219, 223, 229
Stockman, Levi, 52
Stone, Lucy, 185
Stowe, Harriet Beecher, xx
Strychnine, 135, 252
Suffering, 285
Sugar, 174-75, 224
Suicides, Millerite, 54
Switzerland, 244
Sydney, Australia, 245, 247
Systematic benevolence, 92

Takoma Park, Maryland, 249
Taylor, C. L., 350-51, 353, 357, 361-62, 364, 369, 379-80
Taylor, Charles, 141
Taylor, Daniel T., 128, 140
Tea, 83, 84, 88, 89, 100, 102, 115, 125, 134, 219, 224-27, 231, 232, 235, 236, 265, 271
Teetotal pledge, 229
Temperance, 45, 82-83, 96, 97, 100, 102, 105, 107, 120, 121, 132, 227-29, 240, 244; boarding houses, 102
Temple Street Christian Church (Portland), 53
Temporal-lobe epilepsy. *See* Partial complex seizures
Testimonies for the Church (EGW), 93, 389-90, 397, 400
Third angel's message (SDA), 69, 190, 250
Thompson, G. B., 383-85
Thomson, Samuel, 111
Thomsonianism, 110-12, 113
Tiglath Pileser (dog), 235
Time magazine, 7, 30

"To Those Who Are Receiving the Seal of the Living God" (EGW), 77
Tobacco, 83, 84-88, 100, 109-10, 115, 120, 134, 135, 219, 225, 227, 232, 236, 265
Tongue, tinned, 233
Topsham, Maine, 69-70, 136, 137, 296
Townsend's sarsaparilla, 79
Trall, Russell T., 114-15, **116**, 117, 120, 135, 140, 146, 149, 160, 162, 172, 173-78, 207, 208, 224, 240, 242, 322
Trembley, Jennie, 177
Tuberculosis, 235, 237. *See also* Consumption
Tulare, California, camp meeting, 235
Turkey meat, 233
Turner, Joseph, 56, 57, 67-68

University of Illinois, 253
University of Michigan, 179, 252

Vegetarianism, 84, 96, 97, 99, 105, 109, 123, 125, 129, 131, 133, 134, 137-38, 140, 145, 164, 219, 221-23, 230-35, 250, 256-57, 265, 321, 368-71
Veltman, Fred, xv
Visions in 19th-century America, 47, 58-61, 279, 281
Vitalism and vital force, 211-14, 215, 269
Voice of the Prophets, 128, 136, 137
Voice of the West, 128

Waggoner, E. J., 218
Waggoner, J. H., 87, 131-32
Wakeman, W. H., 365, 373, 377
Waldorf, N. J., 371-72, 375
Walker, E. S., 168
Walling, Lou, 241, 319
Washington Sanitarium (Takoma Park, Maryland), 249
Washingtonian Temperance Society, 82-83
Water cure. *See* Hydropathy

412

Index

Water-Cure Journal, 109, 115, 120, 125, 128, 135
Weiss, Herold, xii, xviii, 5, 40
Wellcome, Isaac, 43, 62
Wells, Samuel R., 120
Westbrook Seminary and Female College, 45
Western Health Reform Institute, 155, 156-83, **158**, **182**, 192-93, 198, 216, 230, 243, 276. *See also* Battle Creek Sanitarium
White, Anna, 78
White, Arthur L., xxviii, 4, 12-14, 23-24, 39
White, Ellen G.
Health: chronology, 291-319; ankle injured, 197, 309, 311; anxiety, 281, 283, 285, 292, 297, 299; arteriosclerosis, 264, 319; asthenia, 264, 319; breast cancer, 303; breathing difficulties, 65, 76, 81, 276, 291, 297, 299, 302; broken thigh bone, 264; "cancer" of the eyelid, 81, 297; chronic myocarditis, 264, 319; complex partial seizures, 268, 278-79; consumption, 65, 76, 293; cough, 77; death, 264, 319; depression, 52, 66, 244, 267, 269, 276, 281, 283, 300, 313-14; dropsy, 138, 276, 293, 298; epilepsy, 268; fainting spells, 65, 76, 81, 93, 132, 242, 276, 283, 296, 300, 301; good health, 138, 245; hallucinations, 276; headaches, 134, 276; healed by "shock of electricity," 305, 308; heart problems, 81, 138, 276, 283, 297, 298, 305; histrionic personality style, 269, 280, 282, 283, 284, 289; hysteria, 9, 63, 81, 143, 144, 280; impaired speech, 66, 81, 276, 285, 295; impaired vision, 276, 283; inflammation of the brain, 276; influenza, 304; injuries, 44-45, 76, 241, 264, 297, 309, 311; insomnia, 134, 309, 310, 315; lame legs, 93, 276, 299; loss of strength, 153; lungs affected, 242, 276, 293, 297, 301, 302, 305, 310; menopause, 242-43, 302; mental health, 37, 76, 267, 268, 274, 276-90, 292, 295; miraculous healings, 77, 81, 287, 296, 297, 301, 304, 305, 306, 308, 310-11, 314, 315; nosebleeds, 276, 300; paralysis, 81, 138, 276, 286, 298, 303, 307; pleurisy, 276, 309; pneumonia, 278-79; pressure on the brain, 276, 300-301, 305; rheumatism, 245, 276, 312-13, 317; shattered nerves, 76, 287, 310; skin cancer, 318-19; somatization disorder, 269, 279-80, 282; sore throat, 76, 305; spot on forehead, 249; "strokes," 81, 82, 138, 319; tenderness of the stomach, 276, 300, 310; trembling hands, 45, 67, 292, 295; unconscious, 276, 297; undergoes water treatments, 150; weak back, 93, 299; x-ray treatment, 318-19
Life: photographs, **vi**, **46**, **142**, **194**; influence, xxx, 72-74, 89-90, 265-66; antimeat pledge, 13, 234-35; birth, 44; diet, 13, 152, 220, 231-33, 238; early travels in New England, 37, 66, 68; childhood accident, 44, 45, 210, 278, 282-83, 288, 291, 317; first reads about end of the world, 43, 51; education, 44, 45-47, 282-83, 291; hatmaking, 47; conversion at Buxton camp meeting, 51; baptism, 51; hears William Miller, 50-51; religious anxiety, 52-53, 283-85, 292; religious dreams, 52, 292-93; first public prayer, 53, 283, 293; early public ministry, 53; dis-

413

missed from Methodist church, 54; first visions, 52, 56-58, 61-64, 65; and Dammon trial, 326-43; fanaticism, 274, 326; and Satan, 298, 299, 309, 314; interactions with angels, 294, 296-97, 298, 299, 303, 308, 315, 317; interactions with Jesus, 311-12, 317; accepts seventh-day Sabbath, 58; meets James White, 68; marriage, 69, 243, 303-4; in Gorham, Maine, 69, 296; warrants for arrest, 69; birth of Henry, 69; in Topsham, Maine, 69, 70, 136, 137; birth of Edson, 70; in "exile" in the 1850s, 73-74, 75, 286; in Rochester, New York, 74-75, 81, 141, 150, 152, 154; birth of Willie, 75; in Battle Creek, Michigan, 75, 92-93, 138, 145, 215, 228, 238, 240; healing power, 79-80; birth of John Herbert, 93; hydropathy, 94, 126, 130, 135, 145; and J. C. Jackson, 94, 126, 130, 135, 136-37, 141-45, 150, 152 153, 208, 225; in Otsego, Michigan, 132; and H. S. Lay, 133, 150, 160, 167, 171, 322; and R. T. Trall, 135, 172-74, 178, 208, 240, 322; struggle with vegetarianism, 137, 145, 231-33, 256-57, 368-71; adopts health reform, 137-38, 219-20; visits Dansville, 141-45, 150-54, 156, 188, 191-92, 206, 210, 320-23; and J. H. Kellogg, 148, 181, 229-30, 232, 234, 238, 249, 251, 253-55, 316; nurses James White, 150-51, 154-55, 300; in Greenville, Michigan, 154, 198; in Wright, Michigan, 193; in Oakland, California, 228, 241; temperance lectures, 228-29, 240, 244; death of James White, 243, 307; in Australia, 233, 235, 245-46, 312-15; in New Zealand, 245; alleged misconduct, 172, 239-40; national recognition, 240; in Colorado, 240-41; in California, 228, 241; change of life, 242-43; in Europe, 244; in St. Helena, California, 233, 246-47; in Santa Rosa, California, 241; promotes sanitariums, 246, 247-49, 265; death, 264, 319

Views on: abuse of marriage relation, 215-16; alcohol, 219, 225, 227-29, 231, 236, 265; American costume, 144, 190-96, 320-21; amusements, 145, 153, 170-71, 321; blood, 269; Fannie Bolton, 258-59, 287-88, 313; brain, 269, 272; breast-paddings, 203; butter, 219, 223, 224, 231, 236-37, 238, 256, 387; cake, 236; cancerous humors, 143, 210, 272; celibacy, 217-18; cheese, 219, 223, 224, 231, 238; children in heaven, 232-33; Civil War, 93, 145; coffee, 84, 134, 219, 225-27, 229, 232, 236, 265, 271; condiments, 223; contraception, 216-17; corn flakes, 251; cosmetics, 203; creation, xxii; dancing, 145, 153; depression, 275; diet, 85-86, 133-34, 219-38, 272; dress, 51-52, 90, 144, 145, 190-203, 320; drugs, 133, 134-35, 240, 263; eating twice a day, 135, 219-20, 238; Mary Baker Eddy, 200; eggs, 219, 223-24, 231, 236, 237, 256, 387; electrical currents, 214-15, 269, 275; evil angels, 302, 318; exercise, 153, 155, 272; fish, 232; frequency of intercourse, 215-16; frequency of meals, 135, 219-20, 231; germs, 237; gossip, 226-27, 272; hair styles, 204-5; "health foods," 250-51; *Health Reformer,* 164, 175; hoop skirts, 90, 190; humors, 134,

210, 222, 272; inheritance, 271; labor unions, 247-48; male physicians treating women, 264; masturbation, xxiv, xxxi, 207-12, 215, 272, 288; meat, 133, 134, 137-38, 219, 221-23, 228, 235-36, 368-71; medical education, 262-64; medical missionaries, 262; mental health, 269-76; mesmerism, 206, 275; milk, 220, 224, 236, 256; mind cure, 275; use of "Mister" and "Miss," 170; novel reading, 272; opium, 271; phrenology, 143, 146, 205-7, 216, 320; physicians, 77-82, 134-35, 138, 156, 165, 249; pork, 89-90, 134, 223; prayer for healing, 80-81, 246, 275; prenatal influences, 207; psychology, 206, 268, 269-76; reform dress, 184, 190-203; restaurants, 250; rich pastries, 219, 223, 236; salt, 219, 224, 225, 236; sanitariums, 246-50; SDA church, 91; SDA water cure, 155; sex, 184, 207-18, 288; shut door, xxiv, 56-57, 60, 70, 71-72, 80; slavery, 93; snuff, 219, 236; spices, 219, 223, 236; spiritualism, 190-91; sugar, 224; tea, 84, 134, 219, 224-27, 231, 232, 236, 271; temperance, 83, 132, 227-29, 244; time of Christ's coming, 36, 71; tobacco, 84-85, 134, 219, 225, 227, 232, 236; University of Michigan, 252; vital force, 211-14, 269; wages of physicians, 170, 263-64; water, value of, 138; Western Health Reform Institute, 156, 165-72, 181-83; James White, 168, 169-70, 241, 243; wigs, 204-5; the will, 275-76; wine, 227-28, 271; women physicians, 264; women's rights, 190; x-rays, 249, 318-19

Visions: 276, 294; authority of, 344-401; as a test of fellowship, 73-74, 261, 262; attitudes toward, 8-9, 58; cause of, 63, 66-68, 281; cessation of, 73, 242-43, 286, 298, 306; compared with those of biblical writers, 73; controversies about, 63, 72-74, 135-37, 172, 193-202, 254-61; descriptions of, 61-64; early, 52, 56-58, 61-64, 65, 294-98, 326; as Imitation of Christ, 326, 329-31, 333-38; independence of, 65, 135-37, 254-56; of Chicago building, 255-56; of Satan, 64; on astronomy, 58; on cancerous humors, 134, 210, 237, 272; on cause of disease, 134; on cleanliness, 86, 132; on coffee, 84, 88, 134; on December 25, 1865, 154, 157; on diet, 86, 89, 132-33; on dress, 51-52, 193, 195-98; on drugs, 133-35; on eating meat, 133; on fever-producing miasma, 134; on fresh air and sunshine, 133; on the "Great Controversy," 286, 298; on a health institute, 154, 157, 166-68; on hydropathy, 132, 135; on importance of October 22, 1844, 57; on intemperance, 132, 134; on June 5, 1863, xxxi, 133-35, 141, 160, 190, 195-96, 208, 219-20, 227; on narcotics, 133; on physicians, 135; on pork, 89-90; on the seventh-day Sabbath, 58; on sex (1868), 215, 216; on shut door, 57; on stimulants, 133; on tea, 84, 85, 134; on tobacco, 84-85, 134, 227; on the use of medicines, 79; re Battle Creek critics, 254, 257, 260-61; re rebuilding Battle Creek Sanitarium, 247, 256; re James White, 132, 154-55; re Willie White, 138, 244; similarity of early visions to Foy's and Foss's,

INDEX

60-61; visions of the night, 64, 242, 301-2, 306

Writings: An Appeal to Mothers, 14, 208-11, 212, 216, 272; *Christian Temperance and Bible Hygiene,* xxxii, 217, 233; *Counsels on Diet and Foods,* 265; *Desire of Ages,* xv, 34, 387, 389; "Disease and Its Causes," 146; divinely guided, 65, 239; *The Dress Reform,* 201; "Duty to Know Ourselves," 164; *Early Writings,* 398; *Education,* 394; *The Great Controversy,* 34, 389, 392, 394, 395, 397-98; *Health; or, How to Live,* 146-49, 191-95, 215-16, 257, 288; inconsistencies in, 38, 254, 256-57; letter in *Day-Star,* 70; manipulation of, 239, 255, 258-59; *The Ministry of Healing,* 217, 235, 265; parallels with other authors, xiv-xv, xxxii, 11-12, 34-35, 129, 134-35, 146, 148-49, 160, 200, 211, 212, 213-15, 216, 257-58, 261, 289-90; *Patriarchs and Prophets,* 363, 390; *Prophets and Kings,* 34; in *Review and Herald,* 72-74; role of James White, 70-71, 168, 259; *Sabbath Readings for the Home Circle,* 229; *A Sketch of the Christian Experience and Views of Ellen G. White,* 72, 80; *Sketches from the Life of Paul,* 33, 257, 356, 388-89, 390-91; *Solemn Appeal,* 216; "Special Department," in *Health Reformer,* 175; *Spiritual Gifts,* vol. II, 80-81; *Spiritual Gifts,* vol. IV, 133-34, 134-35; *Testimonies for the Church,* 93, 389-90, 397, 400; testimonies on tobacco, 87; testimonies of medical missions, 246; *Testimony No. 10,* 190, 193, 195; *Testimony No. 11,* 166-68, 193, 197; *Testimony No. 12,* 168, 197; "To Those Who Are Receiving the Seal of the Living God," 77. *See also* Bible Conferences of 1919

Ellen G. White Memorial Hospital (Los Angeles), 264

White, Henry, 69-70, 79, 138, 297

White, James, xvi, 62, 68, **142**, 385-86; and J. H. Kellogg, 13, 177, 179, 181, 243; mental health of, 13, 132, 154, 169-70, 276; travels with Ellen Harmon, 37, 69; early life and education, 68; Millerite preacher, 68-69; marriage, 69, 243; in Topsham, Maine, 69-70, 136; itinerant preaching, 70; publishing activities, 70-71, 72, 92, 149, 241, 243, 286; influence on EGW's writings, 70-71, 168, 243, 259; on EGW's shut-door testimonies, 71-72; on EGW's visions, 8, 73-74, 220, 262, 388; poor health, 73, 75, 79, 132, 138, 149-54, 175, 243, 276; as a health reformer, 83, 175, 224; on money, 13; on tea and tobacco, 85, 88; on pork, 89-90; organization of SDA church, 8, 90-91, 243; income, 92; and Civil War, 93, 149; and hydropathy, 130; interest in health reform, 131, 136-37, 172, 219; and J. C. Jackson, 130, 136, 137, 141, 150, 324-25; visits Dansville, 141, 144, 146, 149-54; buys fresh fish, 145; and the Iowa rebellion, 149-50; stroke, 150; recuperation in Greenville, Michigan, 154-55, 157; on physicians, 165; in the trial of Israel Dammon, 37, 328-31, 335-41; and the Western Health Reform Institute, 168-70, 181-82, 243; and the *Health Reformer,* 175-76; and need for SDA physicians, 176, 177, 181; death, 182, 243; on the American costume, 191-92; on two meals a day, 220; on meat, 223; on domestic wine,

227-28; reputation, xi-xxv, 239-40; letter-writing, 241; character, 243; and Battle Creek College, 243; influence, 243; on the need for a medical school, 252

White, James Edson, xvii, 13, 70, 78, 141, **142**, 143, 177-78, 210, 232, 242, 259-60, 197, 320

White, John Herbert, 93, 138

White, Willie, xvii, 8, 13, 75, 133, 138, 141, **142**, 143, 175, 177-78, 179, 232-33, 235, 237, 242, 244, 254, 259-60, 261, 320, 323-34, 344, 388, 391, 395, 397

White Estate. *See* Ellen G. White Estate

The White Lie (Rae), xiv

Whittier, John Greenleaf, 49-50

Whorton, James C., 32

Wigs, 204, 205

Wilcox, F. M., 354, 361, 367, 369, 377-78, 381, 386, 391-92, 395

Wilcox, Roger, 4

Wilkinson, Jemima, 59, 217, 257

Will, exercising the, 275-76

Williams, Flora Lampson, 358, 370-71, 389

Williams, Peter W., xx

Wilson, Neal, 18, 29

Wine, domestic, 227-28

Wirth, W. G., 358, 365, 367

Women and health reform, 106, 113, 114, 115, 173, 184-204. *See also* individuals

Women physicians, EGW's views on, 264

Women's Christian Temperance Union, 228, 250

Women's rights, 190

Woodward, Samuel B., 211

World's Health Association, 121

Wright, Michigan, 193

X-rays, 249, 318-19

Yates County Chronicle, 94, 126

York(e), Mrs. Dr. George W., 321, 322

Young Men's Guide (W. Alcott), 105

www.ingramcontent.com/pod-product-compliance
Lightning Source LLC
Chambersburg PA
CBHW021814300426
44114CB00009BA/163